Pregnancy
after a Loss

Pregnancy
after a Loss

---

*A Guide to Pregnancy
after a Miscarriage, Stillbirth or
Infant Death*

CAROL CIRULLI LANHAM

Berkley Books, New York

THE BERKLEY PUBLISHING GROUP
Published by the Penguin Group
Penguin Group (USA) Inc.
375 Hudson Street, New York, New York 10014, USA
Penguin Group (Canada), 90 Eglinton Avenue East, Suite 700, Toronto, Ontario M4P 2Y3, Canada
(a division of Pearson Penguin Canada Inc.)
Penguin Books Ltd., 80 Strand, London WC2R 0RL, England
Penguin Group Ireland, 25 St. Stephen's Green, Dublin 2, Ireland (a division of Penguin Books Ltd.)
Penguin Group (Australia), 250 Camberwell Road, Camberwell, Victoria 3124, Australia
(a division of Pearson Australia Group Pty. Ltd.)
Penguin Books India Pvt. Ltd., 11 Community Centre, Panchsheel Park, New Delhi—110 017, India
Penguin Group (NZ), 67 Apollo Drive, Rosedale, North Shore 0632, New Zealand
(a division of Pearson New Zealand Ltd.)
Penguin Books (South Africa) (Pty.) Ltd., 24 Sturdee Avenue, Rosebank, Johannesburg 2196,
South Africa

Penguin Books Ltd., Registered Offices: 80 Strand, London WC2R 0RL, England

The information contained in this book is not a substitute for professional medical advice. While the advice and information in this book are believed to be true and accurate at the date of going to press, neither the author nor the publisher can accept any legal responsibility for any errors or omissions that may be made. The publisher makes no warranty, express or implied, with respect to the material contained herein. Readers should consult their physician or midwife before acting on any of the information contained in this volume. The publisher does not have any control over and does not assume any responsibility for author or third-party websites or their content.

PREGNANCY AFTER A LOSS: A GUIDE TO PREGNANCY AFTER A MISCARRIAGE, STILLBIRTH OR INFANT DEATH

This book is an original publication of The Berkley Publishing Group.

A Berkley Book / published by arrangement with the author

Copyright © 1999 by Carol Cirulli Lanham
A continuation of copyright credits appears on page 377.

PRINTING HISTORY
Berkley trade paperback edition / October 1999

Berkley trade paperback ISBN: 978-0-425-17047-2

PRINTED IN THE UNITED STATES OF AMERICA

25   24   23   22

For Patrick

Contents

Foreword by Dr. Uel D. Crosby, M.D.   ix

Acknowledgments   xiii

Introduction   xvii

1   The Search for Answers   1

2   Are You Ready to Try Again?   41

3   Trying Again   75

4   Pregnant Again: The First Trimester   113

5   Pregnant Again: The Second Trimester   167

6   Pregnant Again: The Third Trimester   219

7   Pregnant Again: The High-Risk Pregnancy   255

8   Labor and Delivery   297

9   After the Next Baby's Arrival   329

10 The Father's Perspective on Pregnancy after a Loss 355

Resources   371

Permissions   377

Foreword

THE EXPERIENCE OF pregnancy is very personal and unique to each individual woman. Although we have come to expect that every pregnancy will be uneventful and perfect, the reality is that one out of four pregnancies ends in some kind of loss. In many cases, those losses are due to random problems that are not likely to recur in a future pregnancy. And generally speaking, the odds of having a healthy baby in a subsequent pregnancy are very much in a woman's favor. But that is of little comfort to someone who has experienced the tragedy of pregnancy loss. For her, the loss was 100 percent.

As a woman contemplates another pregnancy after a miscarriage, stillbirth or the death of an infant, she needs more than a simple reassurance that the odds of giving birth to a healthy baby are in her favor. She needs to know that it is not unusual for her to have feelings of loss, helplessness, guilt, anger, resentment and isolation. She also needs to know what to expect during the next pregnancy, from paralyzing fear to unbridled joy. *Pregnancy after a Loss* provides that much-needed guidance.

Carol Lanham, who has been a patient of mine for many years, writes about pregnancy after a loss from firsthand experience. She came to our office in 1994 after experiencing a late pregnancy loss.

In the ensuing years, she had two subsequent full-term pregnancies and gave birth to two healthy baby boys. She has combined her own personal experience with that of nearly one hundred other women who have experienced loss, from early through late pregnancy to shortly after birth. But this book is much more than a chronicle of personal experiences.

In these pages, the author has extensively researched the benefits of prenatal education and prenatal care. She has recognized the need for excellence in these areas. She has made practical suggestions on how to select an obstetrician and other health team members, and has provided information that will lead a woman to realize that she is her own best health care advocate. There are no easy solutions to the problem of pregnancy loss, but these pages do provide guidance and hope on how to approach a subsequent pregnancy.

Though this book is primarily for the patient who has experienced a loss, it also has a great message for physicians and health care providers. Obstetrics is usually a very happy and positive specialty, and those who got into the field are typically caring, sensitive and compassionate individuals. But because the majority of pregnancies do end happily, we sometimes lose sight of the special needs of women who have experienced a pregnancy loss. Although we, as physicians, feel a sense of loss ourselves when a pregnancy ends badly, it is easy to get caught up in our busy practices and overlook the needs of women who require more time and attention. This book underscores how important it is that we, as health care providers, make a more concerted effort to maintain a sensitivity to women experiencing a subsequent pregnancy.

This need for sensitivity is of greater importance today than ever before. The incidence of pregnancy loss has been on the rise in recent years as more women put off childbearing until later in life, when the associated medical risks are higher. Reproductive technology is also allowing women to get pregnant who otherwise might not have been able to conceive, and puts some in the position of experiencing multiple losses before ultimately achieving a healthy pregnancy. Modern testing also makes it possible to detect pregnancies earlier than ever before, which means women may now know they suffered a miscarriage when they previously might not even have been aware they were pregnant.

In the nearly forty years since I delivered my first baby, we have come a long way in addressing the concerns of women who have experienced a loss at any point in their pregnancy. Whereas a woman might once have been told to forget what happened and simply get pregnant again, there is now an awareness among medical professionals that we must acknowledge the loss and provide emotional support. Unfortunately, though, misperceptions remain. It is not uncommon for a woman who has experienced a loss to be comforted with the words, "You can try again." This reflects the widely held, but erroneous, belief that a woman who has suffered a loss is magically healed once she becomes pregnant again.

Of course, as anyone who has conceived again after a loss knows, pregnancy is not a cure-all. Often, it only serves to resurrect the grief as the tragedy of the last pregnancy is replayed over and over in a woman's mind. And the nine months' gestation can seem unusually long when coupled with the anxiety that is associated with a subsequent pregnancy. It is for all these reasons and others that I will encourage each of our physicians, nurses, health/education professionals and associates to become increasingly sensitive to the needs of the individual patient who has experienced a loss and is pregnant again. I feel these pages will provide that guidance.

Uel D. Crosby, M.D.
Professor, Department of Ob/Gyn
The University of Texas
Southwestern Medical Center at Dallas

Acknowledgments

I AM SO grateful to the many people who made it possible for me to write *Pregnancy after a Loss* by sharing their time and expertise and giving me much-needed support over the nearly five years it took to complete the book. Specifically, I'd like to thank: Ginny Robinson and Diane Galloway of the Healing Matters support group in Plano, Texas, who were among the first to help me see the value of this book and continued to encourage me every step of the way; the many experts who shared their knowledge about subsequent pregnancies including Joann O'Leary, of the Pregnancy after a Loss Program at Abbott Northwestern Hospital in Minneapolis; Fran Rybarik, executive director of Bereavement Services/RTS; Dr. Peggy Morton, adjunct associate professor of social work at New York University; Sherokee Isle, author of *Another Baby? Maybe* and numerous books on pregnancy loss; Andrea Seigerman, a licensed clinical social worker in the high-risk obstetrics clinic at Yale–New Haven Hospital; Donna Jeane Pappas, a licensed professional counselor in the Department of Obstetrics and Gynecology at the University of North Carolina at Chapel Hill; Sister Jane Marie Lamb, founder of SHARE Pregnancy and Infant Loss Support; Dr. Judith Lasker, coauthor of *When Pregnancy Fails*; Melissa Swanson, director of Pen-Parents Inc.; Donna Roehl, of the Pregnancy and Infant Loss Center; and Molly A. Minnick, coauthor of *A Time to Decide, A Time to Heal*; those who provided spiritual advice that will benefit so many readers, including Rabbi Nina Beth Cardin, author of *Out of the Depths I Call to You: A Book of Prayers for Married Jewish Women*; Rabbi Stephanie Dickstein, a chaplain and educator in New Jersey; and Rev. Richard B. Gilbert, executive director of The World Pastoral Care Center; those who gave insight into the unique challenges faced by women pregnant with multiples, including Maureen Doolan Boyle, founder and executive director of MOST (Mothers of Supertwins); and Janet Bleyl, founder and president of The Triplet Connection; William Reinhart, a member of the national board of directors of SHARE Pregnancy and Infant Loss Support, who helped me understand the special challenges faced by fathers during the subsequent pregnancy; Dr. Charles Corr, who offered advice on how to deal with the needs of surviving children during the subsequent pregnancy; those who took time out of their busy schedules to patiently explain complicated medical information, including Dallas perinatologist Dr. Michael Cavenee, M.D., and Dr. Michael R. Berman, M.D., founder of Hygeia, an online journal for Pregnancy and Neonatal Loss; those who shared inspirational stories of how they have chosen to remember their babies who died, including Diana Sundwall, founder of Infants Remembered in Silence (IRIS); Becky Thompson, founder of Our Precious Angels; and Gail Fasolo. I'd also like to extend my special thanks to those who read all or portions of my manuscript and gave me suggestions that made the book so much better: Candace Hurley, executive director of Sidelines National Support Network; Cathi Lammert, executive director of SHARE Pregnancy and Infant Loss Support; Perry-Lynn Moffitt, coauthor of *A Silent Sorrow: Pregnancy Loss*; Cathleen Church-Balin, director of education services for the March of Dimes; and genetic counselor Jill Sawyer. My appreciation also goes to Uel Crosby, M.D., who will forever be dear to my heart for safely bringing my two healthy boys into this world and for not only reading the manuscript but also writing the foreword. Although I cannot recognize them individually by name, I'd like to express my sincere gratitude to the dozens of women who opened their hearts to me and shared not only the trials and tribulations, but the joys of their subsequent pregnancies. This book could not have been written without them. I'd also like to thank my editor, Hillary Cige, and my agent, Carol Mann, for recognizing the need for a book on pregnancy after a loss. And thanks also to Scott McCartney, who helped get the ball rolling. In addition, there are many, many people who gave me the personal support that I needed as I faced the ups and downs of my own subsequent pregnancies and the challenges involved in writing this book. Thanks to Lynn Kennedy, whom I consider an angel on earth, for her counseling and spiritual support after my loss and during my subsequent pregnancy; Christina Pantin, who was not only a compassionate boss but a prayerful companion during my subsequent pregnancy; Patty Ramirez and Charlotte Smith, who took such good care of my children and made it possible for me to write without guilt; my mother, Maria G. Cirulli, who not only helped me care for my children but taught me what it means to be a good mother; my sons, Andrew and Michael, who are the incredible blessings that resulted from my subsequent pregnancies and put all the pain in perspective; and my husband, Sean Lanham, who is my biggest advocate and greatest supporter. Were it not for his love and encouragement, this book could never have been written. Finally, I am grateful for my son, Patrick, the true inspiration for this book. Although his time on this earth was brief, the impact he had was tremendous. I love you.

Introduction

FOR MOST COUPLES, the nine months leading up to the birth of a child is one of the most exciting times of their lives. From the moment they get the results of the pregnancy test, they begin making plans for the baby's arrival, telling family and friends, preparing the nursery and anticipating how everything will change once the child is born.

But for those of us who have lost a baby during pregnancy or shortly after birth, the mere thought of trying to conceive again unleashes a wave of emotions. While we may desperately want another baby, the idea of going through another pregnancy fills us with dread. So instead of making plans, we ask questions: Why did my last pregnancy end in a loss? What could have been done to prevent it? Could it happen again? How long should I wait before getting pregnant? Should I keep the same doctor, go to the same hospital or use the same baby things? What will I do when I don't feel the baby move? Will I ever be able to love another baby as much as I love the one I lost?

I asked all of these questions and many others when I considered getting pregnant again after losing my son Patrick to an umbilical cord problem late in my first pregnancy. Like other women who have suffered a pregnancy loss, I vacillated between wanting to try again right away, and fearing that I would never be able to endure another pregnancy. As I struggled to make a decision, I talked to my husband, my doctor and other women who had lost babies. And as I always do when I'm looking for answers, I searched for books that would offer guidance.

What I discovered was that while there were many books available to help women cope with the pregnancy loss itself, most included only one chapter on the subsequent pregnancy. There were other books on preventing miscarriage and coping with a high-risk pregnancy, but they were written by doctors and focused almost exclusively on medical issues. Even though the medical information was important to me, my interest went much deeper. I needed to know how to respond to strangers who asked me whether I was expecting my first baby, and what to do when my anxiety, no matter how irrational, overwhelmed me. And as for all the other popular pregnancy books, I felt that they were written for women who had never experienced the devastation of a loss and would only serve as a painful reminder of how different my next pregnancy would be from the last one.

Since I was a journalist and was soon going to experience my own pregnancy after a loss, I decided that I would be the one to write the book I wanted. I thus embarked on a journey that lasted nearly five years, included months of research, interviews with nearly one hundred women and experts, and two more pregnancies of my own. The result is *Pregnancy after a Loss*.

It is a guide to every aspect of pregnancy after a loss, from the search for what went wrong the last time, to the decision to try again, to the birth of the next child. It focuses on the feelings that are unique to women who have suffered a pregnancy loss, and offers tips on reducing anxiety. It also describes the medical aspects in simple, straightforward language. But most important, it is a book filled with hope because it contains the stories of dozens of women who have made it through a pregnancy after a loss, and who now have one or more healthy babies.

Because I wanted this book to speak from the heart, I have tried to keep it conversational. It is for that reason that I opted not to use the formal terms like health care provider or medical professional, even though they are technically more correct than saying doctor or obstetrician without also referring to general practitioners and mid-wives. I also refer to all doctors as he, even though I know many of you are under the care of qualified female physicians. It is also worth noting that this book should not be used as a substitute for profes-sional medical advice. I, like you, am a layperson and intended the information to be used only as a guide that you could use to discuss issues of concern with your own health care provider. As I say throughout the book, the better informed you are, the better equipped you will be to take a proactive role in your care and ensure you get the very best medical treatment. Again, it simply seemed too cum-bersome to always say he or she. As you read through the book, you also might notice that I do not use words like fetus and embryo. That's because I believe that the vast majority of women who experience a pregnancy loss feel in their hearts that they lost a baby, not a fetus.

A few experts in the field of grieving and bereavement suggested that I also avoid using the term "lost" because it implies something that can be found. While I appreciate their concerns, I believe that it is common for women to say they "lost" their babies. Avoiding that phrase would have meant changing the quotes of many of the women who talked to me.

Finally, I'd like to point out that I changed the first names, and in some cases identifying details, of the women I interviewed. I did this to protect their privacy, which in turn enabled them to share intimate details of their pregnancy that they otherwise might not have. And it is their honesty and insight that will make this book so helpful to you. After hearing from the voices of experience, you will realize that if we could survive a pregnancy after a loss with our sanity intact, you can too. That should make your difficult journey just a little bit easier. I wish you the very best.

Carol Cirulli Lanham
Dallas, March 1999

chapter one

The Search for Answers

A FEW SHORT years ago, I was envisioning a life without children. I had suffered a pregnancy loss on my due date, just one day before labor was scheduled to be induced. I was devastated. Not only did the idea of another pregnancy fill me with dread, I also had trouble imagining giving birth to a healthy baby. For other women, it seemed to be so easy. They spent their pregnancy worrying about little more than the color of the nursery or which names to pick, and, before they knew it, they were bringing a healthy baby home from the hospital. It seemed that none of them ever thought to question whether everything would be all right. They just assumed that it would be. For me, things were different. Even though I had started out like those other women, something had gone horribly wrong, and on the day that I should have been bringing my first-born home, I was attending his funeral. I knew all too well that nine months of pregnancy would not necessarily produce a healthy baby. In my case, pregnancy only resulted in heartbreak and despair.

If you have recently had a pregnancy end in miscarriage, stillbirth or the death of your newborn, you're probably feeling as I did then. It may be difficult for you to envision making it through another pregnancy, much less having a healthy baby. All you feel right now is grief and disappointment. And yet you desperately want a child, not to replace the one you lost, but to fill your empty arms and heart.

Even if you have other children—living proof that a successful pregnancy for you is possible—you may have deep-seated doubts about your ability to conceive again and carry to term. Although you have given birth to a healthy child before, your perspective is different now. You may feel that your body has somehow betrayed you, and it may be difficult to believe that your life can ever be the way it once was.

All of these feelings are quite natural. You have lost a part of yourself, a baby that you dreamed about from the moment you found out you were expecting. You had hopes and plans for your baby. Then you suddenly had to say good-bye before you even had the chance to say hello. That's not how a pregnancy is supposed to end, so it's no wonder that after such a traumatic experience you are fearful of going through it again. Your concerns may be compounded by not knowing anyone else who has suffered a pregnancy loss. It's very likely that you are surrounded by other women who seem to have it so easy. This means that as you face the prospect of what doctors call a "subsequent pregnancy," you may not have anyone to talk to about issues that most women would not even begin to understand: your desperate search to understand what went wrong; your anxiety over when, or even whether, to get pregnant again; and your all-consuming fears about the nine months that would follow.

Aside from your doctor, women who have experienced a loss and have had the courage to try again are in the best position to give you the encouragement and advice you need. You will meet many such women in this book. They, like you, have experienced the heartbreak of pregnancy loss. But each of them has also gone on to have a subsequent pregnancy that ended with the birth of a healthy baby—proof positive that, contrary to how you may be feeling now, a successful pregnancy is possible after the devastation of a loss. Yes, for some there were roadblocks and setbacks along the way. A few even had to endure more than one loss. But ultimately, each of them brought home the baby they so desperately wanted. If you did not think the same was possible for you, then you probably would not even be considering another pregnancy.

In my case, I conceived again four months after my first son, Patrick, died. It was a difficult pregnancy, not so much physically as emotionally. Although I tried to maintain a positive attitude, I was continually scared that something would go wrong. I held my breath each time the doctor checked for my baby's heartbeat. And anytime the baby didn't move, I panicked. It was only when I was finally able to hold my newborn son, Andrew, in my arms that I finally began to relax.

A year and a half later, I got pregnant again, and this time things were a little easier. I had a toddler to care for and didn't have as much time to worry. Besides, I knew that it was possible for me to have a healthy baby. I could see proof of it before my eyes. Still, I was tense before every checkup and spent many sleepless nights fearing the worst. Thankfully, on May 15, 1997—the very day that Patrick would have celebrated his third birthday—my husband and I brought our third baby home from the hospital, a boy named Michael. It was bittersweet to welcome a new baby home on the anniversary of our loss, yet it was a vivid reminder of how wrong I had been to think that I would never experience such joy.

In some respects, I might be considered one of the lucky ones. My loss was the result of a rare problem with the umbilical cord that was unlikely to ever recur. Otherwise, my pregnancy was altogether healthy. But in the course of researching this book, I met woman after woman who had to beat incredible odds to have another baby.

Nancy, for example, suffered the loss of twin boys after spending thousands of dollars on fertility treatment over several years. For her, having another child not only meant the stress of making it through the subsequent pregnancy, but also another stressful round of hormone shots, blood tests and in vitro fertilization. It took Nancy more than a year to conceive again after her loss, and early on she had problems that landed her on bed rest for the entire pregnancy. But she is now the mother of a rambunctious sixteen-month-old girl and says that while her pregnancies were the hardest experiences of her life, they were also, by far, the most worthwhile.

And then there was Lynn, who had a rare genetic defect that made her odds of having a healthy baby only fifty-fifty. Although perfectly healthy by all appearances, Lynn discovered that she had a chromosomal problem shortly after suffering a miscarriage. She was then faced with the dilemma of whether or not she should try again. She knew that it was just as likely as not that she would miscarry again in the first trimester. After much soul-searching and prayer, Lynn and her husband decided that they were willing to brave the odds. Today, they have two healthy boys.

I also met Rita, who had given birth to her daughter Natalie nearly sixteen weeks prematurely. The baby was given a slim chance of surviving beyond the first three days. But she ended up fighting for her life for months in the neonatal intensive care unit. During this stressful period, Rita discovered to her horror that she was pregnant again. She was convinced that she would miscarry because of the tremendous strain she was under. Things only got worse when Natalie died when Rita was twenty-four weeks pregnant—the same point when she had gone into early labor the first time. Although it wasn't easy, Rita did not let grief overwhelm her. Naturally she mourned, but she also did her best to stay calm and follow her doctor's orders. She eventually gave birth to a full-term healthy boy and has since had two other children.

My hope is that by sharing our experiences, those of us who have successfully completed a subsequent pregnancy can help you through the journey that awaits you. If you know what to expect—from the paralyzing fears to the unbridled joy—the prospect of another pregnancy can be much less daunting. You will realize that your feelings are not all that different from others who have walked down the same path.

But this book will offer you much more than just personal experiences. You will also learn about the latest medical procedures available for prenatal monitoring and testing and get pointers on how to cope if your doctor confines you to bed rest. You'll find answers to some of the most common questions about pregnancy after a loss, everything from the mixed feelings a positive pregnancy test is likely to evoke to the pros and cons of finding out the gender of your next baby.

We'll also consider the father's perspective on the pregnancy, especially those feelings that he may have difficulty sharing. And we will discuss some ways that both you and your partner can ease your anxiety during what are likely to be some of the most difficult months of your lives. We'll discuss the feelings you may experience when you bring a healthy baby home from the hospital and tell you how other parents have chosen to remember the children they have lost. We'll begin by exploring the reasons for your loss, because if you can understand what went wrong the last time, you will be in a better position to ensure that it does not happen again.

The Search for Answers

In the weeks following a loss, every woman grieves for what might have been. The empty crib, the closet full of tiny outfits and the carefully prepared nursery are all reminders of the baby who won't be coming home. Going out usually isn't much help because there inevitably seems to be some well-meaning coworker, bank teller or store clerk who hasn't heard the news. Even your own body offers no respite. One look in the mirror at your enlarged breasts and deflated tummy and you'll feel that life is at its cruelest.

If your loss came very early in the pregnancy, you may not have any visible reminders of your baby, and that can be difficult too. Perhaps you and your partner had not told anyone that you were expecting, and so have no one with whom to share your grief. And since there was no memorial service or funeral for your baby, you may feel like you never had a chance to say goodbye. These are some of the reasons why pregnancy loss has been described as a silent sorrow.

Although all of us who have suffered a pregnancy loss share a common grief, emotions can run the gamut when it comes to thoughts about another pregnancy. You may have left the hospital determined to get pregnant again as soon as you are physically able. Or you may have a completely different perspective and feel that you could never go through it again, at least not for a long while. Neither attitude is unusual.

Since you were ready to welcome a baby into your family, it's not surprising that you would want to find a way to make that happen again as soon as possible. Melinda had not even delivered her baby who had died in utero when she started talking about trying again. "As soon as they said the baby was dead—he was still in me—I was saying I want another one." On the other hand, you've experienced a major tragedy, so who can blame you for not wanting to get pregnant again? It took Diane six months after the death of her newborn son before she could even think about another pregnancy. "It hurt so bad, I couldn't imagine going through it again. But over time I realized that the four days that I had with my son were worth everything that I had been through, so even if things did not turn out okay the next time, I still wanted to try."

Regardless of how you're feeling right now, keep in mind that the period immediately following your loss is a critical time for gathering information that will help you decide if and when to get pregnant again. Doctors can begin the search for what went wrong by investigating what caused the baby's problems, and, if necessary, putting you through a thorough physical exam to isolate any medical condition that may have been a factor in your loss. Obviously, your physician will play an important role in this process, but you should not hesitate to seek a second opinion. Often, another doctor will simply confirm what you already know, but in the process, will give you the reassurance you need to face another pregnancy with some confidence.

"I think the need to know what went wrong in the pregnancy that ended in a loss is related to the fact that if a woman knows what happened, then she might have some control in the next pregnancy," says Joann O'Leary, who has helped run the Pregnancy after a Loss program at Abbott Northwestern Hospital in Minneapolis for the last ten years. "Not knowing makes the next pregnancy even more scary because then she really doesn't have a sense of control."

For some couples, the search for answers brings devastating news, but for the vast majority, it brings new hope that enables them to try again. Laura is a case in point. She was thirty-five years old and had been married six years when she became pregnant for the first time. In the early months, there were no indications of any problems, but late in her second trimester she began having contractions. Although she was only twenty-three weeks along, she went into early labor and delivered a baby who died shortly after birth. From the baby's appearance, the obstetrician suspected he had died as a result of a heart defect, but since no other details were available, Laura and her husband Tom agreed to an autopsy. Unlike smaller hospitals where autopsy results are available within a few days, test results at the large Chicago medical center where Laura delivered were not due in for at least two months. In the meantime, the couple decided to talk to their doctor about their prospects for a subsequent pregnancy. According to Laura:

> *The doctor had a little bit of information about what had happened with David, but not enough to be very specific. So she told us that the risk of it happening again could be anywhere from very slight to a 50 percent chance. Of course, all we focused on was the 50 percent, so we left feeling absolutely devastated. When we had a chance to talk about it, we decided that for our own peace of mind, we were not going to get pregnant again until all the results of the autopsy were in.*

Fortunately, the autopsy revealed that the baby's heart condition was rare and unlikely to recur in another pregnancy. So, with that information in hand, Laura got pregnant again two months later and went on to deliver a healthy baby girl. But Laura and Tom's experience illustrates how important accurate information can be when making a decision about another pregnancy. If they had not discovered that the pregnancy loss was the result of a rare condition, they either might have decided not to try again or faced another pregnancy with unnecessary anxiety. Although there were still plenty of tense moments during Laura's next pregnancy, she and her husband were able to reassure themselves with facts.

Another important reason to search for the causes of your loss is that it may help alleviate any irrational guilt that you may be feeling. If your doctor was like mine, one of the first things he said after the loss is that there was absolutely nothing you did to cause your baby's death, and there was nothing you could have done to prevent it. You might have nodded your head in agreement at the time, yet found it difficult to believe later.

Perhaps you reviewed everything you did or did not do right around the time the baby died. Melinda blamed herself for going out on a boat when she was thirty-five weeks pregnant. "I wonder if all that bumping around caused the cord to twist." Christine had made a cross-country trip to California and ended up miscarrying while she was out of town. "I felt so guilty for traveling so far when I was pregnant." Some women even see the pregnancy loss as punishment for something they have done in the past. That's how Sharon felt when she first learned the news. "My mom said the first thing I said to her when I got to the hospital that Monday was 'What have I done?' And I really meant it. I thought I must have done something to deserve this and this is payback time."

Although there are things women can do to trigger a pregnancy loss, the kinds of actions that most of us tend to feel guilty about are not among them. "It is normal for women to wonder whether they were somehow responsible for their loss," says Cathi Lammert, executive director of SHARE Pregnancy and Infant Loss Support in St. Louis, Missouri. "They think, 'Maybe I took something that I shouldn't have,' or 'Maybe I was too stressed out at work,' or 'Maybe I shouldn't have picked up the other children.' But over time, they reflect and know that they didn't do anything wrong." Did you feel like you worked too hard, didn't exercise enough or ate too much junk food? Chances are that the things that you worried about had nothing whatsoever to do with your loss.

Nevertheless, some of us can only rid ourselves of guilt by discovering exactly why our pregnancy ended in a loss. It is only when we have the facts in hand that we are finally able to come to terms with the idea that our loss was not anybody's fault. And what about those couples who are never able to pinpoint the cause? We'll address that situation later in this chapter. For now, let's focus on all of the things you *can* do to get some answers.

The Follow-up Visit

Typically, the follow-up visit, which takes place anywhere from two to six weeks after the pregnancy ends, will be your first chance since your loss to talk to your obstetrician about what happened and why. If you agreed to genetic testing or an autopsy on the baby, all the test results are usually in by this time, and you and your doctor can discuss them in depth. But the weeks leading up to the visit can be agonizingly long.

In my case, I waited six weeks for an appointment, only to have it rescheduled at the last minute because the doctor had been up all night delivering a baby. I cried all day, bitter at the thought that he had been busy bringing a healthy baby into this world while I had to wait one day longer to understand why mine had died. In retrospect, I realize that I should have been more assertive about getting the information I wanted. Although my doctor had explained some things to me before I left the hospital, I had a long list of unanswered questions. Yet I just took it for granted that I had to wait another six weeks to talk with him again. Those turned out to be some of the hardest weeks of my life. Not only was I mourning my baby, I was also wondering if I would ever have another one. Instead of basing my fears on the facts, I relied on my imagination, which conjured up scenarios that were far worse than reality. I now know that I could have avoided some of that pain by picking up the phone and insisting that I meet with my doctor sooner.

I hope that you can learn from my experience. If you think six weeks is too long to wait for an appointment, let your doctor know how you feel and ask that your follow-up visit be scheduled in two or three weeks or whenever you want it to be. You have already been through enough suffering; there is no reason why you should have to wait any longer than necessary to get the answers to your questions.

Keep in mind that it usually takes less than two weeks to get the results of an autopsy or blood work, and chromosomal analyses are usually available within four weeks. Even if the results prove inconclusive, it is still helpful to meet with your doctor sooner rather than later. When there is no obvious cause for a loss, the biggest key to figuring out what happened is simply to review every detail of the pregnancy from beginning to end. You will want to do that while the memories are still fresh. Your doctor may not have all the answers at the follow-up visit, but the appointment can be an important start. You can leave armed with a strategy for resolving unanswered questions and can then do everything in your power to ensure a successful pregnancy the next time.

But as much as you and your husband may be anticipating the follow-up visit, the meeting itself can be very painful. Simply stepping inside the doctor's office will bring all the memories of your pregnancy flooding back. It is an experience that would be difficult even several months or years after your loss. But coming as it does only weeks later, it can be heartbreaking. The hormonal changes taking place inside your body only compound the pain. You may also be fearful of the news you may receive. I worried that my doctor would advise me not to get pregnant again for months. Or worse still, that I would find out there was a strong possibility that I would suffer another pregnancy loss.

How your physician and his staff react to you during this emotional time will give you an indication of whether you will want to keep the same doctor during your next pregnancy. If they are sensitive to your feelings now, there is a good chance that they will be closely attuned to your needs when you return for your next round of prenatal care. That was the case with Mary, whose first baby died six hours after birth:

My doctor was in a practice with five or six others, so they saw a lot of patients. But when I walked in the door for my postpartum visit, they immediately whisked me away so I wouldn't have to sit in the waiting room. Then, he and the nurse sat down with me and spent a long time answering

all my questions. I found out that day that the nurse had lost a baby, too,
so she really understood how I was feeling. They were so good to me, and
I think that was 100 percent of my recovery. My doctor, the nurse and
everyone associated with my case were so wonderful, not only to me, but to
my family.

Not surprisingly, Mary stayed with the same doctor during her next pregnancy. But unfortunately, not everyone's follow-up visit is such a positive experience. Suzanne's appointment was enough to convince her that she could never go back to the same doctor for a future pregnancy:

When I arrived at the office and saw all those pregnant women in the
waiting room, I wanted to scream. I started crying and just kept thinking,
"Why did this have to happen to me?" I went into the bathroom and tried
to pull myself together, but I couldn't, so I went to the nurse and asked if
I could go into a room by myself. She acted like she didn't want to deal
with it, but she did take me to the nurses' station. Then she sat down and
started talking to me about her grandkids. I was thinking to myself, "I
don't want to hear about your grandkids. I either want to sit here and be
quiet, or I want to talk about what happened." When the doctor finally
came in, he said, "I don't want you thinking about this baby. What hap-
pened was just a fluke. You can wait a year or two and get pregnant again."
That was not what I wanted to hear either.

For Suzanne, who lost her baby at thirty-five weeks, the idea of waiting a year or two to get pregnant again sounded interminable. Physically, she was fine, and she knew from her baby's autopsy results that the problems she had in her previous pregnancy were unlikely to repeat. Upon reflection, she decided that the doctor had given her advice without taking into account her despair over her loss and her strong desire to have another baby. After seeking a second opinion and doing some soul-searching with her husband, Suzanne got pregnant again six months later.

If your doctor seems as indifferent as Suzanne's, it may help to remember that obstetricians are not accustomed to dealing with death. Early pregnancy losses are fairly common, but unless a doctor specializes in high-risk pregnancies, he generally will only rarely see a late pregnancy loss. That means that when it does happen, he may be unprepared to handle it. Complicating the situation is that the doctor may feel guilty, angry or resentful about what happened. He may also feel a sense of failure or helplessness. Researchers have found that doctors often cope with these feelings by trying to block the loss out of their mind. That obviously makes them extremely insensitive to the needs of those who had suffered the loss. In their defense, doctors point out that they receive virtually no training, either in medical school or through further study, to deal with pregnancy loss. This may help explain why so many women feel that their doctor said all the wrong things after the loss.

When faced with a loss, many doctors struggle with what they see as a paradox: their job is to relieve suffering, but discussing the loss with their patient inflicts pain. Some physicians even admit that they chose ob/gyn as a specialty because they were uncomfortable with death and dying. While their aversion is understandable, you will need to find a doctor who can discuss your loss openly and help you deal with the fears that will be an inevitable part of your next pregnancy. That means choosing someone with the right combination of good bedside manners and medical expertise.

For most of us, the follow-up visit is neither as pleasant as Mary's nor as traumatizing as Suzanne's. My appointment might have been tolerable were it not for no one in the office even bothering to mention my loss until I had been there for nearly an hour. In fact, the same nurse who had visited me in tears at the hospital greeted me six weeks later as if I had come in only for a routine visit. She went about the business of weighing me, taking my blood pressure and asking general questions about my physical condition, never once asking how I was coping with my loss. The doctor behaved similarly in the examination room. He looked at my c-section incision, performed a pelvic exam and pronounced me fit. Although they both shifted gears and were quite sympathetic when we went into his office to talk, I was put off by the way they had treated me earlier. I wondered if they took such a matter-of-fact approach because they were afraid of upsetting the other patients. Once again, it seemed that the women who were expecting babies were given priority over me.

Obviously, there is no way to control how your doctor and his staff will treat you during your follow-up visit, but there are some steps you can take to reduce your stress. For starters, call ahead and emphasize that you will need some extra time with the doctor. Ask if you can be the first or last appointment of the day. That way you can avoid sitting in a waiting room full of pregnant women. Or simply request that they allow enough time between appointments so that you do not feel rushed. Having done that, put the issue out of your mind. Even if the waiting room is full when you arrive, insist on taking all the time you need. Another advantage to calling ahead is that it will serve as a reminder to the staff to prepare for your arrival. As difficult as it is to believe, some of those who work in your doctor's office may not be aware or may have forgotten that you suffered a loss. That was the case when Cynthia went in for her follow-up visit only two weeks after being told by her doctor that her baby had died:

> The same nurse who had been handing me tissues to dry my tears two weeks before asked me as she was escorting me into the examination room, "So, how many more weeks until delivery?" I didn't expect her to necessarily remember me because I know it's a very busy practice, but she had my chart in her hands. If she had just opened up the chart, she would have known.

Cynthia was all the more shocked at the nurse's insensitivity because her doctor specialized in high-risk pregnancies. "In an office like that where they probably deal with a lot of losses, you would think they would try to familiarize themselves with what the visit was about," she says.

It may also help to write down your questions ahead of time. That will guard against the risk of returning home only to realize that there were important things you forgot to ask. You also may want to bring along a tape recorder and record the conversation so that you can replay it when your head is clearer. As you compose your list of questions, keep in mind that some information may be potentially painful. If you are unprepared, these questions may be better left unanswered. Janice wanted to know whether her baby, who was stillborn two weeks after her due date, suffered when he died. She was relieved when the doctor told her that the end came quickly and was likely painless. But if the answer had been different, it very well may have haunted her for years.

If the doctor is unable to answer your questions, you may consider asking him to closely review your chart one more time to see if there was anything out of the ordinary that might explain what happened. Was your blood pressure high? Was the baby measuring according to dates? Did the sonogram indicate any areas of concern? How much amniotic fluid did you have just before your loss? Did your placenta look healthy? All of these questions could provide valuable insight and help to unravel the mystery.

You could also try reversing roles and letting your doctor be the one to ask the questions. As discussed earlier, the circumstances surrounding the loss are extremely important when there are no clear-cut reasons for the baby's death. A good doctor will be like a detective looking for clues. By closely reexamining the course of your pregnancy along with your medical history, he may be able to determine what went wrong. Start at the beginning and reconstruct everything that happened after conception. Ask your doctor to prompt you with appropriate questions. How was your overall health? Were you taking any medications? Did anything out of the ordinary happen? Upon reflection, was there anything that seemed insignificant then that now takes on new meaning?

It is particularly important to discuss in detail what was happening in the hours and days just before your miscarriage or stillbirth. Did you have any bleeding? Were you having contractions? Was the baby's movement good? One doctor I know starts asking these questions even before he gives a woman the news that her baby has died. While this may seem cruel on the surface, it enables him to gather critical clues before the shock sets in and details become hazy. Even if you covered a lot of the same ground with your doctor immediately after your loss, go over it again. There may have been something you missed that will prove to be significant.

In some cases, the reasons for your loss are so clear-cut that there is really not a lot of new information to discuss at your follow-up appointment, other than if and when you can safely get pregnant again. That was true of Beth, whose baby was diagnosed at birth with a rare genetic disorder. But that didn't make her visit any easier. "It was hard because I had my baby weight, I was hurting and I had nothing to show for it," she said. "I felt like the only thing I got out of my pregnancy was pain."

Other Sources of Information

If you and your partner are among the many couples who decided against genetic testing or an autopsy on the baby, and the doctors you consulted were unable to pinpoint why the pregnancy ended in a loss, the search for answers will be more difficult. But there are plenty of other avenues you can explore. Keep in mind that even if you were too devastated in the weeks following the loss to seek any sort of explanation, it is never too late to begin. In some cases, genetic counseling might be in order. Or if your own health is suspected in the loss, there may be medical procedures that you can undergo to improve your chances of carrying a baby to term. Doctors will usually begin with the simplest, least expensive test and proceed to whatever else is necessary to try to determine the reason for your loss.

One word of caution: it helps to be informed about all your testing alternatives, since the approaches that doctors take in investigating pregnancy loss vary widely. If the loss came after twenty weeks in your pregnancy, the search for answers is likely to be relatively thorough. But if your loss was early (even if it was your second miscarriage), your obstetrician might just chalk it up to bad luck and simply tell you to go home and try again. Only about 15 percent of women who miscarry once go on to suffer a second consecutive loss—about the same percentage as those who have never miscarried before. Put another way, between 80 and 90 percent go on to have a term pregnancy. After two successive miscarriages, the risk of subsequent loss increases to about 25 percent. That means 75 percent of women go on to have a successful pregnancy without any treatment at all. This may help explain why some doctors are reluctant to begin looking for the cause of a pregnancy loss until after the second or even third miscarriage.

But while the "wait-and-see approach" may have been standard medical practice in the past, there has recently been a change of thinking on this issue. If you look at the statistics again, you'll see that the risk of a miscarriage nearly doubles after the second miscarriage. That's one of the reasons why the American College of Obstetricians and Gynecologists now recommends testing after a second successive loss—especially for women over the age of thirty-five. That is welcome news for women like Cynthia who have had to endure multiple losses with no explanation whatsoever:

To make a woman suffer through three miscarriages before [doctors] start looking for answers is crazy. I knew after I lost my first at sixteen weeks that something was wrong. You don't just lose a baby at sixteen weeks. But everyone kept saying, it's just bad luck and sometimes things just happen. Then, when I lost the second, I said, that's enough. You've got to start looking for something.

When your doctor does decide to study further to determine what may be causing your losses, it is important to remember that some physicians take a more aggressive approach to testing than others. You may have one or all of the following tests and procedures depending on your particular doctor and your individual circumstances. The evaluation may turn up several factors that alone or together may be responsible for the loss.

Immunologic Testing

In recent years, there has been mounting evidence that immune problems are involved in pregnancy loss, especially recurrent losses. There are three types of antibodies commonly linked to problems in pregnancy: antiphospholipid antibodies, antithyroid antibodies and antinuclear antibodies. Despite their long and complicated names, they all work in a similar fashion. To understand exactly what role they play, it helps to know a little about the body's immune system.

The immune system, our body's first line of defense against disease, is made up of antibodies that help fight foreign organisms like bacteria and viruses. In some cases, otherwise healthy women produce antibodies that go haywire and start attacking normal cells. This phenomenon is commonly known as an autoimmune disorder. The most common of the autoimmune disorders linked with pregnancy loss is antiphospholipid antibody syndrome. The disorder gets its name from the body mistakenly recognizing phospholipids—part of a cell's membrane—as foreign and producing antibodies against them. It is not clear how these antibodies complicate a pregnancy, but one theory is that they may cause clots in the blood vessels of the placenta. Since the placenta serves as the baby's life-support system, anything that affects the flow of nourishment and oxygen between the mother and her baby can cause serious problems. Antiphospholipid syndrome has been linked to a variety of pregnancy complications, including a higher risk of miscarriage, poor fetal growth, pre-eclampsia and placental abruption. Often the losses occur late in the first trimester or in the second trimester, but the syndrome has also been associated with third-trimester pregnancy losses.

Doctors who suspect an autoimmune disorder in their patients routinely test for the antiphospholipid antibodies most often associated with recurrent pregnancy loss—anticardiolipin antibody and lupus anticoagulant. But actually other antiphospholipid antibodies can also cause problems in pregnancy. A full work-up would include checking for every known type of antiphospholipid antibody. If the results of these tests come back normal, your doctor may also decide to test for other antibodies associated with complications in pregnancy, such as antinuclear antibodies and antithyroid antibodies.

Treatment for a woman who tests positive for an autoimmune disorder is usually based on her medical history. If you have suffered only one loss, and perhaps have even given birth to a healthy child before, your doctor may recommend that you simply take one baby aspirin a day, beginning one month before you start trying to conceive again and continuing throughout your pregnancy. Aspirin thins the blood and helps prevent the formation of clots. For women who have a history of recurrent pregnancy losses or blood clots, the therapy of choice is usually heparin in combination with low-dose aspirin. Heparin, a more powerful blood-thinning drug, is typically injected twice a day, but it can also be administered with a portable pump. Studies have shown that therapy with a combination of heparin and aspirin is more effective than aspirin alone. Since heparin does not cross the placenta, it has not been linked to any problems with the baby, but it may sometimes cause nose bleeds or other minor side effects in the mother. While research on the best treatment options are still ongoing, some studies have reported a 75 to 93 percent success rate in the subsequent pregnancy with the heparin/baby aspirin therapy.

For women who have unusually high amounts of antiphospholipid antibodies in their bloodstream, doctors sometimes prescribe the steroid prednisone in addition to heparin and baby aspirin. This steroid is believed to suppress the activity of the errant antibodies. But since recent studies have suggested that prednisone could have significant side effects in both the mother and the baby, this treatment is somewhat controversial. The decision to take any medication in pregnancy is never an easy one, so the best approach is to discuss all of the pros and cons of the various treatment options with your obstetrician. Your doctor will make the final decision after weighing the associated risks and benefits.

A new but extremely expensive method for treating autoimmune disorders is intravenous immunoglobulin (IVIg), a process whereby the mother is infused with antibodies from donors in the general population. The donor immunoglobulin distracts the harmful antibodies, thus keeping them away from the developing baby. The cost for IVIg treatment throughout pregnancy ranges from $10,000 to $30,000, but does provide an alternative for women who continue to suffer losses even with the heparin and aspirin therapy.

Regardless of which course of treatment is prescribed for you, your doctor will want to closely monitor your baby throughout your pregnancy for problems typically associated with autoimmune disorders. You may have monthly sonograms to check your baby's growth. Beginning at thirty-two weeks of gestation, you may also have weekly biophysical profiles and non-stress tests.

Rh incompatibility is another type of antibody problem, which was once a leading cause of pregnancy loss, but today can usually be easily managed. It occurs when the mother's blood is Rh-negative and the father's is Rh-positive. If the baby also has Rh-positive blood, the mother can became Rh-sensitized. That means that if the baby's blood mixes with hers, as often happens during birth or following a miscarriage, she develops antibodies that attack the baby's red blood cells. This can cause anemia in the baby as well as a host of other life-threatening conditions. Rh-sensitization rarely occurs in first pregnancies but is of concern in subsequent pregnancies.

Fortunately, a vaccine has been developed that can prevent this problem from occurring. If you are Rh-negative and your partner is Rh-positive, you were probably given an injection of Rh Immune Globulin after your miscarriage or delivery. This was done to prevent you from producing antibodies to Rh-positive cells that could cause problems should you decide to get pregnant again. You would receive additional injections at twenty-eight weeks gestation in your next pregnancy, and after each amniocentesis, chorionic villus sampling or any other time when there is a possibility that maternal and fetal blood may have mixed. Occasionally, a mother can develop the dangerous antibodies to the Rh factor before the vaccine is administered. In that case, doctors monitor the next baby closely for signs of anemia, and, in extreme cases, do a blood tranfusion in utero.

Uterine Exams

Abnormalities of the uterus are a significant cause of miscarriages and stillbirths. One of the most commonly seen problems is a misshapen uterus. It may be too small or have two chambers rather than the usual one. Many women have a septum running down the middle of the uterus, giving it a heartlike shape. In certain cases, this may mean that the baby does not have enough room to grow. Less frequently, fibroid tumors can be a source of complications. Depending on their size and location, these benign growths can interfere with implantation of the embryo or the blood supply reaching the baby.

Since sonograms and old-fashioned X rays can miss subtle but important abnormalities, doctors are increasingly using a more sophisticated technique called a hysterosalpingogram to detect uterine problems. In this procedure, a radiologist injects dye into the uterus and then uses high-resolution ultrasound imaging to conduct an examination. If the imaging is inconclusive, the next step is to directly view the inside of the uterus using a hysteroscope. In this procedure, the cervix is dilated, and a flexible fiberoptic telescope is inserted, enabling the doctor to look at the cavity of the uterus. Carbon dioxide gas may be used to expand the uterus for better viewing. Minor abnormalities, such as fibroids, can be removed during this out-patient procedure. The removal of a septum, on the other hand, usually requires surgery.

Even if doctors find and correct a uterine problem, there is no guarantee that it was the cause of the miscarriage. However, it will be one less thing that can interfere in the course of the next pregnancy.

Genetic Testing

Genetic testing may offer some clues as to what caused the pregnancy loss, or perhaps may simply reassure you that you are at no greater risk than anyone else of having a baby with a particular problem. A chromosomal analysis of the baby, for example, can sometimes determine whether a genetic problem was a factor in the loss. If the results indicate that it was, your doctor or a genetic counselor can discuss the possibility of that particular defect recurring in another pregnancy. Often, however, genetic testing of the baby proves inconclusive either because there is not enough fetal tissue available for analysis or because it is not possible to culture the baby's cells in the laboratory. In that case, you may want to consider having your own chromosomes checked for abnormalities. You and your partner can be completely healthy but still carry a defective chromosome or gene that combines to cause problems for the baby.

In a procedure, known as a karyotype, blood is taken from both you and your partner and sent to a laboratory where both sets of chromosomes are analyzed. About 2 to 3 percent of the population have a chromosomal problem known as a balanced translocation. That means that even though they are perfectly healthy, their chromosomal material is arranged incorrectly. When this rearranged genetic material is passed on to an offspring, the pregnancy may end in a loss or with the birth of a baby who has congenital abnormalities. But it is also possible for a parent with a balanced translocation to have a healthy baby.

As part of your genetic screening, a counselor will ask you to fill out a questionnaire on any family history of birth defects. This is done to determine whether a baby you conceive could be at any greater risk for a particular type of defect. You will also be asked about your ethnicity, since some genetic problems are more prevalent in certain ethnic groups. For example, Jews of central and eastern European descent are at greater risk for having a baby with Tay-Sachs disease, while African Americans can be carriers of the gene for sickle cell anemia.

We will further examine different types of genetic problems later in this chapter, but keep in mind that because karyotyping is expensive—costing around $600 per person—it is usually only recommended for couples considered to be at high risk. If you are among those that will not be genetically tested there is little reason to dwell on the possibility of birth defects. Despite your history of pregnancy loss, it is important to remember that 98 percent of babies born to women under forty are born without any inherited diseases.

Laboratory Studies

Suffering minor illnesses during pregnancy, such as the common cold, has not been associated with complications in the developing baby. But there are a wide range of infectious diseases that can damage the baby growing in the womb, although a direct link is sometimes difficult to establish. For example, several infections are believed to cause congenital malformations or pregnancy loss. These include rubella, also known as German measles; cytomegalovirus, the most common cause of intrauterine infection; parovirus, which causes an infection known as fifth disease; toxoplasmosis, a parasite found in cat feces; mycoplasma, an infection linked to recurrent miscarriages; and sexually transmitted diseases, such as chlamydia, gonorrhea, syphilis and HIV. Other common infections that cause problems are genital herpes, mumps, chicken pox, hepatitis A and B, and Group B Streptococcus.

If your baby was not tested at the time of your loss, your doctor can check to see if you have any evidence of these infections either through a blood test or a culture taken from your cervix and vagina. Urine samples and sperm specimens from the father can also reveal infections. If the results show that you have a bacterial infection, such as mycoplasma, you probably will be treated with antibiotics. Treatment for viruses may vary. The good news is that infections rarely tend to recur in subsequent pregnancies.

Hormone Tests

The hormone progesterone plays a very important role in early pregnancy. Among other things, it helps to build up the lining of the uterus after ovulation so that the uterus can provide vital nutrition for the baby. Progesterone is produced by the ovaries until the placenta assumes this function sometime between the seventh and tenth week of pregnancy. But some women produce such low levels of progesterone in early pregnancy that they miscarry shortly after conception. The medical term for this problem is luteal phase defect.

If your loss occurred before the tenth week of pregnancy, your doctor may want to perform an endometrial biopsy, a procedure in which the lining of the uterus is analyzed to determine whether it is developing normally. The biopsy is done by inserting a narrow catheter through the cervix and into the uterus. A small sample of tissue is scraped from the uterine lining and sent to a lab for analysis. If the lining has not properly developed, it may indicate a hormonal problem. Another way to test for low levels of progesterone is through a series of blood tests. Blood samples are taken at regular intervals beginning at ovulation. The levels of progesterone in the blood should be rising. If they are not, it may indicate a hormonal deficiency. But checking for a hormonal deficiency is not as easy as it sounds. Since the amount of progesterone needed to sustain a pregnancy varies from woman to woman, it is difficult to determine exactly what level of the hormone should be present in the blood. Similarly, some suggest that the endometrial biopsy is only as good as the pathologist reading the results.

Once a diagnosis of low progesterone has been made, the fertility drug clomiphene citrate is often prescribed. Marketed under the brand name Clomid, this drug enables a woman to keep producing the hormones the ovaries need to manufacture progesterone throughout early pregnancy. Hormone supplements, in the form of suppositories, injections, pills or a combination of the three, are another option. Doctors usually prescribe supplements before conception to enable women to get a healthier start on their pregnancies. Under one approach, vaginal suppositories of natural hormone progesterone are used three times a day, beginning at ovulation. If a pregnancy test at the end of the cycle shows that a woman has not conceived, she would discontinue the use of progesterone until ovulating the following month. If she is pregnant, she would continue taking the hormone through the first trimester of pregnancy, usually until about the tenth week. During this time, a doctor would continue doing hormone-level tests to ensure that progesterone levels remain high.

Although the effectiveness of progesterone therapy has not been clinically proven, it is routinely prescribed since the natural hormone used by doctors today is similar in chemical structure to the progesterone produced in a woman's ovaries and is therefore believed to be safe. Since progesterone levels can vary from month to month, some doctors even prescribe hormone supplements when the level appears to be normal. But as with any medication taken during pregnancy, it is a good idea to discuss the inherent risks and benefits of hormone replacement therapy with your own obstetrician.

In rare cases, hormonal problems in pregnancy can be caused by disorders of the thyroid. If your doctor suspects that a thyroid disorder may be the cause of your loss, he can perform a thyroid function test to determine if you have an imbalance or deficiency of the hormone thyroxin.

Getting a Second Opinion

Sometimes, despite your doctor's best efforts to find the reason for your loss, you will feel dissatisfied. Cynthia was frustrated by her doctor's seeming lack of interest in figuring out what had caused her loss.

We expected to go in and have him take a "take-charge" type of attitude and be aggressive about figuring out what we could do to rectify the situation. But he expressed absolutely no concern in helping us find out what the problem was; none whatsoever. I asked him, "What do you think this was?" and he said, "I have no idea." I said, "What can we do?" and he said, "I have no idea." So, needless to say, we parted ways. The next doctor I found took an entirely different approach to the problem. The very first time we met with him, he said "I just want you to know, this is war." It

made me feel like someone else was genuinely, compassionately concerned
about helping me figure this out.

The second doctor tested Cynthia for the full range of antibody problems, one of which turned out to be the cause of her losses. She then went on to give birth to twins. As Cynthia's experience illustrates, sometimes a second opinion can make the difference between suffering multiple losses and having a healthy baby.

Most of us are reluctant to challenge an authority figure, but you should not hesitate to trust your instinct even if your doctor reassures you that there is no need for a second opinion. Sheila's obstetrician had told her that although tests revealed that her uterus was misshapen, there was no reason why she should not be able to carry a baby to term. Or, as he put it, "If it ain't broke, don't fix it." While that news was reassuring at first, there was something about it that didn't ring true in Sheila's mind. So, she decided to go see a specialist. As it turned out, he had an entirely different take on the problem.

"I could tell as soon as he looked at my medical records that he had an idea," Sheila says. The second doctor believed that Sheila's two previous miscarriages had been caused by a septum that ran down the middle of her uterus, essentially dividing it in two. The only way for her to have a viable pregnancy, he said, was to correct the problem through surgery.

I remember going back to him for my post-op visit, and he said, "You're
ready to go. You're fine." And I asked, "Are you sure?" And he looked at
me and said, "That was the problem. It will not happen again because of
that." This time I really felt like that was the case. And that's what I needed
before I could try again.

Even if you were satisfied with the reasons you were given for your pregnancy loss, a second opinion is still a good idea. Although some women are fearful of offending their physician by going to someone else, most doctors will understand your desire for more information.

If your physician is part of a large practice, he may not even know what you are doing. "I was just a number," says Sheila, whose doctor was in practice with six other partners. "I don't think they cared." Another doctor can confirm the diagnosis or perhaps offer additional insight into other factors that may have come into play. During the consultation, you can also get tips on special measures to take during your next pregnancy. If, like Sheila, you get conflicting opinions when you go see a specialist, you might even consider going to a third doctor.

Initially, I didn't want a second opinion for the same reasons you may have decided against one. I trusted my doctor implicitly and was confident that the explanations he had given me were completely accurate. Plus, the last thing I wanted to do was make him question my loyalty. Like most women, I had developed a close relationship with my obstetrician and felt I would be betraying him by seeing someone else. It was my sister who persuaded me to reconsider. She pointed out that the loss of my baby was one of the most serious things that would ever happen to me in life, so why not get some answers from the very best medical professionals in the field? Chances were, she said, that they would only confirm what I already knew, but wouldn't it be nice to have that extra reassurance? After thinking about it, I agreed.

Since my local medical school had a well-known maternal-fetal medicine department with doctors who were regularly quoted in newspaper and magazine articles on pregnancy loss, I decided to start there. When I called to describe my situation, they suggested that I make an appointment with the head of the department, who regularly consulted with women like me. That was the easy part. Now I had to work up the courage to tell my obstetrician what I had planned. It turned out to be relatively painless. I just called his office and told the nurse what I was doing. She, in turn, asked me to send in a written request for my medical records and suggested that I also contact the hospital for records pertaining to the delivery. Everything was sent to me, and I then forwarded copies to the medical school. By the time I arrived for my appointment, the doctor had everything he needed to assess my case, including the baby's autopsy results.

It should be just as easy for you to obtain your own medical records. Doctors and hospitals will usually release them to you upon written request, and there is absolutely no reason why you should be shy about asking. Offices are used to dealing with these requests all the time. You may even find your records to be interesting reading. Although they will be filled with medical jargon, you may discover details that your doctor did not mention that give you a clearer picture of what happened. Anything that you don't understand you can discuss with your specialist.

Just as before my postpartum visit, I was a nervous wreck before my appointment at the medical school. Even though I trusted my obstetrician, I feared that this new doctor would give me devastating news that would call into question everything I believed. In fact, just the opposite happened. The doctor confirmed that my particular problem was usually not detectable with ultrasound; therefore, nothing could have been done to prevent it. He also reiterated that what happened to me was extremely rare and assured me that the chances of the same thing happening again were remote. Even more reassuring to me was his advice about what I should do in the second pregnancy. He suggested that I keep a chart of the baby's movements beginning at twenty-eight weeks. He also advised that I undergo non-stress tests twice a week toward the end of my pregnancy. Since those were all things that my obstetrician had recommended the first time, I was convinced that I was receiving the best possible care.

Chances are that you, too, will learn that your obstetrician did everything right and that your loss was an unpredictable event. But if the news is not as good, keep in mind that your newfound knowledge can make a difference in your next pregnancy After discussing her case with a specialist, Charlotte realized that her doctor had been wrong to dismiss her concerns when she called to tell him the baby didn't seem to be moving as much. "He just told me to drink some juice and jiggle my stomach. He really wasn't concerned at all. I'm not sure that my baby could have been saved even if he had taken a more proactive approach, but I would have felt better knowing that he had tried harder." There have also been cases when doctors put off delivering a baby at the first sign of complications because it wasn't convenient or because they weren't on call that day. Perhaps your own doctor reassured you that things were probably going to be all right and that there was no need to worry. But as one physician I interviewed put it, obstetricians should not even have the word "probably" in their vocabularies; there simply is no room for maybes in obstetrics.

If you come to believe that your doctor could have acted more effectively to prevent the loss, find someone who will be more vigilant in your subsequent pregnancy. That won't necessarily help ease your bitterness about your loss, but it will improve your chances of bringing home a healthy baby next time. I'm a firm believer that knowledge is power, even when the information is bad. Another benefit that I derived from seeking a second opinion was hearing how optimistic the perinatologist was about a subsequent pregnancy for me. And when I told him that I didn't think I could cope during those periods when my second baby didn't move, he said, "But think how wonderful it will be when the baby *does* move." That lifted my spirits more than anything else I had heard.

Whom to Consult

If you decide to get a second opinion, you most likely will want to consult with a perinatologist, an obstetrician who specializes in high-risk and problematic pregnancies. When deciding who specifically to meet with, you may want to ask for a referral from your obstetrician. If that makes you uncomfortable, consider asking a nurse who works in a hospital labor and delivery ward, a friend who has lost a baby or the organizers of a pregnancy loss support group. Or, you could do as I did and call a medical school in your area. In some cases, consulting with a specialist might mean that you have to travel for hours to the next town or even the next state. That was true for Sydney, whose husband was stationed at a military base in North Carolina. "We had to drive over an hour to see one doctor and more than two hours to see another one." Like Sydney, however, you probably will find that the consultation is more than worth the effort.

When There Are No Answers

Unfortunately, in as many as half of all pregnancy losses, there is no explanation for what went wrong. Like Sudden Infant Death Syndrome, which inexplicably claims the lives of babies under the age of one, many pregnancies end in miscarriage or stillbirth for no apparent reason. In fact, recent research has suggested that the two phenomena may actually be linked. In both SIDS and unexplained stillbirth, babies die for no apparent reason. But the similarities do not end there. One study found both occur more often to boys than to girls and tend to be more common in fall and winter than spring and summer. These similarities have led some researchers to question whether some babies may have an unidentified susceptibility to sudden death that is programmed at a very early stage in their development.

If you have been unable to find an explanation for why your baby died, it may be more difficult to face the prospect of another pregnancy. The unknown can be much more painful and frightening than the known. You may tend to blame yourself for the loss and carry the heavy burden of guilt into your next pregnancy. "Human nature being what it is, most women can cope better if they know the reason for their loss," says Fran Rybarik, executive director of the national pregnancy loss organization Bereavement Services/RTS in La Crosse, Wisconsin. "It's much harder to cope when you don't know."

But the good news is that doctors generally agree that when there is no known cause for a pregnancy loss, the chance of suffering another loss is no greater than the odds faced by anyone else. Nevertheless, your doctor will probably want to see you twice as often as a regular OB patient to be sure that the baby is growing normally and that you have a good level of amniotic fluid. If he has an ultrasound machine in the office, he may perform a sonogram at every visit. All of this should serve to reassure you that your pregnancy is progressing well.

Coming to Terms with Your Loss

Often, women who have suffered a loss continue to search for causes long after doctors have put the issue to rest. This seems to be true whether or not they were given a reason for the loss. Despite reassurances to the contrary, women continue to wonder what they could have done to prevent the tragedy, or if there was anything they did to cause their baby to die. The feelings of guilt and the seemingly insatiable need to understand what caused the loss lead many women on a desperate quest for answers.

Katie, for example, found it impossible to take her doctor at his word when he assured her that there was nothing she could have done to cause her baby's stillbirth at forty weeks. Sensing her skepticism, he photocopied pages of information from his medical books describing the rare condition that caused her loss. Still, Katie was unable to accept the medical facts at face value. In some strange way, she felt that knowing she was responsible for the loss would make her feel that she could do something to ensure a successful pregnancy the next time around. On a mission, she went to the local medical school library and pored over articles looking for the magic formula that would ensure the success of her next pregnancy. "I absolutely knew it was my fault. In fact, I was wishing there was something I had done so that I could make sure that I didn't do it again," she says.

The searching can be even more intense when there is no explanation for the loss, as with SIDS. Matthew was twelve weeks old when he died on his third day at an in-home day care. After an exhaustive investigation that included a complete autopsy, examination of the death scene and a review of the baby's clinical history, the medical examiner ruled SIDS as the cause of death. Not surprisingly, Matthew's mother, Terri, was initially unable to come to terms with her son's mysterious death. The first person she looked to for answers was the woman who had been caring for her baby on the morning he died:

On the day of my son's funeral, I couldn't sleep, so I just got up and left my husband a note saying "Don't worry. I've gone to get some answers." Even though it was only 5 o'clock in the morning, I headed for her house. To be honest, when I drove up, I didn't know what I was going to do. I just knew I hated her. She didn't answer her door at first, so I just sat on her porch and cried.

Eventually, the babysitter let Terri in, and they talked again about the events that led up to her son's death. A few minutes into their conversation, another mother arrived to drop off her child. As chance would have it, she, too, had lost her first baby to SIDS but he had died at the home of a different daycare provider. "She was a big help to me," Terri says, "because I thought surely if she trusts this babysitter to care for her child, then she must be okay."

Still, Terri's search for answers was only just beginning. After she had ruled out the babysitter's role in her son's death, she began looking for medical explanations:

I started calling research centers and getting information on SIDS. I went to the library and got tons of articles from all kinds of medical journals. That's how I dealt with it—I read and read and read. Every time I found something that seemed related to what happened to Matthew, I'd go into my pediatrician's office and say "what about this?" He'd always bring me back down to reality. I also called the medical examiner on several occasions and asked him to review the autopsy results just one more time. I just wanted to be sure that there was nothing he might have missed that might explain why my son had died. He always took my calls, but I never learned anything new. After a while, everything was starting to sound the same.

This type of desperate search for answers is part of the natural grieving process. Researchers who have identified the different stages of grief say that searching and yearning typically follow the shock and numbness that we feel when we first find out about a loved one's death. After a pregnancy loss, we yearn for the baby who died, but we also yearn to know why.

Common Reasons for Pregnancy Loss

We've already discussed the role that immunologic problems, hormone deficiencies and infection can play in miscarriage and stillbirths. Now we will turn to some of the other common reasons for pregnancy loss, as well as the likelihood that the problem could recur in another pregnancy. Rather than perusing through this list casually, use it as a resource once you have isolated what caused your own loss. You will have enough to worry about in your next pregnancy without reading up on all the things that can possibly go wrong.

Genetic Problems

Genetic defects are the number-one cause of miscarriages, especially those that occur very early in pregnancy. They are responsible for more than half of all first-trimester losses and about 15 percent of miscarriages that occur in the second trimester. In some cases, a baby with a major genetic defect will survive the pregnancy, only to die a few hours or days after birth. Older mothers are more prone to pass on certain types of chromosomal problems, such as Down syndrome, but anyone can have a child with a genetic defect.

If your loss was attributed to a genetic problem, you undoubtedly want to know what caused it and whether it could happen again in a subsequent pregnancy. As discussed earlier in this chapter, you and your partner can undergo genetic counseling to determine whether you have a chromosomal problem or are carriers of any inherited diseases. In some cases, a chromosomal analysis can be done on the baby to determine what went wrong. However, it is important to keep in mind that the vast majority of genetic defects are random and unlikely to recur in a future pregnancy.

To understand why these random problems occur, it helps to know a little bit about how the reproductive process works. When a baby is conceived, a man and a woman each contribute twenty-three single chromosomes to create the new life. These forty-six chromosomes carry all of the child's genetic material—everything that determines the color of his hair to the size of his feet. Since these chromosomes duplicate themselves and divide many thousands of times during the course of a pregnancy, the possibility exists that problems will occur.

In the case of Down syndrome, for example, children have forty-seven chromosomes instead of the normal forty-six. Since there is an extra copy of the twenty-first chromosome, the abnormality is known as Trisomy 21. Although Down syndrome is the most common chromosomal abnormality, Trisomy 13 and Trisomy 18 are also caused by an extra chromosome and are almost always fatal to the baby. The vast majority of these cases are isolated occurrences; however, about 3 percent result from the parents being carriers of a chromosomal problem known as a balanced translocation. Although the parents appear normal, the genetic code they pass on to the baby is not.

Still other genetic defects, such as muscular dystrophy, sickle-cell anemia and cystic fibrosis, are the result of an abnormal gene on a chromosome. These defective genes can be recessive. That means a baby can inherit that particular defect only if both parents happen to be carriers. In this case, the chances of passing the disorder on to a child is 25 percent. Occasionally, an abnormal gene dominates over a normal one. For example, the gene for Huntington's disease, a degenerative disorder of the nervous system, is dominant. That means even if only one parent is a carrier of the disease, the baby has a 50 percent chance of inheriting it.

The chance that a particular type of genetic defect will recur in a subsequent pregnancy may range from no greater than average, when neither parent has an abnormal gene or balanced translocation, to a 50 percent chance in the case of a "dominant defect." The risk of having a baby with a chromosomal abnormality, such as Down syndrome, increases with a mother's age. For example, the risk of having a baby with Down syndrome is 1 in 1,667 at age 20, but increases to 1 in 378 by age 35. At age 40, the risk is about 1 in 106.

Once you have conceived, you can have prenatal testing for certain types of genetic problems. The most common forms of prenatal screens and tests include the maternal alpha-fetoprotein test, chorionic villus sampling, high-level sonograms and amniocentesis. We will discuss all of these procedures in depth later in the book.

Neural Tube Defects

Neural tube defects, such as spina bifida and anencephaly, are among the most common causes of pregnancy loss. In spina bifida, the spinal column does not completely enclose the spinal cord, which may result in paralysis, mental retardation or even death. Babies born with anencephaly have a severely underdeveloped skull and brain, a condition that is nearly always fatal. These conditions occur when the tube that forms the brain and spinal cord in a baby does not close completely by the end of the sixth week of pregnancy.

Researchers believe that neural tube defects are caused by a combination of genetic and environmental factors. Recent studies have indicated that diet may also play a significant role. In a landmark British study, doctors found that increased intake of folic acid at least one month before conception and in early pregnancy reduces the risk of neural tube defects by as much as 70 percent. We'll talk more about the role of folic acid in chapter 3.

Placental Problems

Placental problems are responsible for somewhere between 15 and 25 percent of all stillbirths and early infant deaths, making them one of the most common causes of pregnancy loss. The placenta serves as the baby's life-support system and begins to form from the moment an egg is fertilized. Oxygen and sustaining nutrients pass from the mother to the baby through this vital organ, while carbon dioxide and waste products cross through the placenta in the opposite direction, where they are disposed of by the mother. Not surprisingly, problems with this vital system are often life-threatening to the baby.

Placental abruption occurs when the placenta separates from the wall of the uterus before or during birth. Normally, the placenta does not separate from the uterus until after the baby is delivered. When it happens prematurely, it can deprive the baby of the nourishment it needs to survive. It can also cause internal bleeding in the mother, which can put her life at risk. Although placental abruption can occur at any time during the pregnancy, in nearly half of all cases the condition develops after the thirty-seventh week.

Researchers are not sure what causes the placenta to separate prematurely from the uterus, but they have identified several risk factors. One of the most significant is high blood pressure. Hypertension, whether pregnancy-induced or chronic, is thought to weaken the blood vessels that connect the placenta to the uterus, resulting in separation. Other factors that have been linked to placental abruption include cigarette smoking, abdominal trauma and preterm rupture of the fluid-filled sac surrounding the baby. Women who have had several D & Cs also are thought to be at higher risk for placental abruption because the procedure, which is sometimes done after a miscarriage to remove any remaining tissue in the uterus, can weaken the uterine wall.

If your loss was caused by a placental abruption, your next pregnancy will be considered high-risk since the condition tends to recur in about one in eight subsequent pregnancies. Although there is nothing you can do to guarantee that the problem will not happen again, you can try to minimize the risks. Be sure to monitor your blood pressure closely, both at home and during frequent visits to the doctor. If you smoke, quit. Also, keep in mind that when placental abruption is diagnosed early and the separation is minimal, the condition can be controlled through a combination of bed rest and medication. Your doctors will closely monitor the baby and schedule a delivery as soon as his or her lungs are mature enough.

Another potentially life-threatening problem with the placenta is placenta previa. This occurs when the fertilized egg implants in the lower portion of the uterus rather than in the upper portion as in a healthy pregnancy, and when the placenta grows over or very near the internal opening of the cervix. When this happens, heavy vaginal bleeding can occur, which can result in premature delivery or pregnancy loss.

Umbilical Cord Problems

So-called "cord accidents" are a relatively rare cause of pregnancy loss and typically are only cited as a cause after all other possibilities have been ruled out. For example, true knots in the cord are found in about 1 percent of all pregnancies. But in the vast majority of cases the knot causes no serious problems for the baby. On occasion, the cord may become wrapped around the baby's neck or may twist with devastating consequences.

There also are many types of cord abnormalities that cause pregnancy loss. My own loss was caused by an abnormality of the cord known as velamentous insertion. Normally, the cord inserts firmly in the center of the placenta. But in about 1 percent of pregnancies, the cord inserts at some distance from the placenta, leaving the blood vessels relatively unprotected. Usually, the pregnancy progresses well and the doctor only identifies the problem once the baby is born and the placenta is expelled. But in rare cases like mine, the vessels rupture, causing the baby to bleed to death. It only takes a small amount of blood loss to be fatal to an infant, which explains why my baby slipped away before I even realized it.

Vasa previa is a similar condition. In this case, the unprotected blood vessels cross the cervix. When a woman's water breaks, the vessels sometimes rupture, causing the baby to hemorrhage. Another type of umbilical problem is the two-vessel cord Normal cords contain three vessels—one vein and two arteries. When one of those arteries is missing, there is a higher chance of congenital abnormality, intrauterine growth retardation (IUGR), preterm delivery and miscarriage. Cords also can be too long or too short. If a cord is too long, it is more likely to prolapse through the cervix before delivery, impairing blood flow to the baby, while a cord that is too short can cause placental abruption.

Incompetent Cervix

About 15 percent of all second-trimester losses are caused by what is known as an incompetent cervix. In a healthy pregnancy, the cervix, which is the opening to the womb, is strong enough to withstand the pressure that a growing baby places on it. But in some cases it is too weak to support a pregnancy and dilates and thins prematurely, leading to preterm birth and pregnancy loss. Anyone can have an incompetent cervix, but certain women are at greater risk. These include anyone who has had previous miscarriages and D & Cs, and the daughters of women who took DES, a hormone given from the 1940s to the 1970s to prevent miscarriages, but is now known to cause reproductive problems in offspring. Women who have undergone multiple second-trimester abortions are also at greater risk since repeated dilation of the cervix can weaken the muscles and connective tissue fibers causing them to lose their elasticity.

If your pregnancy loss was caused by an incompetent cervix or if you had an unexplained mid-trimester loss, it is important for your doctor to examine you early in your subsequent pregnancy to diagnose a possible recurrence. If the cervix appears to be dilated or thinned, your doctor can perform a cervical cerclage, a procedure in which stitches or a band is placed around the cervix to close and reinforce it. The cerclage is most commonly put in place just after the first trimester, strengthening the already weakened cervix. In some cases, women are required to rest in bed afterward and possibly take medication to prevent contractions and infection. When the procedure is done in time, the outlook is good for a healthy pregnancy.

Illness in the Mother

Certain chronic illnesses in the mother can cause pregnancy loss. For example, women with diabetes, epilepsy, systemic lupus erythematosus, certain heart conditions, kidney disease and severe hypertension are at a higher risk for miscarriage and stillbirth. The actual risk depends on the type of illness and its severity. Often, babies whose mothers are battling a serious illness simply do not grow adequately, resulting in a condition known as intrauterine growth retardation.

Common Reasons for Early Infant Death

When an infant dies shortly after birth, the cause can often be linked to prematurity; many babies die simply because they were born too early and did not have a chance to fully develop in the womb. In fact, prematurity is a leading cause of early infant death. Of those preterm infants who survive, many suffer from serious disabilities, such as brain damage and blindness.

Sometimes babies are born prematurely because of an infection. But in more than half of all cases, doctors cannot determine why a baby is born before thirty-seven weeks' gestation, the point when a pregnancy is considered full-term. Regardless of whether the cause was clear in your case, there are some things that you can do to minimize the risk of preterm labor in your next pregnancy. In particular, you can ask your doctor about new diagnostic tests designed to identify those women at risk for preterm labor and delivery. You can also learn to detect the onset of labor as soon as it occurs, significantly improving your chances of stopping it and carrying the baby longer. Once the cervix has started to dilate, it is difficult if not impossible to prevent the onset of labor. However, if detected early, preterm labor can be treated with medication that reduces uterine contractions. We will discuss this issue in more depth in chapter 7, which addresses high-risk pregnancies.

Congenital Problems

Congenital problems are another common cause of early infant death. While most unions that result in genetic abnormalities end in miscarriage, about 3 percent of all newborns have some form of congenital abnormality. This can range from minor imperfections to major defects that are eventually fatal to the baby. Among the major defects, congenital heart disease is one of the most common.

In early pregnancy, the heart starts out as a single, straight hollow tube. It then divides into two sides and folds over on itself twice to reach its final form. Because this process is extremely complex, there are many ways in which the heart can develop abnormally. Newborns with congenital heart disease may appear healthy for the first few hours after birth, but later their color may begin to change or their breathing may become labored. Since newborns with infections and lung immaturity often exhibit the same symptoms, it may take several hours for doctors to diagnose a heart problem.

Certain groups of pregnant women have been identified as being at higher risk of delivering a baby with a heart problem. In particular, women who have had one child with heart abnormality have a 2 to 3 percent chance of having another one. If the woman herself was born with heart disease, the risk increases to as much as 5 percent. Some medications and very high doses of Vitamin A can also damage the developing heart.

If you are at high risk of having a baby with a cardiac problem, you can have a prenatal test called a fetal echocardiogram. Using the same technology as an ultrasound, the entire heart can be examined for normal development. Any potentially abnormal areas can be evaluated in detail by using Doppler ultrasound, a technique that measures the direction and speed of blood as it flows through the heart.

Group B Streptococcus Infection

As many as 800 babies die every year in the United States as a result of Group B Streptococcus infection (GBS), the leading cause of life-threatening infections in newborns. Of the other 7,000 babies who become infected with GBS annually, many are left mentally or physically handicapped. Although the bacteria causes few or no symptoms in healthy, adult pregnant women, it can be transmitted to the baby during delivery (and occasionally even in utero.) When it enters the baby's bloodstream, it can cause serious complications such as shock, pneumonia and meningitis.

The good news is that testing and treatment are available that can prevent GBS infection. The American Academy of Pediatrics recommends that all pregnant women be screened for GBS bacteria between thirty-five and thirty-seven weeks gestation. Those who test positive can be given antibiotics intravenously during labor. Through these two procedures, it is estimated that more than 75 percent of all cases of GBS in the first week of life can be prevented.

SIDS

Nearly 3,000 infants die of Sudden Infant Death Syndrome every year in the United States. SIDS is defined as "the sudden death of an infant under one year of age, which remains unexplained after a thorough case investigation, including performance of a complete autopsy, examination of the death scene and a review of the clinical history." As its name suggests, SIDS is unpredictable. Some babies are thought to be at higher risk for SIDS than others. These include those with low birth weight and those born to parents who smoked or used drugs during pregnancy. But the majority of babies who die do not fall into any known risk category. Most babies die of SIDS between the ages of one and four months. The risk drops dramatically at six months of age and diminishes completely after one year.

After years of research, scientists still have not been able to determine exactly what causes SIDS, but they have found some factors that can help reduce the risk. As most of us know by now, the number-one way to reduce the risk of SIDS is by putting your healthy baby on her back to sleep. According to the American Academy of Pediatrics, the rate of SIDS has decreased in the United States by 42 percent since 1992 when the organization issued the recommendation that babies sleep on their back. Other things that are believed to reduce the risk of SIDS include preventing babies from getting too warm, creating a smoke-free environment around the baby and breastfeeding.

chapter two

Are You Ready to Try Again?

WHEN I FIRST found out that my baby had died, one of my first thoughts was *never again*. There was no way I was ever going to put myself in a situation where I would experience that much pain and sorrow. I thought that for me, another pregnancy was out of the question. Although I truly believed in those panic-filled moments that my decision was final, it literally only took a few hours before I had changed my mind. I remember that as they were wheeling me into the operating room to do a c-section, I was begging my husband to stay by my side and make sure that the doctors didn't perform a hysterectomy. There was no real reason to believe that they would, but I feared it nonetheless. Despite the enormousness of my loss, I suppose that was the first indication of how strong my desire to have another baby actually was. That desire grew over time, and by my postpartum visit six weeks later, one of the main things I wanted to know was when I could safely get pregnant again.

As you contemplate the possibility of becoming pregnant again, you, too, may find that your feelings fluctuate from one day to the next and even from one moment to another. Sometimes you may think that all you want is to get pregnant again, while other times you are convinced that you could not possibly live through another nine months of pregnancy. This kind of uncertainty, combined with intense feelings of grief, may make you wonder at times if you are losing your mind. Rest assured, you're not. It is completely normal to be unsure at a time like this. In fact, nearly every woman who has had a pregnancy loss goes through a period of very mixed emotions.

When they first receive news of their loss, many women react as I did. Says Diane, "Right at first, we were so shocked. Daniel was our first child, we didn't know anything was wrong, and he only lived for four days and had three surgeries during that time, so it was very stressful. At that point, I didn't know if I could ever try again." Allison was even more resolute. "I remember as I was sitting in the doctor's office after they couldn't find the baby's heartbeat, I just wanted everything removed. I kept telling my doctor, take the uterus, take everything, I don't ever want to do this again. It's obviously not in my future to have children and I just want it over."

A few weeks or a couple of months after your loss, you may find yourself obsessed with the idea of getting pregnant again. During this period, you also may develop a fear that you will not be able to have another baby, even if there is no physical reason that would prevent it. If you have other living children and your last pregnancy was not planned, you still may desperately want to try again, since most women do not want to end their child-bearing years with a loss. Says Leslie, "I was way overboard. I ate, drank and slept getting pregnant again. It was very obsessive, very unhealthy." Beth went so far as to ask her doctor for fertility pills even though she had never had a problem getting pregnant. "I knew I was missing something in my life, and it hurt so bad, and knowing that I could have another baby helped me through it. My doctor said, 'Are you sure that's what you want?' And I said, 'Yes I'm sure. Give me fertility drugs, give me something.' But of course he wouldn't."

Those women who make it through this period without getting pregnant usually find that their desire wanes a bit over time. Barbara ended up waiting more than a year before trying again. "At first I wanted to get pregnant again right away, but as time passed I realized that mentally I wasn't ready. I knew I was going to be a mom again some day, but I didn't want to jump into anything. I wanted to deal with all the emotions of grieving for my baby. I didn't have a whole lot of control over what had happened, but I did have control over how I dealt with it."

Complicating this roller coaster of emotions is the fact that you will probably be getting a lot of advice, both solicited and unsolicited. Your doctor will obviously have his opinion, which should be a valued one. But well-meaning relatives and friends will also have their views, some of which might not be so welcome. "Get pregnant again right away. It will help you forget all about the one you lost. Look ahead, don't look back." "Wait at least a year before getting pregnant again. It's much too soon to even think about having another baby." "Maybe you should consider adoption. In your case, pregnancy is too risky." Even if your loss was recent, you no doubt have already heard some variation of all of these.

There may be people who try to give you a formula for knowing when you're ready. You may be told that you are ready to try again if you can hold someone else's newborn baby or look at another pregnant woman without feeling resentful or walk through a baby department without crying. Those of us who have suffered a pregnancy loss may always have trouble coping with certain reminders of our tragedy. That does not, however, mean that we are not ready for another pregnancy.

It can be confusing to be bombarded with so many opinions, especially at a time when you are already so emotionally vulnerable. That's why it's important for you to remember that once you are physically healed, the decision to get pregnant again is an intensely personal one that only you and your partner can make. And unfortunately, there is no easy formula for knowing what to do. It will depend on your emotional well-being, your past experiences, your current situation and the amount of support you received in the weeks and months following your loss.

In the final analysis, it doesn't matter what your mother, sister, best friend, or, within reason, even your doctor says. It is your body and your baby, and you and your partner are in the best position to determine what is right for you and your family. Some couples decide to try again as soon as they are physically able, while others wait for years. A few opt never to try again. The best way to decide what is best for you is to review the facts, both about physical and emotional readiness, and then to examine your own heart to determine if you are ready to move ahead. Diane described her decision-making process this way:

> After about six months, I came to terms with the fact that I never was going to know anything for sure. I didn't know if I got pregnant that it would happen again or that I would ever come home with a healthy baby. But we just really wanted to be parents, and we felt like we wanted to keep trying even if it meant going through those terrible things. In that six-month period, somewhere along the way, I got enough strength to go through it again.

Physical Readiness

Barring any health problems, you are physically ready to handle another pregnancy after two or three regular menstrual cycles, or about three to six months after the end of your last pregnancy. If you had an early loss, your doctor might give you the go-ahead to try again after you have had only one period. If, like me, you had a c-section, the recommended waiting period may be slightly longer, but generally ranges from four to eight months. Remember that it may take a couple of months or more before you get your first period, especially if your baby died late in your pregnancy or shortly after birth. During that time you may alternate between fearing that you may not be able to bear any more children and worrying that you might have become pregnant again by accident. When Katie still had not had a period two months after losing her baby at term, she felt disappointed in herself. "Not only did my baby die, but my body had just shut down." What she did not realize is that it was very normal for her not to have a period, especially given that she was under so much stress.

Doctors generally recommend waiting to try again until you have had at least two or three normal cycles to ensure that the uterus has returned to its normal shape and size, and that the lining is thick enough to allow for a good implantation of the placenta. It will also give your doctor the ability to accurately date your pregnancy. Accurate dates will enable your doctor to closely monitor your baby's growth and to intervene at the first sign of trouble.

In some cases, extenuating factors may prompt your doctor to suggest that you will need more time to heal physically. If you lost a lot of blood during your delivery, for example, your iron levels may be poor and you may need more time to rebuild your strength. Or if you have a chronic illness that contributed to your loss, you may need to receive treatment before becoming pregnant again. And if your loss came after a full-term pregnancy, you should be aware that some evidence suggests becoming pregnant again within six months significantly increases the risk that the next baby will be premature or small.

Even if your doctor tells you that it's all right to get pregnant again after only two or three periods, you may feel it will take you longer before you feel physically ready. For example, it may take several months for you to lose the extra weight you gained while you were pregnant and to get back into shape. While this may be important for your self-esteem, researchers have discovered that it is also critical for the well-being of your baby. One recent study found that obese women are two to four times more likely to have a baby with a neural tube defect, such as spina bifida or anencephaly, than women who are not significantly overweight. Even if you are not obese, it makes sense to lose the extra weight now since you cannot go on a diet once you are pregnant. You will also want to be sure to start taking folic acid supplements beginning two or three months before conception, since research shows that this vitamin can dramatically reduce the risk of neural tube defects. Unfortunately, there was no risk reduction seen in heavier women who took the recommended levels of folic acid, which is one more incentive to lose extra weight.

Obviously, your physician is in the best position to advise you when you will be physically ready to handle another pregnancy. But he also may try to tell you how long your emotional healing will take. For example, you may be advised to wait at least six months, or maybe even a year or two, until you have had a chance to work through your grief. Or your doctor may recommend that you get pregnant again right away. If you get this kind of advice, keep in mind that you are probably better able to judge your emotional readiness than your physician is. In fact, a study on this topic found that most women surveyed were resentful if their doctor told them precisely how long to wait before getting pregnant again, and they usually ignored the advice anyway. They preferred if their physician simply assessed physical readiness, gave them the pros and cons of getting pregnant again right away and left the final decision up to them.

Laura's experience illustrates how doctors can alienate their patients by being too specific about what to do:

> The day after we lost David, my doctor came into my hospital room and said, "I expect to see a baby picture this time next year." I think that was her way of reassuring me that what happened with David would not happen with another baby. But then a few weeks later when we went back for the postpartum visit, she suggested that we wait at least six months before trying again. That really confused me. I started thinking, "Am I in worse shape than I thought I was, or am I not handling this as well as I think I am?" Now I realize that she probably shouldn't have said what she said the first day. I think she was a good clinical doctor, but she didn't handle the emotional side very well.

Emotional Considerations

As you try to make the decision of when to try again, remember that you can be physically ready for another pregnancy before you are emotionally able to handle one. By now, you have probably realized that you will never completely get over the loss of your baby, even though over time the intensity of the pain will lessen. If you are still in the throes of grief—crying most of the day, eating very little and spending lots of sleepless nights thinking about the baby—it probably is not the best time to get pregnant again, especially since the hormonal changes of pregnancy may only deepen your grieving. Here's how Diane described her feelings during the period after her pregnancy loss:

I felt like there were clouds of darkness over me. For literally a year, I felt like I couldn't enjoy anything in life. I don't think I was clinically depressed, but there was just that overriding feeling that we thought we'd be parents and what if we're not going to get to be again? It was all I'd ever wanted.

While it is no doubt difficult to know the difference between sadness over your loss and clinical depression, there are some questions you can ask yourself to determine whether you have worked through the most intense stages of grief. Have you reached a point where your baby no longer occupies your every thought? Are you back in your regular routine? Is your appetite normal again? Are you able to sleep at night? Have you worked through any feelings of failure or guilt? Researchers have found that it usually takes anywhere from six to twelve months before women who have lost a baby can answer "yes" to those questions. In a few instances it can even take two years or more for women to make the slow progression through the stages of grief and mourning.

"People grieve the loss of a baby for a long, long time in many different ways, but that doesn't mean they shouldn't consider having another child," says Andrea Seigerman, a licensed clinical social worker in the high-risk obstetrics clinic at Yale–New Haven Hospital. "If they are able to function again in daily life—function at work, function at home, function with other children—then that's an indication that they're ready for another pregnancy."

In many ways your grieving process will be no different than that experienced by anyone who has lost a loved one. In some respects, however, it can be more complicated. For starters, pregnancy and childbirth are in themselves stressful events. Combining these with the task of mourning your baby's death can be physically and emotionally draining. Studies show that this can be even more difficult when you have suffered multiple pregnancy losses. Since your friends and family may have never seen or held your baby, they may have trouble understanding the depth of your sadness. If your baby died before birth, there may be an even greater tendency for people to see the child as replaceable. This is especially true of women who suffer early losses. The lack of emotional support can make it difficult for you to work through your grief.

You may also find that the loss has strained your relationships with some of the most important people in your life. You may be angry at your partner if he is not grieving the way you expected. Or maybe your doctor has disappointed you, either because he was not as sympathetic as you would have liked or you thought he could have done more to prevent your pregnancy loss. You may be upset with family and friends who seemingly have no clue as to what you are feeling. Perhaps they get quiet when you try to talk about the loss or change the subject, or maybe they stay away from you altogether. This can contribute to feelings of isolation and may lead you to see your own grief as the primary way of remembering your baby. In that case, the grieving process may be prolonged since you may consider any resolution of your feelings as a betrayal of your baby.

Researchers have found that women who get pregnant again before working through these complex issues may put their grief on hold during the subsequent pregnancy only to see it come back with a vengeance once they have had another baby. At this point, the grief is so unexpected that it may be more difficult to handle. Studies show that women who get pregnant again less than five months after their loss are more likely to experience so-called "inappropriate grief."

Researchers have identified another risk to getting pregnant again before you have worked through this intense grief. They call it "the replacement child syndrome." If you conceive again too soon, you may have unrealistic expectations for the next child and be unable to welcome the baby in his or her own right. In her book *Empty Cradle, Broken Heart*, Deborah L. Davis describes how this can happen:

According to psychological and medical literature, the replacement child syndrome occurs when parents idealize their dead child and seek to "re-

place" that child by having a new baby. When the new baby is born, the parents may have difficulty focusing on this child as an individual separate from the child who died, even imposing expectations for the new baby to be like the dead child. This new baby then grows up in the shadow of the dead sibling.

Davis goes on to explain that there are other replacement feelings that are benign and very common among bereaved parents. These include wanting a baby to fill your empty arms and wondering if your dead baby might have been similar to the new one. There is nothing wrong with comparing your babies as long as you do not idealize the one that is gone.

It is only in the past twenty years or so that women have been warned about the dangers of trying again too soon. In the past, mothers were told just the opposite. They were encouraged to get pregnant quickly so that they could forget the loss and resolve their grief. Barbara's comments show how far women have come in their thinking since then. "I knew I was going to be a mom again, but I didn't want to jump into anything. I wanted to deal with all the emotions. I felt I owed it to my child to honor his memory and not confuse him with another child." Virginia expressed similar sentiments:

I knew getting pregnant again would help the pain somewhat, but I didn't want to short-circuit the process. I didn't want to rush right into it in order to stop feeling how I felt. The pain was hard. It was agonizing. But I wanted to walk through it and come out on the other side. I felt like getting pregnant right away would have been like trying to put a Band-Aid on the pain by trying to replace my baby.

Another advantage to waiting is that it might give you a chance to work through your fear that the same thing could happen again. This fear can be overwhelming, even if the odds are clearly in your favor. Since statistically you were not expecting to lose your baby the last time, you may not be reassured by favorable odds. Barbara, whose pregnancy loss was due to a rare genetic defect, was told that the chances of the same thing happening again were about one in five thousand. But in the course of attending support group meetings, she met three other women who had experienced the same problem. "I thought something's wrong with these statistics. I don't know twenty thousand people, and I know of four women right now who have had this problem." Barbara found that one of the best ways of coping with her fear was talking with other women who have suffered a loss and have gone on to have healthy babies. "Being able to see other people who have healthy children makes me feel deep-down inside we can have that too," she says.

As you've probably realized by now, your emotions in the months following the loss will run from grief to anger to guilt to fear. Sometimes it is only in retrospect that women understand that making it through this period is a long and complicated process. Trisha describes it this way:

> *We kind of convinced ourselves that we were over it, so we started trying to get pregnant again three months after we lost the triplets. But looking back I was very glad that I didn't get pregnant until all of the intense grieving was done. My subsequent pregnancy was emotionally and physically difficult, but had I not worked through the grief the way that I had, I think it would have been much worse.*

Keep in mind, however, that you should not expect to be completely over the loss before you seriously consider another pregnancy. To some extent, you will continue to grieve for the rest of your life, since unlike the death of an elderly parent or grandparent, the loss of a child affects your future and not just your past. Fran Rybarik, who has worked with thousands of women who have suffered pregnancy losses in her role as executive director of the national pregnancy loss organization Bereavement Services/RTS, explains that there used to be a tendency for people to view the loss of a baby as a "snapshot in time." Today, there is a growing awareness that losses build on each other over time. If the pregnancy loss is not the couple's first experience with death, they may be grieving not only for the death of their baby, but all their past losses as well.

"Sometimes people in nursing homes will do a life review and they will remember the baby who died many years before," Rybarik said, "so I'm real uncomfortable with saying that anyone 'gets over' a pregnancy loss. It may not always be as hurtful or as emotionally devastating, but it's still part of our lives."

There may come a day when you realize that you feel normal again, but it will be a different kind of normal. Your life is never going to be the same as it was before the pregnancy loss. In fact, you may always view things in terms of before the loss and after the loss. "What I tell people is that grief is part of the package of the next pregnancy," says Joann O'Leary, who runs the Pregnancy after a Loss program at Abbott Northwestern Hospital in Minneapolis. "You will still be mourning the loss when you get pregnant again, and, in fact, a new layer of grief emerges during the pregnancy—the fear that this baby is going to die too."

Advantages of Waiting

We've already touched on some of the disadvantages of getting pregnant again too soon. Namely, that you may be putting your grief on hold only to have to come back with even more intensity later. Or that you may see your next child as a replacement for the baby who died. But there are other issues to consider as well that might encourage you to wait six to twelve months before trying again, as many professionals recommend.

If you get pregnant three months after the loss, when your physical recovery is complete, the birth of your next child will coincide with the anniversary of the loss. If you suffered a full-term loss, as I did, you will be pregnant again at the same time of year. While some do not consider that to be a problem, others find the prospect disconcerting. Says Mary, "I just didn't think I could go through another pregnancy at the same time, especially since the baby could be born on the same day. I'm strong, but I don't know if I could deal with that."

Others feel like they cannot even consider getting pregnant again until after they have made it past the due date of their previous pregnancy. "I had to get through my due date," says Brooke. "That was part of my mourning." Melissa Swanson, director of Pen-Parents Inc. and editor of the *PAILS of Hope* newsletter (which stands for Pregnancy and Parenting after Infertility and/or Loss Support) for parents going through pregnancy after a loss, believes that the best way of coping is to wait a full year before trying again.

When you wait a year, you go through all of the anniversary marks. You go through your first holidays after the loss, your first Mother's Day after the loss, all of the memories of the times of the year that you were pregnant. I can remember Valentine's Day when I was pregnant with my triplets. I had gone to the Hallmark store and made my husband a personalized card from me and the triplets, and it's something he still treasures. So the following Valentine's Day, all of the memories of how fun that was and how special that was were overwhelming to me. I think if you give yourself that year, you give yourself permission to grieve at all of those times. Then the grief isn't lost in being pregnant or thinking about another baby.

By waiting to get pregnant again until you have given your mind and your body every chance to heal, you can also avoid the guilt that can come with getting pregnant again too soon. Danielle never even had a period between the end of her last pregnancy and the beginning of her next one. When she developed complications that put her subsequent baby's life in jeopardy, she felt guilty. "I thought, if my son dies, it's all my fault because I didn't wait long enough." Her son was born prematurely—but healthy—only nine and a half months after her pregnancy loss.

In some cases, the waiting is not by choice, but many of those who were forced to wait are happy they did. Heather is a case in point.

She found out that her baby had anencephaly about halfway through her first pregnancy, but she decided to carry to term anyway. Her baby only lived a few hours. Although she and her husband started trying to conceive again right away, Heather later realized that during the seven months it took her to get pregnant again, she went through an important grieving process that better prepared her to welcome the next child.

I had started a cross-stitch blanket when I was pregnant with Anna, and I was trying to get it done so she could be buried with it. It was about six weeks before she was scheduled to be born that I realized I wasn't going to be able to finish it in time, so in a fit of hysteria, I thought, "Since I'm not going to get it done, I'm going to do without it." After she died and the doctor said we could start trying again, something made me pull the blanket out and start working on it again. I thought, when I'm able to finish this blanket and I can pack all her stuff away, then I will be ready to go on and have another baby. I finished the blanket and a week later I found out that I was pregnant. I realize now that finishing the blanket was my way of grieving for Anna. Until I did that, I was not mentally prepared to get pregnant again, even though I wanted to with a passion.

Pam, who lost twins in her first pregnancy, says she only realized after several months of trying to conceive again that she initially had been trying to replace one pregnancy with another:

I was ready to pretend like the first pregnancy never happened. I was twenty-two weeks pregnant when I lost the twins, so I was thinking if I could get pregnant right away it would be like an extra long pregnancy. That's something it took me a long time to recognize. I wanted to be a mother so bad after going through a year of infertility, and I was upset that I couldn't do it. I felt really angry at my body for denying me that chance, and I felt bad that two human beings died because of me and I wanted to make things right. So I was trying to get pregnant again for all the wrong reasons.

Advantages of Getting Pregnant Right Away

Although postponing another pregnancy for a while has many advantages, it is by no means the right decision for everyone. Waiting a year or more, as some experts recommend, will be close to two years before you'll have another baby. Given your feelings right now, it may seem unacceptable to wait that long, especially since you had planned to be mothering a baby very soon. Perhaps you are in your thirties and feel that you should try again sooner rather than later. Or maybe the ages of your living children are a factor in your decision. It could be that you are facing the prospect of fertility treatments and know that another pregnancy might take months or even years to achieve. Or maybe you want to try again just because you feel you are ready to have another baby. All of those are valid reasons for following your own timetable if you feel you are emotionally prepared for what lies ahead.

Often it is only after the birth of a healthy baby that women realize they made the right decision of getting pregnant again right away. Martha says, "I don't know if it would have been any less stressful if I had waited a year, but I do know that being pregnant again gave me hope at a time when I had none. And I sort of felt like if I didn't do it right away, I would never do it again. Obviously, I don't regret it now because I have Mark."

Some of the women who were forced to put off the pregnancy because they were unable to conceive again right away believe, in retrospect, that waiting was not in their best interest. Melinda, who did not get pregnant for a year and half following her loss, wishes things had turned out differently. "Waiting was very hard for me. I had those empty arms, and that just about drove me crazy. I just wanted to hold babies. I didn't care whose babies they were. It was a very painful time. And once I did get pregnant again, I was still scared to death. Waiting didn't help me at all."

As Melinda's example shows, waiting a predetermined number of months is no guarantee that the next pregnancy will be any easier. If you spend the months following your loss simply counting down the days until you are pregnant again, you may not make any progress toward resolving your grief. The time between pregnancies is not as important as what you do with that time. Your subsequent pregnancy can also be an important time of healing. But if you do decide to try again before the generally recommended six-month waiting period, it can be difficult to go against conventional wisdom. I know this from first-hand experience.

When I talked to my doctor at my postpartum visit, he gave me the standard advice about getting pregnant again: From an emotional standpoint, he said, it was up to me. But he cautioned that most experts believed it was better to wait at least six months to guard again seeing the next baby as a replacement child. Physically, he added, I would be ready after two or three regular cycles. I had already read several books that discussed the emotional side of pregnancy after a loss and was convinced that I would not see my second child as a replacement for Patrick but rather as his little brother or sister. So I focused instead on the news of when I would be physically ready. I was elated that even though I had had a c-section, I would be able to try again so soon. I left my appointment convinced that I would start trying again as soon as I was physically able.

A couple of weeks later, I started having doubts, as this entry from a journal I was keeping reveals:

It's been nearly two months since Patrick died, and it's only in the last week that I've begun to understand why all the experts suggest waiting a few months before trying to get pregnant again. I still am having trouble sleeping, I cry a lot, and I'm so very, very sad. Is that the kind of environment the next baby deserves? No, I know now that only after I have worked through my grief will I be able to be a good mother to the next baby from the moment of conception. Pregnancy is stressful enough without making grief a part of the process. I don't want this next baby to suffer any ill effects because of my love for Patrick.

Two months after I wrote that journal entry, I had the requisite two periods and was feeling much better emotionally. But I was still ambivalent about getting pregnant again. On the one hand, I was desperate to have another baby growing inside me. I would see pregnant women walking down the street and think to myself how lucky these women are. On the other hand, I was dreading the idea of enduring morning sickness and the other physical problems that pregnancy causes, especially since I was finally feeling good again. I also did not look forward to all the anxiety that I was certain I'd experience.

After my husband and I discussed these issues and did some serious soul-searching, we decided that even though we were not 100 percent ready, we would start trying again. Part of our reasoning was that we had no idea how long it would take to conceive again: it could take six days or six months. As it turned out, I got pregnant again during the very first month we tried. Although I was ecstatic to have the hope that comes with expecting a baby, there was a downside that I had not anticipated: I felt overwhelmingly guilty. Here I was a well-read, educated person and yet I was ignoring all the experts' advice. I felt that I was the only woman in the world who had not waited at least six months to get pregnant again, so I was haunted by doubts. Would the pregnancy be harder emotionally because I had not waited long enough? Would my sadness rub off on my next baby? Was I just trying to replace one child with another? Would everyone think I was crazy for having another baby so soon? Since I had no answers to these questions, one of the ways that I coped was by not sharing my news with anyone.

Imagine my surprise when I started researching this book and found woman after woman, who, like me, had gotten pregnant only three or four months after her pregnancy loss. What this helped me to understand is what we have been saying all along: there is no right or wrong amount of time to wait before getting pregnant again. Some women choose to wait six months to a year, but many do not. The best decision is the one that is right for you.

In retrospect, I believe that getting pregnant again after only four months was the right decision for me. Yes, my pregnancy was emotionally grueling, but I'm not sure that it would have been any easier if I had waited. And although I was happy to have another child, he in no way is a replacement for Patrick. I think I will always grieve for my first son. As for my fear that my sadness would rub off on my next baby, I think anyone would be hard-pressed to find a happier, better-adjusted child.

It is important, however, to point out that in my case, a number of extenuating circumstances made my decision to get pregnant again the right one. For one, I started interviewing women who had experienced a pregnancy loss within weeks of Patrick's death. While the interviews were technically part of my research for this book, they were also very healing for me emotionally. I retold my story time and time again and listened as other women recounted what had happened to them. I also interviewed support group leaders and counselors. Yes, it was research, but it was another way for me to work through the grieving process.

Perhaps most helpful of all, I started seeing a counselor who specialized in grief therapy. She met with me twice a week and listened to my fears and concerns. Most important, she gave me a shoulder to cry on. Just six weeks after my baby died, I thought I was ready to stop seeing her. Thankfully, she was wise enough to know that I still needed her and urged me to keep coming back. That meant her support was there as I went through my next pregnancy.

My second son, Andrew, turned out to be the anniversary baby that the literature on pregnancy loss warns us about. He was born just one year and three days after Patrick died. It might have been overwhelming to mark the anniversary of my first son's death when I was very nearly at the same point in my subsequent pregnancy, but I'll never know for sure. Fate intervened, and my focus was diverted.

On the first anniversary of my loss, a good friend of mine, who was also pregnant, suffered a seizure and had to be rushed to the hospital. She was later diagnosed with a brain tumor and was operated on while still pregnant. Faced with that kind of emergency, I didn't have time to really grieve for my baby. Instead, I spent hours at the hospital that day trying to lend what support I could.

One thing that the experts were right about in my case, however, was the suspended grief reaction. On the second anniversary of Patrick's death, I felt as though I had been hit by a ton of bricks. That was partly because, by then, I understood just how much I had lost. My year of parenting my second child had taught me that. But I also think that I was grieving twice as much as I would have if the first anniversary had been a true day of mourning. As I already mentioned, fate intervened again on the third anniversary and I brought my third son home from the hospital that day.

To me, these experiences show that the future cannot be predicted when making the decision to try to get pregnant again. I dreaded that the first anniversary would fall in the ninth month of my subsequent pregnancy. Yet the day did not turn out at all the way I had expected. That has been true of nearly everything following my pregnancy loss. So while anticipating the difficulties of getting pregnant again too soon, it is also important to remember that life will take its own twists and turns.

Your own circumstances may be very different from mine. Maybe you have found ways to work through your grief, and maybe you haven't. You may have the same fears that I did, or you may have entirely different ones. Only you can be the judge of your feelings. But if you do decide you are ready to try again after three or four months, do not feel guilty. You are not alone. Let's now take a closer look at some of the other factors that may influence your decision on when to start trying again.

The Biological Clock

If you are over thirty-five, you may feel pressure to try again as quickly as possible. As you are probably all too aware, advancing age increases the risk of certain genetic disorders and decreases fertility. Even if you are still in your twenties or early thirties, you will feel the same type of pressure if your partner is older. In those cases, waiting may not be an option. Lynn, for example, felt like she needed to forge ahead when she miscarried at age thirty-five, since she already regretted waiting so long to get pregnant the first time. "I'm glad I've had my life and done everything that I've done. But in hindsight, I would have started a family when I was much younger." Laura, who was thirty-six years old when her first baby was stillborn and thirty-seven when she miscarried in her subsequent pregnancy, also felt a strong sense of urgency. "We didn't have the luxury of saying we're going to give ourselves a couple of years. I was thirty-seven, and with every pregnancy I was getting a little older."

Younger women can also feel the pressure of the biological clock. Diane was only thirty years old when her baby died, but her decision to try again was based on how long it had taken her to get pregnant the first time:

People say you're young, you have a lot of time. But when I look at it, I say it's taken us five years to get to this point and if I want to have three or four kids and it takes five years for each one, I'm running out of time. I'm not saying that it would necessarily happen that way, but my mind plays that kind of game with me. So even though I realize thirty is not old, I feel like we don't have a lot of time to play with.

Spacing of Siblings

Just as your own age can be a factor in your decision about another pregnancy, the ages of your other living children may influence you as well. Sydney's son was four years old when she suffered a pregnancy loss. Although she waited a year before trying to conceive again, she worried that her children would not be as close in age as she would have liked. "The year that we waited after I lost my daughter, I kept thinking, my son's getting older. The pregnancy is going to take nine months, and he's getting older."

When Sydney finally did get pregnant again, she miscarried eight weeks later. At that point, she decided that she could no longer worry about the spacing of her children, especially since she was fearful about the impact another pregnancy loss might have on her living child. But the decision was heart-wrenching nonetheless. "I think that coming to terms with the fact that my child won't have a close sibling has been one of the biggest disappointments for me. It's almost like raising two only children. It's the loss of a dream."

Virginia, whose subsequent child was born when her other living children were nine and eleven, continues to wonder whether she should get pregnant one more time so that her youngest child will have a sibling who is close to his age.

In nine years, my two oldest children will both be out of the house. So Christopher is going to spend at least half of his life as an only child. I had siblings who were twelve and thirteen years younger than I was, and I know how much we had to remake our relationship with one another once we reached adulthood. Christopher will have to go through that, too. So I'm not sure what to do.

In many cases, mothers who have other living children have the additional pressure of worrying about their own ages. Kelly was already thirty-eight years old when she and her husband started trying again after her pregnancy loss. Her two living children were seven and ten at the time. "It had taken us five years to get pregnant with Joshua, so I started doing the temperature thing and the ovulation tests right away. Nine months later, I still wasn't pregnant, so I called my doctor and said, 'I'm old and my other children are growing up. Isn't there something you can do?' " Kelly ultimately went through a round of infertility treatment and gave birth to a healthy child two years later.

Fertility Problems

If, like Kelly, you have had fertility problems in the past that have made it difficult for you to get pregnant, you may start trying again sooner that you otherwise would. Since it had taken Carla five years to get pregnant the first time, she was back in her fertility specialist's office the month following her miscarriage. "I felt okay with myself and my partner, so even though I was grieving for the other baby, it was good for me to start trying again." On the other hand, your grief over your loss may be compounded by the knowledge of the hardships you will have to endure to conceive again. Depending on the extent of your particular fertility treatment, there will be pills to swallow, injections to take, blood to draw and eggs to harvest, all with no guarantee of success. Still, women often go to extraordinary lengths in an effort to conceive again.

Nancy's story illustrates the tenacity that many women exhibit in the quest to have another baby. She had been through two years of disappointing infertility treatments before she finally got pregnant with twins through in vitro fertilization. Six months into her pregnancy, she suffered a loss due to problems that were wholly unrelated to her infertility. For Nancy, the decision to try again was extremely difficult. She had to overcome obstacles ranging from a fertility specialist with a poor bedside manner to the financial burden of the treatments. But most of all, she had to prepare herself to deal with the fertility treatments themselves. "I wasn't so much thinking about another pregnancy as I was about the disappointment of infertility. I knew I had to be strong enough to go back into the fertility game— going in and giving blood and taking shots every time, and getting all psyched up when they said everything was looking good and then facing the disappointment when they said maybe it wasn't going to be a good cycle."

One of the ways in which she made the process easier was by finding a fertility specialist who would meet her needs. "I went in and said, 'This is what I expect: I want you to tell me what's going on; I want to know what my options are; and I want to know what you recommend; then I'll decide what I want to do.' Before, I'd always say okay to anything that the doctor recommended. I never challenged him. But this time I realized that I needed to know what was going on and take an active part in the decisions."

Since Nancy's insurance plan did not cover expensive infertility treatments such as in vitro fertilization, she also had to deal with the issue of cost. "To me it couldn't be a financial consideration, even though it was a financial burden. One of the ways that I rationalized it is by thinking, if I had conceived way back when, we wouldn't have had my income through these years, so my income was really like extra money. That was just a mind game, but it helped me justify it." She recalls how she got motivated to go through it all again:

> One thing is, I really wanted to parent; I wanted to do the task of parenting every day. Another thing is that I took it one step at a time. I told myself, "Okay, I can take these shots tonight" or "I can go give blood this morning," and if I wake up tomorrow and I don't want to do it anymore, I can get out. So much of the control is taken away from you, down to the intimate parts of your life, that I knew that one thing I did have control over was whether or not I was going to do it again.

Health Considerations

Chronic health problems or a history of difficult, complicated pregnancies may also influence your decision to try again. During her pregnancy, Barbara had severe morning sickness (known as hyperemesis gravidarum) and she was in and out of the hospital. Not only could she not face the prospect of going through that kind of pain again right away, she also needed time to physically recover. "It took me five months to get feeling healthy again," she says.

Women who have experienced multiple miscarriages may want to put off another pregnancy while they try to determine the causes of their losses, despite that in about 50 percent of all cases, no cause is ever found. "I felt like it would have been irresponsible of me to get pregnant again without at least trying to understand why I kept miscarrying," says Sydney. "I needed to pursue all my available options first." Those who do find answers often decide to go ahead at that point, even if the available treatments offer no guarantee of success. Cynthia had been diagnosed with an autoimmune disorder after four losses and knew she was a high-risk patient. But she says her decision about another pregnancy was clear-cut: "I knew that if I didn't try again, I would spend the rest of my life being very bitter and angry."

Women with chronic health problems might also have to delay their pregnancies temporarily for medical reasons, but they too often take extraordinary risks to try again. Sharon, for example, was only twenty-one years old and had a one-year-old daughter when she found out that she had a serious kidney disorder that would require major surgery and years of treatment. Despite a spate of medical problems, Sharon never gave up her dream of having another baby. As the years passed, she gradually became healthier and was finally able to conceive again. But by a cruel twist of fate, her baby died due to a cord accident when Sharon was twenty-four weeks pregnant. Sharon describes how she made the decision to try a third time despite not having any idea what another pregnancy might do to her health:

As devastating as it was to lose Megan, the one thing that pulled me out of the fog I was in was the thought that I could have another baby. That feeling never left me. I had wanted a second baby for so many years, but because of my physical problems I couldn't have one. Now we had gone through so much and still had no baby. So even though I was scared to death about another pregnancy, I still wanted a baby to love and to take care of and to nurture. I needed that. Not as a replacement, but to fill that need that I had for a baby. For all of those reasons, I made the decision that we had to try again. My husband was really unsure about it, but I likened it to climbing this huge mountain and getting three-fourths of the way up. Now which would you rather do? Fight three-fourths of the way back down or go ahead and finish? I felt like we had to keep going.

Some women face medical problems of a different type that influence their decision to get pregnant again. For example, some couples discover after their loss that they are carriers of a genetic defect that could be passed on to their other children. At that point, some decide that the risk is not worth taking, while others opt to brave the odds even when they are clearly not in their favor.

Lynn had been told that because of an abnormality in her chromosomes, her chances of having a healthy baby were about fifty-fifty. While there was a strong probability that she would miscarry in the first trimester if a problem developed, there was also a small chance that she might go to term with a baby that had virtually no chance of surviving. Still, she and her husband decided to try again. "We really wanted to be parents, so what we did is we put ourselves in God's hands. The thing that scared me the most was that I would have to make a decision about aborting a baby who was sick. Thankfully, I never had to do that." Because of her risk factors, Lynn also spaced her pregnancies close together. Her only living child had just turned one when they decided to try again. "Because of my genetic disorder, we didn't know how many times I might miscarry, so we didn't have the luxury of waiting. We didn't know how long it would take to have a healthy baby."

Practical Considerations

Although you will base your decision largely on emotional and physical considerations, it is also important to take practical issues into account. For example, consider the stress that another pregnancy could put on your marriage, especially if your doctor prescribes extended bedrest. Also, determine whether you will be able to take time off from work if either your own health or the baby's is at risk. Your long-term career plans may be a consideration as well. When Kathy was pregnant for the first time, she quit her job because she wanted to stay home with her baby. She suffered a loss and got pregnant again before finding another job, which in some respects made the subsequent pregnancy more difficult. "I just sat on the couch all day watching cooking shows on TV. That might have made it easier on me physically, but it was much harder emotionally."

Some women decide to schedule their pregnancy for a certain time of year. As trivial as it may sound, the weather can have a profound impact on some pregnant women's mental health. Mary, for example, had given birth to her son Austin in the middle of a hot Texas summer and was determined that her next delivery would occur during a different time of year. "I'm very hot-natured, and I swelled up so bad at the very end that I could barely walk. So I thought I'll be damned if I'm going through it again in the summer."

Sometimes practical issues that are beyond your control end up being a factor in the decision. Perhaps you are changing jobs or graduating from school or moving to another city. Any of these major life changes might prompt you to wait awhile before trying again. Sydney, whose husband is in the military, was living in a large metropolitan area when her pregnancy ended in a loss. She decided to put off another pregnancy because she knew her husband was scheduled to be transferred, but wasn't sure where. She could not face the prospect of being pregnant while moving to a new, and unknown, destination. "We just decided to wait to try again until after the move."

When You and Your Partner Do Not Agree

Couples do not always agree on the timing of another pregnancy. You may desperately want to be pregnant again while he is wary of seeing you go through more pain. That was the case with Katie, whose first baby was stillborn one day after her due date. "I kept begging John to have another baby, but the doctor had said to wait six months, and my husband agreed. Now I'm glad that we waited because I understand how far I had to go. If I had gotten pregnant again right away, I would not have had time to grieve and work through my anger. Those things really helped me in my next pregnancy."

Since men and women tend to grieve the loss of a baby differently, it also is possible that the man may be ready to move ahead with another pregnancy while the woman considers herself to still be in deep mourning. Diane and Randy found that the only way they could resolve their differences on when to try again was to see a counselor:

We needed to work on our communication skills because he was wanting to jump right into another pregnancy, and I wasn't anywhere close to being ready. He also tended to just withdraw into his own little shell while I was wanting to talk and cry twenty-four hours a day. The counselor suggested that I pick and choose my times to talk about what had happened and how we were going to face the future. She said I should give him some time to unwind when he first got home from work and also try not to wake him up at three o'clock in the morning to talk. He learned that when I cried, he didn't have to solve all my problems for me. All he had to do was listen and hold me because there was no way he could fix the situation. Eventually, we were able to talk openly enough to reach an agreement.

Just as men and women have different ways of communicating, they also make decisions differently. "Men are more analytical. They'll make column A and column B, and say there are more things in column A so we'll choose this one. Whereas women are much more willing to take risks," says Candace Hurley, founder and executive director of Sidelines National Support Network for women experiencing high-risk pregnancies. "For [women], money is no object, time off from work is no object, even their own health is no object." So while you may go so far as to put your life on the line to have a baby, your partner may have more concerns about your health. Sharon, who had a chronic kidney problem, knew her husband would be reluctant to let her take the risk of getting pregnant again, so she decided to take matters into her own hands:

I actually went off the pill without Greg knowing for a couple of months because I thought if anything happened to me later because of another pregnancy, he wouldn't have to feel any guilt. But after a month or so, I knew I couldn't do that to him because we had too honest of a relationship. When he found out what I had done, he was very upset, but by that time I was into it and very little could have stopped me. He always wanted another baby but he was very low-key about it because, for him, it was not a matter of what we wanted but what was best.

If you have had trouble getting pregnant in the past, you and your partner also might not agree on how much of an effort to put into trying to conceive again, since men are sometimes less willing to undergo the stress of fertility treatments. According to Sharon, "My husband said, 'I don't want to make this our obsession where we spend the rest of our life focusing on getting pregnant.' I wanted to try for six months, but he only wanted to try for three. I said 'fine' to get him at peace with it. The first two months, I started my period and it was just devastating. The third month I was psyching myself up that maybe it wasn't meant to be, but sure enough, I got pregnant."

Some women develop an aversion to sexual intercourse after their pregnancy because they associate it with their loss. In that case, the sexual act simply becomes a vehicle to another baby, causing problems in the relationship. "The last thing I wanted to do was have sex because it somehow seemed like we were betraying our baby by enjoying ourselves again," says Elise. "The only reason I even did it was to get pregnant again."

The best way to resolve any of these types of differences is to talk openly and honestly about your feelings. More important, listen to what your partner has to say. Some couples find that it helps to put off the conversation for a few weeks until some of their emotions have settled down. Others feel they have to get everything out in the open right away. The timing is not as important as actually finding a way to communicate. The subsequent pregnancy will be stressful enough without adding problems from your relationship to the mix.

Making Decisions about Future Pregnancies

The decision of whether or not to try to get pregnant again can sometimes be even more complicated when you are contemplating a second pregnancy after the birth of a healthy baby. While there are some women who go on to give birth several more times after experiencing a miscarriage, stillbirth or the death of a newborn, many of us can't help but feel that we should count our blessings once we have successfully given birth to one healthy child. That was Nancy's feeling when she gave birth to a healthy daughter after battling infertility and losing a set of twins in her first pregnancy.

I feel like I'm finally winning. This is what I've worked for through all the years of infertility and the loss of the boys, and I don't want to push my luck. But even though I'm raising Ashley as an only child, I still feel like I'm the mother of three.

Some women are reluctant to try again for fear of giving birth to a child with special needs. Christine says, "Now I'm not so much afraid of having a baby that dies, but having a baby with Down syndrome." Others worry what another pregnancy would do to their mental health. That was the case with Sharon, whose chronic health problems made pregnancy extremely risky for her. "I don't think I could go through another pregnancy. I think I would be a very disturbed individual if I did."

My husband and I had those fears and others when we were contemplating a third pregnancy. But ultimately we decided that we did not want Andrew to grow up as an only child. Now that I have two living children, the choices are even more complex. Although I would love to have at least one more baby, I cannot help wondering if I would be tempting fate. We've lost once and won twice. What would happen the fourth time? I'm not sure we have the courage to find out.

There are others, like Heather and her husband, who muster the courage to forge ahead. She had given birth to one healthy boy before losing a newborn daughter. Her third pregnancy resulted in another healthy son. As they considered a fourth pregnancy, they disagreed on what to do. Says Heather:

In my mind we were always going to have three kids; in his mind, two. Finally, we decided we would give it a year. If we got pregnant, fine. If not, then we'd make the decision to stop. As it turned out, I got pregnant right away, and I'm so glad I did because now we have another healthy child. But there were plenty of times when we thought, "Are we pushing it here? Are we trying to grasp at something we shouldn't have?"

For women who developed life-threatening health problems during their previous pregnancies, the decision is usually more straightforward. Knowing that there is a possibility that your surviving child would be left without a mother is a powerful incentive to quit while you're ahead. Leslie, who developed a life-threatening syndrome during pregnancy, says she opted to have her tubes tied shortly after giving birth to her son so that she wouldn't risk changing her mind later. "I knew that in a year or two I would want to have another baby because I would start forgetting all the trauma and everything that I had been through. So I made the decision with my head and not my heart. I didn't want Alex to grow up without a mother."

Ultimately, the decision to keep trying is no different than the choice you made to get pregnant again right after your loss. It is a personal decision that only you and your partner can make, and there is never a right or wrong answer. Follow your heart and pray for what is best.

Ways to Facilitate the Decision-Making Process

Seek Spiritual Support

Faith in God is what sustains many people during the most difficult times in their lives. Even if you were angry and turned away from God when you first found out that your baby had died, you may still have a deep desire for spiritual comfort. Although no one can really answer the question of why your pregnancy ended in a loss, a pastor or rabbi may be able to help you come to terms with your loss, and whether you should try again.

"It is important to find a safe, non-judgmental place to talk things out," says Rev. Richard B. Gilbert, executive director of The World Pastoral Care Center, who has written extensively on grief and spiritual issues. "It's okay to be angry at God because God always embraces our feelings." Gilbert says most bereaved parents find it takes time before they can trust God again. "When trust has been shaken in a human relationship it takes time to heal, and so it is with our relationship with God. The important thing is that God is always willing to wait."

Just as couples go through different stages of grief, they may find that their relationship with God changes over time. Virginia describes the stages she went through after her pregnancy ended in a stillbirth:

I struggled with anger at God because I knew that he could have protected my baby. I thought, "How can I entrust my other children to you if I couldn't entrust this one?" But then a friend helped me realize that God is protecting us and will continue to protect us even though we cannot always see it. I don't know why he chose for Haley to go home so soon, but I've come to the understanding that I am just a steward and my children are entrusted to me for a time, and it is not up to me to determine how long that will be.

Some couples rely on their faith to make the decision of when to try again. A few, like Melinda, believe the timing of their subsequent pregnancy was the result of divine intervention.

We had been trying to have another baby for more than a year after we lost Preston. I reached a point where I was finally ready to give up. But before I did that, I sort of made a bargain with God. There was a Sunday school class at church, and I said, "Okay, God. I'll join the group when I get pregnant." And I felt like he clearly said to me, "No, you'll join and then you'll get pregnant." I really felt that. So I got on the phone and I made a call and joined, and within the first week I was pregnant. I didn't even know it at the time but I was. It's not something you can prove scientifically, but I know that God had a hand in what happened.

Your faith can also help you once you are pregnant again. "I've found that it doesn't matter what religion women are," says Maureen Doolan Boyle, who has counseled many women who have suffered a pregnancy loss in her role as executive director of MOST (Mothers of Supertwins), an organization providing support to families with triplets and more. "If they have faith in God, they do so much better."

See a Counselor

A licensed professional therapist can also help you assess when you are ready for another pregnancy as well as help you cope with the anxiety that you feel once you are pregnant again. Remember that it is extremely difficult to mourn the loss of one baby while giving life to another one. Being able to talk openly about your pregnancy loss is often the first step toward healing.

Attend a Support Group

You also may benefit from attending a support group for couples who have experienced a pregnancy loss. It not only will give you a forum to openly discuss your feelings, but will also provide you with the opportunity to learn how others have coped with their own losses. Talking about your fears can help you work through them and give you a clearer idea of when you might be ready to try again. Martha says she benefitted from meeting other women who had been through the same experience. "I felt like women who had not lost babies were aliens. I really couldn't relate to them at all. And I just didn't want to be around women who did not understand."

While Glenda also felt that the support group helped, she saw a negative side to it as well:

I felt like I would have gone to the support group meeting every day if I could. Even though you may have a very best friend who will listen to your fears, the only person who really understands is someone who either has been through it herself or is going through it. So talking with other women like me is what I really liked about the support group. The problem was that every time we went, we would hear about all the other things that

*could go wrong in a pregnancy, so in a way, it was like a Catch-22. It
helped us overcome one set of fears, while giving us a whole new set to
worry about.*

As you consider whether a support group is right for you, you might
want to analyze whether the benefits of talking with other couples who
have been through a loss outweigh the anxiety you feel when you hear
about the many possible complications of pregnancy.

If You Are Not Ready to Try Again

There are many reasons why you may decide that you are not ready
to try again. You may not feel emotionally or physically ready for
another pregnancy. Or you may feel that you cannot run the risk of
another loss. Some couples decide that their family is fine just the
way it is. Others consider adoption.

If you want to try again but are not ready right now, you must
consider birth control. Barrier methods such as condoms or a diaphragm are a good choice if you think you may be ready again in the
near future. Otherwise, you may want to consider going on the pill.
One word of caution: using birth control when you long for a baby
can be difficult. But aside from abstinence, contraception is the only
option if you are not ready for another pregnancy.

Methods of Contraception

Barrier Methods

Barrier methods such as condoms, diaphragms and vaginal sponges
are ideal if you want to try to conceive again soon since you use them
only when needed and can stop using them literally at a moment's
notice. The condom and the sponge have the additional advantage of

being available without a doctor's prescription, making them relatively easy to use.

The diaphragm is a round rubber dome that is inserted through the vagina to cover the cervix. Used with spermicide, it keeps sperm from reaching the unfertilized egg. If you have used a diaphragm before, be sure that your doctor refits it in case there has been a change in the size or shape of your cervix. The vaginal sponge works much the same way as the diaphragm but is believed to be somewhat less effective since it is not specifically fitted to your body. Condoms have the advantage of being inexpensive and easy to use and are also very effective in preventing pregnancy. They are even more effective when used with spermicide. The downside to these methods is that you will be faced with the decision of whether to use them or not each time you have intercourse. Some couples feel that this interferes with the spontaneity of sex.

The Pill

The pill is the most popular form of non-permanent birth control in the United States. It is also effective, and convenient. The pill works by suppressing ovulation and has the notable advantage of not interfering with the spontaneity of lovemaking. But some women report side effects such as weight gain and breast tenderness, and there are also questions about its safety. Since doctors recommend going off the pill and switching to a barrier method of contraception at least three months before trying to conceive, it may not be the best choice if you think there is a good chance you might change your mind about another pregnancy in the near future.

Natural Family Planning

While nearly everyone has heard about the so-called rhythm method, most couples are not familiar with the more widely practiced form of natural family planning—the ovulation method, also known as the Billings Method. This form of birth control relies on using one or more body signs to determine the time of ovulation and then avoiding intercourse from the first sign that ovulation is about to take place until three days after it has occurred. This method is believed to be much more effective than the old rhythm method, which was largely based on counting the days in a woman's menstrual cycle, and avoiding intercourse on certain days. Before attempting to use the ovulation method, however, be sure to seek help from a qualified instructor. Classes on the subject are offered on a regular basis at many Catholic churches.

Simply put, the ovulation method consists of observing mucus changes in your vagina every time you go to the restroom. As you get closer to ovulation, the mucus will change in consistency, becoming more lubricative, clear and elastic—looking a lot like raw egg white and stretching to one inch or more. The last day of this mucus is known as the peak day and is followed by vaginal dryness. By abstaining from intercourse throughout the period when mucus is present and for three days afterward, you should be able to avoid becoming pregnant.

As a back-up plan, you can augment the ovulation method by measuring your basal body temperature with a basal thermometer. Since basal body temperature rises by about one-half a degree after ovulation, a higher temperature for three consecutive days is an indication that the fertile period has passed.

Although the ovulation method may sound complicated, a five-country study by the World Health Organization found that 97 percent of women could identify the mucus that indicates fertility after three cycles of observation. Other studies have rated the method 98 to 99 percent effective when learned correctly. One downside is that some couples are not comfortable with the idea of abstaining from intercourse for several days of the menstrual cycle. A notable advantage to this birth control method, however, is that you can also use it to become pregnant once you are ready to try again.

chapter three

Trying Again

THE SUMMER AFTER my pregnancy loss, I went through not only the emotional changes that every parent experiences when a baby dies, but I also went through a physical transformation. Although I had gained nearly sixty pounds when I was pregnant, I managed to lose all of the extra weight in just a few months. This was partly because I was just too depressed to eat most of the time, but it was also because I was doing everything in my power to get back in shape. I walked three miles every morning and exercised for a half hour each afternoon. When I did eat, I tried to eat healthy foods. I also stayed away from alcohol and kept taking my prenatal vitamins. I had never been interested in fitness before, but I found that looking better helped me to feel better. Somehow, nothing was worse than carrying around the extra pounds from my pregnancy, and having no baby to show for it. What really motivated me, though, was that I was a woman on a mission. I desperately wanted to have another baby, and I wanted to do everything I could to get my body ready for a second pregnancy.

If you are trying to conceive again within a few months of your loss, as I did, it is extremely important to prepare yourself for the stress of back-to-back pregnancies. Even if it has been six months or a year since your loss, there are certain things you should do before getting pregnant again in order to give your next baby every chance of being born full-term and healthy. Pregnancy is hard work, especially when you have the added burden of grieving for a baby who has died and fearing that the worst might happen again. But the pregnancy will be easier if you are in good physical condition and take certain steps to ensure that you do not put your unborn child at risk. Your doctor is the best judge of what special measures you should take both before and after conception, and it is important that you discuss these at length with him. Generally speaking, every woman who is considering getting pregnant should first do the following: schedule a checkup with an obstetrician; get in good physical condition; take folic acid supplements; keep track of her periods and stay away from alcohol, drugs and cigarettes.

Given that you probably did all of these and more for your previous pregnancy, and since it didn't prevent your loss, you may wonder why you should bother doing anything special at all for your next pregnancy. Lynn, for example, was so cautious during her pregnancy that ended in a loss that she never even drank a Coke for fear that the caffeine might harm her baby. "It makes me think that I might be better off if I didn't try so hard in my next pregnancy and just went about my normal business." All of us, no doubt, can relate to that feeling. But since so much about your pregnancy will be beyond your control, you will feel better knowing that once again you are doing everything within your power to take care of your baby.

Schedule a Checkup

The first thing you should do before actually trying to conceive again is to schedule a physical with your obstetrician. This will give your doctor a chance to do a breast and pelvic exam and Pap smear and to ensure that you have no other health problems that could complicate your pregnancy. If you have a chronic illness, such as diabetes, epilepsy or high blood pressure, you can take steps now to bring it under control. In addition to doing a routine checkup, your doctor can also review your immunization records and test you for certain infections and diseases that can be particularly dangerous during pregnancy. The Coalition for Positive Outcomes in Pregnancy recommends such testing before conception since maternal infection, particularly during the first three months, can lead to miscarriage, birth defects or even infant death.

Usually, a simple blood test is all that is required to rule out infections that could cause serious complications during pregnancy. These include hepatitis A and B; rubella, or German measles; influenza; chlamydia, the most widespread sexually transmitted disease in women; cytomegalovirus (CMV), a common cause of intrauterine infection; parovirus, which causes an infection known as fifth disease; chicken pox; tuberculosis; herpes simplex and HIV. Also of concern are toxoplasmosis, a parasitic disease transmitted through eating undercooked meat or fish or through contact with cat feces, and Lyme disease, which is transmitted through tick bites. If the blood test shows that you are not immune to measles, rubella or chicken pox, you should get vaccinated now and avoid getting pregnant for at least three months.

If your pregnancy loss was unexplained, your doctor may also want to test for antiphospholipid antibodies, which are increasingly being linked to miscarriages and stillbirths. As discussed in chapter 1, these are antibodies that go haywire and attack normal cells instead of fighting foreign organisms such as bacteria and viruses. Doctors typically screen for anticardiolipin antibodies and lupus anticoagulant. But there are other antiphospholipid antibodies that can also cause problems in pregnancy. Depending on your history of pregnancy loss, your obstetrician may want to check for every known type of antiphospholipid antibody.

Get in Shape

Like me, you may find that losing any extra pounds you gained during pregnancy will help your attitude. If you can get back into your old clothes and look and feel physically fit, it may make it easier to face the prospect of going right back into maternity dresses in a few months. There also are medical reasons for being near your ideal weight before conceiving. We already talked in the last chapter about the link between obesity and neural tube defects. But women who are overweight when they conceive also have a greater chance of developing a host of other problems that could cause complications in pregnancy, including high blood pressure and diabetes.

As important as it is to lose any extra weight, don't diet if there's a chance that you might already be pregnant. All of your unborn baby's nutrition comes from the food you eat, so it's especially important to eat healthy, well-balanced meals. You should also avoid losing too much weight, since women who are underweight when they conceive tend to deliver babies with low birth weights.

One of the best ways for you to reach your ideal weight is through exercise. Not only will physical activity help you get in shape, it will also raise your sagging spirits and lower your stress. A brisk walk can do wonders for your mental outlook and your health. Walking is a form of exercise, along with swimming, that you can typically continue to do safely once you are expecting. Be sure to check with your doctor before starting any kind of exercise program.

Take Folic Acid Supplements

In the last chapter we briefly discussed the importance of folic acid in reducing the risk of neural tube defects. Specifically, studies have shown that all women of child-bearing age should consume .4 milligrams of folic acid per day to reduce their risk of having a baby with spina bifida—the leading cause of childhood paralysis—or anencephaly, a usually fatal condition in which a baby is born with a severely underdeveloped skull and brain. About two thousand five hundred babies are born with these defects every year, but the U.S. Public Health Service estimates that number could be cut in half if all women in the United States consumed the daily recommended levels of folic acid.

Since neural tube defects occur when the tube that forms the brain and spinal cord fails to close during the sixth week of pregnancy, it is particularly important to take folic acid from at least one month before pregnancy through the end of the first trimester. But there is new evidence that this vitamin continues to play a vital role later in pregnancy as well. Researchers have found that women who have low intakes of folic acid have two to three times more risk of preterm birth and babies with low birth weight.

Folic acid is naturally found in many foods, especially fresh citrus fruits and green, leafy vegetables. Researchers believe, however, that vitamin supplements are more readily absorbed since the folic acid found in food must first be broken down by the body before it can be absorbed. Most over-the-counter multivitamins contain the recommended amount of folic acid. If your baby died from a neural tube defect in your last pregnancy, you may be at higher risk for having another child with the same problem. In that case, check with your doctor about taking a higher dosage of folic acid. You will probably be advised to take 4 milligrams daily, or ten times more folic acid than the normally recommended amount. Most specially formulated prenatal vitamins have 1 milligram of folic acid in addition to a multitude of other nutrients that are important for a healthy pregnancy. Remember, though, that no vitamin can take the place of a well-balanced diet.

Keep Track of Your Periods

It is important to keep track of your menstrual cycles so that your doctor can accurately date your pregnancy. By knowing the exact date of the first day of your last menstrual period, your obstetrician will be able to determine if your baby is measuring according to gestational age and reaching certain milestones on schedule. He can then intervene at the first sign of trouble. Keeping track of your periods will also help you avoid false alarms that can only add to your anxiety. For example, a Doppler ultrasound device can usually detect your baby's heartbeat twelve weeks into pregnancy. If you think you are twelve weeks along when you are actually, say, only in the ninth week of your pregnancy, your doctor may not be able to detect a heartbeat even though your baby is perfectly healthy. Needless to say, this can cause a lot of unnecessary anguish.

Getting accurate dates may be difficult if your periods are irregular or you have recently stopped taking oral contraceptives. If you have just gone off the pill, consider waiting to try again until your periods are regular. One option is to switch to a barrier method of contraception, such as the diaphragm or condoms, in the meantime.

Avoid Drugs, Alcohol and Cigarettes

Once you start trying to conceive again, you will want to avoid all over-the-counter and prescription medications unless they are absolutely necessary. You should also stay away from illicit drugs. Although a few drugs, such as the acetaminophen found in Tylenol, are believed to be safe during pregnancy when taken in small doses, the long-term effects of many medications on a developing baby are still unknown. The problem is that most drugs can pass through the placenta to the baby, so that anything that affects your body has an even larger effect on your baby. There are also instances when *not* taking a prescribed drug can be more dangerous than taking it. If you are ill, for example, the effects of your disease may be far worse for the baby than any drug that you take to treat it. Talk with your doctor before taking any medication and before you *stop* taking any prescribed drug.

The use of antidepressants and tranquilizers is an area of particular concern to women who have been through the trauma of losing a baby. One study found that about one-third of bereaved parents were taking prescribed tranquilizers two months after their loss. If you have been taking antidepressants to help you cope with your grief, you should talk to your doctor about whether you should continue taking them during pregnancy, since most drugs pass through the placenta to the baby. Fortunately, researchers have found that pregnant women who take fluoxetine (Prozac), the most commonly prescribed antidepressant in the United States, are at no greater risk than women who don't take fluoxetine of having a baby with a major anomaly. However, there is evidence that babies who are exposed to fluoxetine in utero in the third trimester have increased rates of preterm delivery, admission to special care nurseries and low birth weights compared to those who were exposed only in the first two trimesters.

If you smoke, you are probably already aware that you should quit before you get pregnant again. But that, of course, is easier said than done, since smoking is one of the most addictive of all habits. Perhaps all the incentive you need for quitting is knowing that cigarettes have been linked to pregnancy loss. And the more you smoke, the higher the risk. One of the reasons that smoking is so bad during pregnancy is that it is believed to dramatically increase the risk of placental abruption, a serious complication responsible for a large percentage of stillbirths and early infant deaths. Smoking also constricts uterine blood vessels and decreases the flow of nutrients and oxygen to the baby in the womb. There is also evidence that cigarette smoke ingested during pregnancy continues to damage your baby after birth. Recent studies have shown that there is a connection between maternal smoking and the risk of Sudden Infant Death Syndrome.

Alcohol also can be extremely dangerous to an unborn child and sometimes results in miscarriage, low birth weight and preterm birth. Chronic heavy drinking can cause a condition known as Fetal Alcohol Syndrome (FAS). Babies who are born with FAS are below average size and usually are mentally retarded. They also have distinguishing facial characteristics such as small eyes, short noses and thin upper lips, and may have limb or heart defects. How much alcohol does it take to cause these serious problems? According to researchers, women who have three ounces or more of alcohol a day during pregnancy (the equivalent of three to four drinks) are at high risk for FAS. But some less serious problems have been associated with as little as one ounce per day (or one or two drinks). This wide range of opinion has led doctors to conclude that there is no safe level of alcohol consumption during pregnancy.

Doctors are still debating the safety of ingesting caffeine during pregnancy. Although researchers have long theorized that caffeine consumption in early pregnancy increases the risk of miscarriage, the data has been largely inconclusive. There is some evidence, however, that women who consume more than 300 mgs of caffeine per day in the first month of pregnancy (the equivalent of three cups of coffee) have a moderately increased risk of miscarriage in early pregnancy. Caffeine consumption in later pregnancy has been associated with low birth weight. Research on the topic is ongoing, but it may be a good idea to keep your caffeine intake low just to be on the safe side.

Choosing a Doctor

One of the most important decisions you will make once you are ready to try to get pregnant again is selecting who you will see for your prenatal care. Your physician can offer advice on how you can get physically ready to conceive again and also provide much-needed encouragement as you struggle with doubts about the outcome of your next pregnancy. As we've mentioned before, so many things about a subsequent pregnancy are beyond your control, but this is one thing you can do that will, to some extent, determine the course of the entire nine months of pregnancy.

For many women, deciding which health care provider to see is easy because there is no question in their minds that they want to keep the same physician. It's difficult to think of another professional relationship that is as intimate as the one that we develop with our obstetricians. And it's no wonder—your doctor was right there by your side to share in all the joy and excitement of your pregnancy. The first time you heard your baby's heartbeat, the day a sonogram gave you the first glimpse of your baby, and when your baby kicked up a storm during an exam. And it was your doctor who shared in your grief the day your pregnancy ended in a loss.

Or then again, maybe your doctor didn't do any of those things. Maybe you had a physician who was cold and aloof, both in good times and in bad. Or perhaps you never developed a close relationship

with your obstetrician because your loss came early in the pregnancy.
Or your doctor may have been part of a large practice and you may
have seen one of the other partners more often than not. Even worse,
you may feel that your doctor didn't do enough to prevent your loss.
Just as there may be many reasons to return to the same doctor, there
may be plenty of reasons not to. Regardless of your decision, there
will be both advantages and disadvantages to your choice.

Advantages of Staying with the Same Doctor

As we just discussed, one of the benefits of staying with the same
doctor is that you may have come to know each other well, and perhaps the two of you even developed a bond during your last pregnancy.
"Usually, if women feel like their needs were met in the pregnancy
that ended in a loss, they will go back to the same doctor," says Fran
Rybarik, executive director of the national pregnancy loss organization Bereavement Services/RTS. If your doctor was compassionate and
sensitive to your needs after your loss, that bond may be so strong
that you would not even consider changing doctors. It may also give
you a sense of confidence to return to someone who has treated you
before and knows your medical history and physical limitations. This
may be particularly important if the complications you had are likely
to recur in a subsequent pregnancy. "It was much easier to stay with
the same doctor than to try to explain everything to somebody else,"
says Leslie, who had a number of pregnancy-related health problems.
"I also felt like if there was anybody on earth who would want to make
sure that my next pregnancy came out all right, it would be him."

It can be gratifying for both you and your doctor to go through a
successful pregnancy together after experiencing a loss. Although it
may be hard for them to show it, most physicians share in their patients' grief when the worst happens and are happy to get the opportunity to share in the joy as well. According to Jennifer,

I considered going straight to the high-risk doctor because I knew that I was going to be seeing him later in my pregnancy, and it definitely would have been more convenient to go to only one doctor. But I figured because of the emotional connection that I had with my obstetrician, I wanted him to see it through to the end with me. I also felt like he could give me more personalized care because the high-risk doctors see a lot of patients and they see a lot of problems, so they don't get as emotionally connected.

As loyal as you may be to your doctor, however, don't let your feelings interfere with your better judgment. If you have any doubts whatsoever about the medical care you received, do not entrust another pregnancy to the same physician until after you get a second opinion to be sure that your loss was not preventable. Going to someone else will not only give you the opportunity to confirm that your own doctor did everything right, it may even convince you that you don't want to see anyone else for your prenatal care. That was the case with Jane, whose pregnancy loss occurred at twenty-three weeks: "I did get another doctor to review my medical records just to be sure there was nothing that could have been done to save my baby. But even as I was talking to the other doctor, I knew it would have terrified me to keep seeing him when I was pregnant again. My doctor knows me, and he knows what I've been through because he went through it with me. And that's very important to me."

Disadvantages of Returning to the Same Doctor

Although there are many advantages to keeping the same doctor for prenatal care, there are disadvantages as well. One of the biggest drawbacks is that returning to the same office may bring back painful memories. At each prenatal visit, you may be reminded of the happier, and perhaps even carefree, times of your last pregnancy. Diane's experience is typical of what can happen. When she returned to her doctor for a routine physical a few months after her newborn son died, she accidentally overheard a conversation that he was having with a couple who was expecting their first baby. "They had just found out they were pregnant, and he was giving them the whole spiel, his whole presentation of what to expect. I think my doctor had forgotten I was there or something. It was so hard for me to hear all of that and remember how I had felt on my first visit." In retrospect, Diane thinks returning to the same doctor was so difficult for her because her pregnancy had gone full-term. "If I had miscarried in the first trimester, and only seen the doctor once or twice, maybe it would not have been so bad."

Another disadvantage to staying with the same health care provider is that family or friends may harbor resentment toward your doctor, especially if they think the loss could have been prevented. They may be vocal in criticizing your decision not to go to someone else. Libby's family, for example, was angry at her obstetrician for letting her go full-term with a ten-pound baby who was stillborn on her due date:

My mother just kept harping on the fact that if the doctor had only realized how big my baby was and delivered her when she was eight or nine pounds, she'd be alive today. I couldn't think that way. All the "what ifs" just made me crazy. I knew my doctor had done the very best he could, and that what happened was just as much of a shock to him as it was to us. Everything is always easier to see in hindsight. So I was happy to keep seeing him when I was pregnant again, but my family was appalled.

Advantages of Switching to a New Doctor

While most of us are like Libby and can forgive our doctors for being human, you will probably not be willing to overlook negligence. There is no question that you should find another health care provider if it is clear that your physician did not do enough to prevent your loss. You will also be better off going to someone else if your doctor has been neither proactive in searching for a cause for your pregnancy loss nor taken steps to ensure it does not happen again. Although no cause is ever found in about half of all miscarriages and stillbirths, you will want to know that your doctor is doing everything possible to ensure a better outcome the next time. If your doctor was not sensitive to your feelings after your loss, that is also a good reason to switch doctors. It will be hard to share your concerns about the subsequent pregnancy with someone who disappointed you at such an important time in your life.

Regardless of your reasons for finding a new health care provider, there are a number of advantages to taking this route. Another doctor may have different ideas on the best course of prenatal care or may notice something that your other physician overlooked. Diane, for example, had been told by her original doctor that her baby's fatal condition was rare and unlikely to happen again. The specialist she met with later had a slightly different opinion of the situation since he had a patient who gave birth to three boys with the same condition. Rather than finding that news disconcerting, Diane found it comforting. "I appreciated hearing that there was the possibility that it could happen again because I would rather know what we were up against than have a false sense of security. I also felt like he was the one person who knew a little bit more about that particular condition than anyone else that I had talked to."

You can also choose a new doctor who specializes in treating women with high-risk pregnancies. These specialists are known as perinatologists. In addition to serving a four-year residency in obstetrics and gynecology upon graduating from medical school, perinatologists spend an extra two years or more in a fellowship program specializing in maternal-fetal medicine. Generally, only your obstetrician can refer you to a perinatologist, and you will see both doctors during your pregnancy. But on occasion, a perinatologist agrees to see a woman as a regular patient. This provides the added advantage of specialized care at every prenatal visit. Laura believes that regularly seeing a perinatologist gave her the confidence she needed to make it through her pregnancy with less stress:

When we first went to him for the initial consultation before I was even
pregnant, he just struck me as a very caring person, and I knew he was

someone who was used to dealing with high risk, if not loss. So it really made me feel good when he said he was willing to take me on as a patient and not have me go to an obstetrician. Now that I'm pregnant again, I like the fact that he does a sonogram at every visit. He looks at the baby from head to toe and tells us everything. And I need that. I don't know that I could just be going to a regular OB who just gives you ten or fifteen minutes.

Any obstetrician, even one who does not specialize in high-risk pregnancies, can arrange to do frequent sonograms and spend more time with you at each prenatal visit. Although you may not be considered "high risk" in the strictest definition of the term, you may still want the closer monitoring that the term implies. The only way to ensure that you get that kind of special treatment is to ask for it. No doctor can read your mind, so it is important to speak openly about what you need to ease your anxiety about your pregnancy.

Even though you may decide on seeing a particular doctor now, you can always change your mind if you later realize that he will not be able to meet your needs. That's what happened to me, and no one was more surprised about it than I was. If you had asked me before I got pregnant whether I would have gone to someone new, I would have told you absolutely not. I trusted my doctor and wanted him to see me through a successful pregnancy. But then, a series of events led me to a change of heart.

First, a good friend of mine who was also pregnant at the time had a miscarriage. She was spotting a bit and discovered that her baby had died when she went in for a sonogram. Within a few days of hearing this, I started spotting myself and was convinced that I was miscarrying, too. My doctor reassured me that the kind of light spotting that I was having was probably nothing to worry about, but said he would check my levels of human chorionic gonadotropin (hCG) just to be sure. In a viable pregnancy, the levels of this hormone tend to rise quite rapidly.

On that same Friday, I went in for a blood test and was told to return the following Monday for the results. I spent the entire weekend either throwing up or lying on the couch feeling nauseated. Some of my symptoms might have been psychosomatic, since I knew that morning sickness was a good sign that I was still pregnant. Needless to say, every day felt like an eternity. On Monday, which also happened to be my birthday, I went in for the second test and was told that my levels from Friday had been high, a good sign. Still, it was important to see if the levels were continuing to rise, so I needed to have one more blood test. On Tuesday, the news wasn't as good. The levels had gone up, but not as much as expected.

At that point, I fell into an absolute panic, certain that this baby had died, too. Since I was only about six weeks along, it was too early to check the heartbeat with a Doppler. So my doctor said he would perform a vaginal sonogram, not because he was overly concerned by my levels, but rather to reassure me since I was, in his words, a "nervous ninny." I began to cry and told him I was too scared to have a sonogram. All I could think about was the night of my last sonogram when another doctor told me that my baby's heart had stopped beating. Since my obstetrician knew full well what I had been through, I thought he would be understanding. Instead, he scolded me. "I told you that you shouldn't have gotten pregnant again so soon," he said.

Actually, he had done exactly what the experts recommend and told me that although the suggested waiting period was four to eight months, the actual timing was up to me once I had two or three regular menstrual cycles. Even as recently as the month before, when I had gone in for a checkup, he had asked me what my time frame was for getting pregnant again. When I told him we were no longer using birth control, he responded that since it had been four months since my loss, I was within the recommended waiting period after a c-section. Now, he was chastising me for a decision that he had told me was mine to make.

Somehow I gathered the courage to follow him back to the sonogram room, but I closed my eyes and kept crying as he took the probe and started looking for a heartbeat. I couldn't bear to look at the monitor. Thankfully, almost immediately he said the words I was praying to hear. "Look, there's the baby's heartbeat." For me, it was a moment of pure joy. I was so incredibly happy to have life growing inside me again. My doctor, on the other hand, seemed rather indifferent, at least in my view. He completed the exam and went back to his office. As I was leaving, he handed me a packet of information that he gave to all his newly pregnant patients. When I had been pregnant the previous time, I had read all the material religiously and almost immediately started making plans for my baby's birth. Now I couldn't wait to get the packet out of my sight. I was far too scared to make plans for the future.

I wish I could say that particular episode prompted me to change doctors, but it didn't. I made excuses for my obstetrician and figured that his reaction was no different than that of a father who was concerned about his daughter. My attachment to him was so strong that I wanted to continue seeing him even after we bought a new house in a city fifty miles away. I thought I could go to a perinatologist in Dallas and continue seeing my obstetrician in Fort Worth. It was my obstetrician who finally persuaded me to switch to a doctor closer to home. He kept insisting that it would be best if I found someone else, and I finally felt that I had no choice but to accept his suggestion.

Although I was devastated at the time, I realize now that it was the best thing he could have done for me. Not only did I not have to drive one hour each way for my prenatal visits, but I found a doctor who was used to dealing with pregnancies after a loss and was extremely compassionate in the face of all my fears and apprehensions. Looking back, though, I think my reluctance to switch doctors, even in light of how I was treated, shows just how attached we can become to our obstetricians, even to the point of being blinded to the facts.

Once you decide that you want to see someone else for your prenatal care, try not to feel guilty about it. Although most of us feel tremendous loyalty to our doctors, they usually have no trouble understanding that you have to act in your best interest. Although you may fear breaking the news, many physicians will react as Sydney's did when she told him she was going to a miscarriage specialist. "He really took it well. He just said, 'All I care about is that you succeed, and I don't care where that happens.'"

Disadvantages of Going to a New Doctor

One of the disadvantages of going to a new doctor is that he will have to become familiar with you and your medical history. You will also want to make sure that the office staff knows about your loss so that they will be aware that you will have special needs in your subsequent pregnancy. You can facilitate this process by briefing your new physician on the details of your situation on your first visit and asking that the staff be apprised as well. Consider writing out your history as well, so that it becomes part of your permanent file. Here's how Diane describes her first appointment with a new doctor. "Before I went into my meeting with him, I filled out all the forms and detailed everything that had happened to me. When we sat down, I said, 'I need to tell you about my history,' and I went through it all with him. He was great. He was very calm about it and gave me the sense that he would have everything under control."

A bigger drawback to switching doctors is that there is no guarantee that your new obstetrician will meet your needs any better than your old one. For example, Cynthia had a difficult time when she started seeing someone else after experiencing three pregnancy losses in a row:

> I just felt like I needed a different face and a different place—the old office had too many bad memories for me—so I went to an OB who was recommended by a very good friend who was also pregnant at the time. Unfortunately, he turned out to be very much not the right doctor for me. He would say things like, "This one is not going to be a problem," "Go home and start decorating the nursery," and "Get ready to set an extra place at the table." Stupid stuff like that which would build me up. And this was when I was only ten or twelve weeks along. Given my history, I felt like he needed to be realistic, not paint a rosy picture like there was nothing to worry about. To me, that showed that he was being complacent. He knew full well what our situation was, and he did not treat me like I was a high-risk pregnancy at all. He actually said to me, "When are you going to stop being nervous?" And I said, "When I take the baby home." But inside, I

was thinking to myself, "How could you not understand that? How could you not understand why I'm so scared?"

Although Cynthia ultimately switched to another doctor, she still ended up losing her baby girl twenty-one weeks into her pregnancy. When she got pregnant with twins a year later, she decided to return to her original obstetrician in addition to seeing a specialist who treated her for an autoimmune problem. "I think going to someone new helped me get a better perspective on my old doctor," she said. "She had been with me through three miscarriages and knew that I had lost a fourth, so she was as invested in the next pregnancy as I was." The fifth time proved to be charm for Cynthia, who gave birth to a healthy baby girl and boy after a complicated pregnancy.

How to Choose a New Doctor

While we all know that referrals are a good way to find a doctor, Cynthia learned the hard way that a referral has to come from the right person:

I was relying on the referral of a friend, and referrals are great if you have similar situations. But she had wonderfully smooth pregnancies and so thought he was a wonderful doctor, and I'm sure he is in a non–high-risk situation. But in my case, I should have pressed the issue more. I was so desperate for a change of pace and change of atmosphere that I didn't interview enough people and ask specifically, "How are you going to handle my concerns? Are you going to be okay with me being a high-maintenance type of patient?"

Rather than asking for a referral from a friend who has never experienced complications during pregnancy, you should instead talk to someone who has had a loss and gone on to have a healthy baby. With her needs being much more likely to be similar to your own, you will improve your chances of finding a doctor who is right for you.

If you don't know of anyone who shares your history, another good option is to ask for a referral from a labor and delivery nurse at the hospital where you plan to deliver. They work with obstetricians on a daily basis and are in a good position to evaluate both bedside manner and medical skills. Suzanne used this approach to find a new doctor when she moved to another city shortly after her baby died at term:

> It was really pretty simple. I just called the labor and delivery ward and said, "I had a baby who died and it was a really bad experience, and I don't want to get another doctor who is a bad egg." I told her I wanted someone competent who also had a good bedside manner. And the nurse said I should choose Doctor X. He turned out to be just what I needed.

Yet another good source for referrals is support groups for couples who have experienced a pregnancy loss. You can talk to women who attend the meetings about their own doctors. Support group leaders can also be helpful. Organizers of the group that I attended brought in local obstetricians and perinatologists on a regular basis to speak on various topics. That these doctors volunteered their time to meet with women who had suffered a pregnancy loss told me that they probably have a better understanding of our unique needs than most doctors would. If you live in a city that has a major medical school, the maternal fetal medicine department is another excellent source for referrals.

If you belong to a managed health care plan, such as an HMO or PPO, you may be forced to switch doctors simply because your coverage changes. Kathy, for example, had to search for a new doctor when she quit her job and obtained coverage under her husband's insurance plan since her old doctor was not on the new list. Usually, there is not much you can do in a situation like this, aside from asking your obstetrician if he might consider accepting your particular insurance plan or paying for your health care yourself. Otherwise, you will have to choose from the doctors on your list. Your choice of doctors might also be limited if you live in an area where there are few practicing physicians. In cases in which you are not able to visit the doctor of your choice, it is all the more important that you state your needs clearly to your health care provider and do your best to make sure that those needs are met.

Meeting the Doctor

After you have narrowed your choices to one or two physicians, the next step is to schedule a consultation. This gives you the opportunity to ensure that you are comfortable with the doctor and his or her staff, and that their thinking on key issues is in line with your own. "Tell them your story. Tell them what you need. See how they react," says Melissa Swanson, editor of the *PAILS of Hope* newsletter for parents going through a pregnancy after a loss. "You can tell whether or not somebody is going to be supportive." The initial consultation will also give you the chance to see whether the doctor is willing to take time to listen to your concerns. If you feel rushed on your first visit, the same thing is likely to happen later.

As you decide who to see for your prenatal care, keep in mind that you will need more emotional support during a pregnancy after a loss, which means that it will not suffice to a have a highly skilled doctor who has a poor bedside manner. As Candace Hurley, executive director of Sidelines National Support Network for women experiencing a high-risk pregnancy, points out, "A lot of times we're told that not all highly skilled doctors have good bedside manners, so we tend to forgive them. But I don't think that's such a good idea. A mom who has had a loss needs more than a good scientist."

You will be able to gain insight into a doctor's bedside manner at the initial consultation, as Sheila discovered when she interviewed two physicians who turned out to have totally different personalities:

When I walked into the first doctor's office, it was filled with Chinese artifacts behind glass cases, and his desk was impeccable and he just looked like he had a nail appointment to go to. I could tell right off that this was not going to be the right doctor for me. The second doctor was so different.

*His office was stacked high with newspapers and medical journals, and I
just had the feeling that this guy is going to take care of us and solve my
problems.*

Even if your next pregnancy is not considered to be high risk, it
will be of high concern, so you will benefit from more frequent visits
and sonograms. You also may need longer appointments so that you
will have the time to discuss your concerns and get answers to your
questions. If your physician is part of a large practice, you may want
to find out whether you can see your own doctor each time you have
an appointment. Barring that option, be sure that everyone involved
with your care is aware of your history.

Because there are so many different factors to consider in your
selection of a new doctor, it is a good idea to write down all of your
questions ahead of time so that you can discuss them at your first
meeting. Following is a brief list of questions that you should consider
asking. Even if you are keeping the same physician, you might want
to ask some of these questions anyway. Since just about everything
about your next pregnancy will be different, these are issues that you
may not have discussed before.

Will you be able to have your doctor check the baby's heartbeat whenever you feel especially anxious about your pregnancy?

Before your pregnancy loss, you may never have even considered
the possibility that your baby's heart could stop beating. I know I
didn't. But in the subsequent pregnancy, that may very well become
an obsession, especially before you are far enough along to feel movement from the baby. Now that you know your baby could die, there
may be days when you can't relax until you have actually heard the
sound of your baby's heart. Fortunately, most doctors will be more
than willing to accommodate your needs. "My doctor told me from the
very beginning that if I wanted to come in and hear that baby's heartbeat every day just to get through the week, to feel free to do that,"

says Lynn. "He was very supportive." Your doctor should be willing to do the same.

Is the doctor willing to see you for all of your prenatal visits even if he belongs to a large practice?

The days of the sole medical practitioner are dwindling as more and more doctors team up with partners in large practices. But what does this mean for you in a subsequent pregnancy? It may mean that you go in for a prenatal visit and see a doctor who knows nothing about you or your history. This can come as quite a shock if you chose your obstetrician because of his bedside manner and end up seeing a partner who is downright unfriendly. Martha, for example, had been accustomed to talking openly with her physician about her concerns and fears. But one day, she had an appointment with a partner who was seemingly clueless about her needs. "Instead of taking time to talk with me, he lectured me. He said, 'You're too big and this baby is too big.' I was just about in tears, I didn't know what to say."

You can avoid that kind of stress by finding out now whether or not you will be able to see your own doctor for each prenatal visit. Prepare to be assertive with the staff when you call for an appointment. Phyllis made it a point to let the receptionist know each time she called that she wanted to be scheduled with her own physician. "The good doctors have huge practices, and I know a lot of women who got really fed up because they could never get an appointment with their own doctor. You get so intimidated, you think you have no right to ask for anything, but that's not true."

Does the doctor set aside time to take non-emergency phone calls? What happens if you need emergency care during non-business hours?

Virtually all physicians have their nurses or other members of their staff available to answer questions over the phone, but there may be times when you feel that you need to talk directly to your doctor. If your obstetrician is tied up in appointments all day, it may be difficult for you to talk to him directly. Some doctors, however, make it a point to set aside time each day specifically for the purpose of returning phone calls. Sharon's obstetrician went so far as to give her his beeper and home phone numbers so that she could reach him directly at any time. You may not need nor want to go that far, but if talking to your doctor from time to time is important to you, be sure to ask whether it's a possibility. You also need to know how your doctor handles emergency calls during non-office hours.

Will you be seeing a perinatologist along with your obstetrician, and who will that specialist be? At what point in your pregnancy will this begin? How often will you be seeing the perinatologist, and what can you expect during those visits?

As we've already mentioned, many women with high-risk pregnancies see a perinatologist in addition to their regular obstetrician. In some cases, the perinatologist simply performs a high-level sonogram in the twentieth week of the pregnancy. But in cases with a history of multiple losses or a problem that is likely to recur in a subsequent pregnancy, a perinatologist may see the patient on a regular basis. It is important for you to know who you will be seeing and when because the perinatologist may end up playing as vital a role in your pregnancy as your doctor, if not more so.

How aggressive does the doctor plan to be in monitoring the pregnancy? How often will you have prenatal visits? Will you be able to have frequent sonograms and non-stress tests, even if your pregnancy is not considered high risk?

Even if your subsequent pregnancy is not considered high risk, you will probably need a lot of reassurance that everything is progressing well. Your doctor can do this by scheduling frequent sonograms and non-stress tests toward the end of your pregnancy, as much for your peace of mind as the baby's health. If he is not willing to do these things, you may want to consider finding another doctor. That's what Cynthia did after her obstetrician made it clear that he would not do sonograms upon request:

> *There was one point when it took him a long time to find a heartbeat, so I begged him to do a sonogram just to be sure everything was all right. And he said, "No, it's not necessary." I said, "Please, I just want to see the baby, my insurance will cover it." He flat out refused. He said, "No I won't do it."*

Is the doctor affiliated with a major hospital that has a neonatal intensive care unit?

In the area where I live, quite a few suburban hospitals have maternity wards equipped with the latest technology, but have no intensive care units for newborns who need special care. Those critically ill babies must be taken either by helicopter or ambulance to one of the many large hospitals in the city. Dozens of women deliver their babies at these smaller hospitals every day and never give the issue a fleeting thought. But those of us who have suffered a pregnancy loss cannot afford to be as complacent.

If you are at risk for pre-term labor, there is no question that you should arrange to give birth to your baby in a hospital with a high-level neonatal intensive care unit. That is the only way to ensure that the baby will get the best possible care as quickly as possible. But even if your baby is not considered at high risk, it is still a good idea. My third son spent eight days in the NICU because of lung immaturity even though I had an uncomplicated pregnancy and he was born at thirty-seven weeks gestation. Thankfully, he was down the hall and not across town. After leaving the hospital the first time with empty arms, I don't think I could have handled it if my sick baby had been miles away from me. Since you will be doing everything you can to safeguard your baby in the womb, be sure you also make every effort to ensure that your baby has access to the best possible care following birth, too.

Will your doctor be present at your delivery?

For practical reasons, most obstetricians do not deliver all of their patients' babies. If they did, they may never get a decent night's sleep. But given your history, it is not unreasonable to ask your doctor to make an exception and arrange to be present at your delivery. Barring that option, you can discuss alternatives with your doctor so that you can be prepared for whatever happens. Sandy had not thought to ask whether her doctor would deliver her baby, but she was devastated nonetheless when she arrived at the hospital and was told that someone else was on call that night. Fortunately, when she was wheeled into the delivery room, she was happily surprised. "A man came in wearing a surgical mask and scrubs, and I didn't recognize him at first. But then he pulled down his mask and smiled, and I saw that it was my doctor. I've never been so happy to see someone in my entire life." You may not be as fortunate as Sandy, so you can avoid unnecessary disappointment by finding out ahead of time what your doctor plans to do.

The initial consultation is also a good time to ask about other issues related to the delivery. At what point during labor should you go to the hospital? What kind of pain relief will you receive? Will electronic fetal monitoring be done? Will you be able to have anyone besides your partner in the delivery room with you? Knowing what to expect ahead of time will ease some of your fears. It will also help ensure that the joy of giving birth to a healthy baby will not be marred by unexpected problems.

What are the doctor's views on early delivery?

Forty weeks is a long time to be pregnant. It feels even longer when you are pregnant after losing a baby either close to or shortly after your due date. Even those women whose pregnancy loss occurred earlier usually cannot wait for their subsequent pregnancy to be over so that they can finally hold their baby in their arms. Unless there are medical reasons for doing so, most doctors will not deliver a baby before thirty-eight weeks, which is considered full-term. If early delivery is important to you, be sure to ask whether your physician plans to induce labor at thirty-eight weeks or prefers to wait until you go into labor on your own. You may also want to discuss whether there are any reasons to consider inducing labor before thirty-eight weeks.

If your baby was born too soon, how does the doctor treat preterm labor?

Prematurity is a leading cause of early infant mortality. If your baby was among those who was born too early to survive, it is particularly important for you to know the signs of preterm labor and the treatment your doctor would use to stop it. The earlier that preterm labor is detected, the better the chances are that it can be stopped. Under what conditions will your doctor prescribe bed rest? If he does prescribe bed rest, are home visits a possibility? Under what conditions would you be hospitalized? When would preterm labor *not* be stopped? "A very important issue that we are seeing more of is the policy of *not* treating preterm labor before viability, in other words before twenty-four weeks gestation," says Sidelines' Hurley. Fortunately, still a large number of perinatologists do not accept that a premature baby is "God's will" or just "nature taking its course." Hurley recommends choosing a physician who is a proponent of preterm birth prevention efforts such as early identification of women at risk, bedrest and medication to reduce uterine contractions. You also should ask if you will be given a home monitor to check for contractions. All these are questions you will want answers to if there is a possibility that your next baby might come early.

Based on the medical aspects of your pregnancy loss, what does the doctor think about your prospects for having a healthy baby?

This is the question that you would probably most like to have answered. Although there is no way to predict the outcome of your pregnancy, it is possible to estimate whether your chances of having a healthy baby are as good as anyone else's or somewhat less than average. If your chances are good, it will be one more reason for you to calm your shattered nerves; if they are not that good, you can prepare yourself for what may lie ahead.

A Word of Caution

Asking your prospective doctor these questions and others before you get pregnant again will reduce your chances of receiving unhappy surprises later. Your initial interview will give you insight into whether or not you feel comfortable talking with the doctor, as well as whether he answers your questions adequately. But the amount of legwork you do will not guarantee that you find the perfect health care provider. Even the best doctors are not always able to calm every fear and answer every question. The physician you chose so carefully may even at times be insensitive to your needs.

Lynn's obstetrician, for example, went on vacation the week that her amniocentesis results were due. That meant that Lynn had to wait an extra five days to find out whether her baby had major health problems. This was especially trying for Lynn because she had a history of genetic problems and knew that she was at high risk for a pregnancy loss. But because her doctor was so helpful and compassionate in other ways, Lynn forgave him for the oversight. "You realize that no matter how hard your doctor tries, we're not their entire life. They're so busy and they see so many people, and I understand that."

It may also help to remember that your physician and staff are far more accustomed to dealing with women who are happy and relatively carefree during pregnancy than with those, like you, who may be ambivalent and scared and perhaps still grieving the death of another baby. That means that one of them may occasionally say or do something insensitive or inappropriate. But if you believe that their intentions are good, you may be more willing to forgive them.

Considering a Midwife

Certified nurse-midwives are registered nurses who are specially trained to care for women throughout their pregnancy, labor and delivery. They typically deal only with low-risk, uncomplicated pregnancies and have an arrangement with a qualified physician who will provide back-up support should complications arise. To be certified by the American College of Nurse-Midwives, midwives must be licensed registered nurses who have completed an accredited graduate-level program in midwifery. They must also pass a national certification exam. Sometimes, women who select midwives for their care also choose to deliver their babies in a birthing center or at home rather than at a hospital.

Given your history, you may want to give the issue careful thought before choosing a midwife for your prenatal care. Although it is true that most women who suffer a pregnancy loss are under the care of a physician at the time, obstetricians and perinatologists have far more training in obstetrics than midwives and are therefore in a better position to identify and address problems that may arise in your subsequent pregnancy.

If you feel it is important for you to be under the care of a midwife in your next pregnancy, consider seeing one in addition to a doctor. Many midwives are now affiliated with OB practices, and have the time and personality to offer the extra counseling, education and emotional support that you may need. Some physicians will arrange for your midwife to be in the room with you during delivery so you can have the best of both worlds—all of the advantages of a fully equipped medical facility along with the personalized care of a midwife. If you had your heart set on a home birth, keep in mind that a growing number of hospitals are making an effort to create home-like atmospheres in their labor and delivery rooms. Instead of simply having a lone hospital bed illuminated by harsh lights, the rooms now feature easy chairs, sofas, lamps and Chintz curtains.

When You Don't Get Pregnant Right Away

Once you decide that you are ready to try again, it can be very stressful if it takes longer than you had expected to get pregnant. It will be even more difficult if you conceived quickly the last time and did not expect to have any problems with conception. You may find yourself depressed every time your period starts, especially if you suspected that you might be pregnant. In some ways it will be like experiencing a loss all over again, only this time it's the loss of hope. You may even start to worry that you may not be able to have another baby. This will be especially true if your loss occurred in your first pregnancy. In that case, you have no way of knowing whether you really are capable of giving birth to a healthy, full-term baby.

As you wait month after month for signs that you might be pregnant, you will likely be getting news that friends or relatives are expecting a baby. Within three months of my loss, three of my very best friends called to tell me they were pregnant. For two of them, it was their third child. While I only wished the best for them, I couldn't help but be a little envious, considering that they would have three living children to love and nurture before I had even one. In the meantime, all the women I knew who were pregnant at the same time I was had their beautiful and healthy babies. Again, I was happy for them, but also extremely sad for myself.

Because the stress associated with not getting pregnant is so great, some women rearrange their lives to ensure that they are able to have intercourse during their most fertile periods. This might mean that women ask their partners to postpone a business trip or to have sex on a day when they really rather wouldn't. This kind of pressure can only add to the disappointment each time another month passes without conception. Melinda describes what her life was like during the eighteen months it took her to get pregnant again after the loss of her full-term baby boy:

I was obsessed with getting pregnant. I knew the exact minute I was ovulating and that is when we had sex. It ruled my life, and it was awful. I couldn't understand it either because the first time I had gotten pregnant right away. What made it even worse was that there were quite a few women at work who had gone on maternity leave at the same time that I did, and now we were all back in the office again, but they had a baby to talk about and I didn't. I felt like an outcast. They'd be talking and then if they knew I was around, they'd all get real quiet. I'm sure it was hard on them, too. It seemed like I just couldn't get away from it. Even when I went to church, there would always be a young couple with a baby sitting right in front of me. So after a while I said, why bother? I went through a period when I was really mad at God. It just seemed that until I was finally pregnant again, I couldn't get away from all the anger and frustration that I felt.

Some women believe that the stress felt from not getting pregnant again right away is the very thing that prevented them from conceiving. Says Leslie, "It took about eight months for me to get pregnant again, but it felt like years. I'm convinced that it took that long because I was so desperate to have another baby. I remember being very obsessed and very focused and very irrational. I just kept thinking, 'I am a woman and I should be able to get pregnant, and I should be able to do it right this time.' It was just craziness." Glenda also believes that she made it too stressful on herself. "While I was in the midst of all this grief, I was obsessed with becoming pregnant. I had never taken my temperature before, and now I was charting it every day. So I think stress probably had a lot to do with not getting pregnant."

Medical experts have long theorized that stress and infertility may be linked since they are so often seen in tandem. But research suggests that infertility leads to stress and not the other way around. In fact, there is very little evidence that psychological factors interfere with conception. Rather, it is infertility that causes stress because a couple so often feels isolated and frustrated over their inability to have children. Couples also feel as though they have lost control over their lives, especially when their day-to-day routine is disrupted by the evaluation and treatment of infertility.

Given that stress is a result and not a cause of infertility, it's not surprising that even those women who are *not* stressed over their inability to conceive still sometimes find that it takes time to get pregnant again. Mary, whose baby boy died of an infection within hours of his birth, was philosophical when several months had passed and she was still not pregnant. "I feel that I could walk away from this knowing that I've had a baby, and I've gone through the experience. I don't know if I would go through the fertility thing. If it's going to happen, it's going to happen." After six months of trying to conceive, Mary got pregnant again and gave birth to a healthy baby girl.

Infertility Problems

If a year or more passes and you are still not pregnant again, you may be a candidate for infertility treatment. Only about 15 percent of normal, fertile couples are unable to conceive within the first twelve months of trying, so it will be to your advantage to find out if either you or your partner have a problem that is preventing you from getting pregnant again. Infertility problems have been on the rise in recent years, as women increasingly delay pregnancy until later in life. That's because fertility begins to decrease at age thirty-five and then drops sharply after age forty.

The best way to find out whether you have a problem is to ask your obstetrician to refer you to a reproductive endocrinologist. These are obstetricians who have done a two-year fellowship in infertility. They devote their entire practice to treating fertility problems and typically have staff on call seven days a week, including holidays. This ensures that you can receive treatment during the appropriate times in your cycle, even if it happens on a weekend. Most fertility practices of this type are located in large cities, so if you live in a small town or rural area you might have to drive a long distance to receive treatment.

In order to determine why you are having trouble getting pregnant again, your endocrinologist will conduct a rather thorough investigation. It will not be unlike when your obstetrician searched for the cause of your pregnancy loss, only this time the focus will be on your reproductive system. The first vital clues will come from your menstrual cycles and pattern of ovulation. We've already talked about the importance of keeping track of your periods when you are trying to get pregnant again. This information is critical to a fertility specialist. Not only will you be asked to chart your menstrual cycles, you will also be expected to do home ovulation predictor tests to determine exactly when or if you are ovulating. Your doctor will use that information to determine your next course of action.

Since your partner may be just as likely to be the cause of infertility as you are, the endocrinologist will do a semen analysis as well. Some men have abnormal sperm that is immature or unable to move. Others have normal sperm but don't have enough of it. Both of these problems can reduce the chance that sperm will fertilize an egg. You and your partner will also have to take blood tests to check for everything from hormonal imbalances to infections.

Assuming that the cause of your problem is not obvious from the first round of tests, you will then proceed to round two. This includes what is known as post-coital tests. As the name implies, these tests are done after intercourse to determine whether your partner's sperm can penetrate and survive in the cervical mucus. An ultrasound will also be done so the doctor can inspect the condition of your uterus and ovaries and check the thickness of the uterine lining. A thin lining could indicate a hormonal problem. The ultrasound can also reveal potential problems like fibroid tumors, ovarian cysts and abnormalities in the shape of the uterus.

Other tests may include a hysterosalpingogram, a procedure in which dye is injected into the uterus and fallopian tubes, which are then examined using high-resolution ultrasound. This procedure will reveal problems that may not have been visible with ultrasound alone. If a uterine problem is detected, your doctor may decide to directly view the inside of the uterus using a hysteroscope. If problems with the ovaries are suspected, a laparoscopy may be done. Another option is an endometrial biopsy, a procedure in which a small amount of tissue from the uterine lining is scraped off just before menstruation. This can show whether you have a hormonal imbalance that causes you to miscarry early, possibly even before you know you are pregnant. Blood tests also probably will be done to check your hormone levels. The search for the cause of your infertility problems may continue until answers are found, since a successful diagnosis is essential for determining the right course of treatment.

Infertility Treatment

A wide range of treatment options are available to infertility patients, and the choice of treatment depends on the type of problem that has been diagnosed. Ovulatory disorders are the number-one cause of infertility in women. Irregular periods may be a sign of either infrequent or a total absence of ovulation, but some women with ovulatory problems have perfectly normal periods. Fortunately, these types of disorders can be treated fairly successfully using drug therapy that triggers ovulation. In fact, more than 80 percent of women undergoing ovulation induction get pregnant within a year.

If your doctor determines that a hormonal imbalance is inhibiting ovulation, the first treatment of choice will probably be a drug called clomiphene citrate. Sold under the brand names Clomid and Serophene, this fertility agent jump starts the reproductive system, causing a woman to ovulate more often and thereby providing additional opportunities to conceive. Since clomiphene is administered in pill form, the drug treatment alone will not disrupt your sex life or your daily routine. In most cases, the initial diagnosis is one tablet daily for five days beginning during the menstrual cycle. A couple then has intercourse when an ovulation test shows the woman is fertile.

If you are still not pregnant after six or more cycles of taking clomiphene, the next step is usually to add fertility drugs called menotropins, more commonly known as Pergonal, Humegon and Repronex. Administered through injections, this drug therapy tends to disrupt more of your day-to-day life. The timing of the injections is critical, so you basically will have to plan all of your activities around your infertility treatment. To stimulate ovulation, you will also have to inject the pregnancy hormone hCG thirty-six hours before insemination. Much of your time will be spent in doctors' offices. You will be seeing your fertility specialist frequently—sometimes even daily—so that you can be evaluated through blood tests, ultrasounds and cervical mucus exams. Pergonal treatment can be expensive, too. Each vial of medication costs $50 or more, and you may need two or more vials a day for seven to ten days in each treatment cycle. Humegon and Repronex, however, typically cost less.

In addition to the intrusion in your life and the dent in your pocketbook, another drawback to this type of therapy is the increased risk of multiple pregnancy. As the birth of the Iowa septuplets showed, fertility drugs can sometimes give you more than you bargained for. The risk of becoming pregnant with three or more babies while using this type of therapy averages about five percent, but regular ultrasound scans and blood tests can reduce this risk to two percent or less. The results will largely depend on your fertility specialist's ability to determine the amount of medication that will stimulate ovulation without overstimulating the ovaries. This can be extremely difficult, since the dosage can vary from woman to woman, and even from one cycle to the next.

When drug therapy alone fails, the next step is to move to what are known as "assisted reproductive technologies." These include sophisticated procedures such as artificial insemination and in vitro fertilization. In artificial insemination, a large number of healthy sperm are injected directly into the uterus, giving them easy access to the fallopian tubes. To maximize the fertility of the sperm, they are specially prepared in a laboratory before being injected. This is a good treatment when a man's sperm count is low. With in vitro fertilization (IVF), a woman's eggs are removed after ovulation and fertilized in a laboratory. The fertilized eggs are then placed in the uterus a few days later. If implantation is successful, the pregnancy progresses as it usually would from that point on. Although once a headline-making event, IVF is fairly common these days. Gamete intra-fallopian transfer, better known as GIFT, is another common form of assisted reproductive technologies.

The Emotional Impact of Infertility Treatment

We just explored the clinical side to infertility treatment, but there is an emotional side as well. Infertility therapy can be extremely stressful on both you and your husband, especially coming as it does in the midst of your grief. The treatments will not only change your daily routine, they will affect your marriage and your pocketbook. Kelly, who had two healthy children before losing her third to an umbilical cord accident, is a case in point. She was already thirty-eight years old when she started trying to conceive again, and was concerned when fourteen months had gone by and she was still not pregnant. Worried that time was running out on her biological clock, Kelly sought help from a reproductive endocrinologist. The next several months were extremely stressful, as Kelly and her husband went through a series of infertility treatments:

You think you're crazy now, try infertility treatment. At certain times in the month, I was in my doctor's office every single day getting vaginal sonograms. And when you have other kids, that can really get complicated. I remember being at a camp in Missouri with my children and having to stay awake until one in the morning so that a friend could give me a hormone shot to release the egg. Then my husband and I had to be back in the doctor's office thirty-six hours later so that I could be artificially inseminated. My husband hated it. He would moan and groan about having to give a [sperm] specimen, and here I was being poked and prodded and shot, so I didn't like it much either. As it got more and more difficult, his interest really started waning. He was not against it, but he started thinking, "Is this really meant to be?" You get to a point where you really want to give up.

This pressure was compounded by family and friends who could not understand why Kelly and her husband were trying so hard for another pregnancy when they already had a boy and a girl. They seemed to think that the couple was pushing their luck. But even though Kelly knew her age put her baby at greater risk for chromosomal problems, she believed it was a risk worth taking. "I finally got to the point where I thought, 'Get out of your fairy-tale world. Not everyone lives happily every after. It is a fact that every X number of pregnancies go bad, but if you want a child bad enough, it's worth the risk.' " After seven months of working with a fertility specialist, Kelly got pregnant and ultimately delivered a healthy baby boy.

Feelings about a Positive Pregnancy Test

Women who are under the treatment of a fertility specialist are monitored so closely that they find out immediately when they are pregnant again. But those of us who buy home pregnancy tests to know for sure sometimes put off getting the news because of the fear of what another pregnancy could bring. Some women who have experienced a loss delay buying a home pregnancy test until well after they suspect they are pregnant, while others buy the kit only to leave it sitting on a shelf. Says Laura, "I bought a pregnancy test when my period was one day late, but I couldn't bring myself to use it for about two weeks. Of course, we were thrilled when we saw it was positive, but it only took about fifteen minutes before the fear set in."

In addition to the fear that nearly every couple feels when they find out they are expecting again after a loss, a whole range of emotions may come flooding in once you get the news, ranging from elation over the new beginning, to anxiety at the thought of going through another pregnancy, to sadness over how the last pregnancy ended, and perhaps even guilt that you are moving on with your life. Cynthia, who had experienced multiple losses, recalls her reaction when she found out from her endocrinologist that she was expecting again:

I had a panic attack when I first got the news. I was literally shaking. The thought of what lay ahead for us was almost immobilizing, I was so scared. So for the whole first day and most of the second day I was pretty upset just worrying about the enormousness of it all. But after that, I adopted an attitude that worrying about it wasn't going to make me or the baby live two minutes longer. And if, God forbid, something bad happened, I would have plenty of time afterward to be devastated.

Glenda, whose second child died at birth, says the hardest part for her was realizing she had absolutely no control over what happened next:

My husband and I are both type A personalities, and this was something that we could not control. The first time you get pregnant it's almost like blissful ignorance. You just don't realize how unbelievably fortunate you are to have a trouble-free pregnancy and have a perfect child. But when your baby dies, you just feel like it's going to happen again. You never feel that unrestricted joy again as you did the very first time you found out you were pregnant. You are always going to have that hesitation that you didn't have the first time.

When my own pregnancy test came back positive four months after my loss, I literally fell to my knees and begged God not to let this baby die, too. Then I cried for the baby who had died, for myself, for my husband and for the future that we had lost. But at the same time, I was grateful for a second chance. I knew I could not have Patrick, but I could have his little brother or sister.

When the Pregnancy Is a Surprise

You won't have to make the decision to try again if your next pregnancy is unexpected. This often happens to women with a history of infertility problems who were under the mistaken impression that they could not get pregnant again. Other times, birth control simply fails. In the book *Angelic Presence*, Chuck Lammert describes how he and his wife, Cathi Lammert, executive director of SHARE Pregnancy and Infant Loss Support, found out they were expecting again a few months after their newborn son had died.

> *We unknowingly conceived our fifth child. I say unknowingly because we attempted to insure our decision to prevent a pregnancy by using two different methods [of birth control]. When Cathi first started to experience all of her previous pregnancy symptoms, we did not recognize them. It wasn't until the home pregnancy test confirmed her suspicions that we knew for sure. We shared mixed emotions, happy for what might be but scared about what could happen. Through it all we both felt a certain peace that we could not explain.*

Although Cathi and Chuck had medical reasons for trying to prevent another pregnancy, and despite the prognosis for both the mother and baby being grim, she ended up giving birth to a perfectly healthy baby girl. Given the odds that they were facing, the Lammerts were thankful that the decision had not been theirs to make. "We are grateful that the decision to have another child was taken out of our hands and placed in God's with a little help from our son."

The news of another pregnancy is not always as welcome, however. Diane unexpectedly became pregnant three months after her baby died, which meant that her due date would coincide with the anniversary of her pregnancy loss. "We were going to wait and give my body some time to heal before we were even going to try again, but I got pregnant anyway. At first, I was really upset. I thought I don't want to be pregnant this month. But over time, I gradually came to terms with it." For Rita, the news of another pregnancy was even more upsetting because her premature daughter was still fighting for her life in the neonatal intensive care unit of a hospital.

Natalie was seven months old, and I had still not had a period, but I was under so much stress that I really didn't give it a whole lot of thought. I figured it was just because I wasn't taking care of myself. When I finally decided to go see the doctor about it I found out that I was thirteen weeks pregnant. We hadn't been trying. In fact we had hardly even had sex. When my doctor told me that I was pregnant, I was absolutely hysterical. I didn't think I could go through it again. And I felt like there was no way the baby could be healthy because I hadn't been taking care of myself at all. Sometimes I'd even go twenty-four hours without food.

Adding to Rita's concerns was that she had an incompetent cervix and knew that she would be facing surgery in a few weeks. Although her baby girl, Natalie, died two months after Rita found out she was pregnant again, she gave birth to a full-term baby son and has since had two more healthy children.

chapter four

Pregnant Again: The First Trimester

IT'S THE MOMENT you have been looking forward to—and dreading. You're pregnant again. Now what do you do? If you're like most women who are pregnant after a loss, you prepare yourself for nine months of contradictions. There's elation over knowing that you're expecting another baby, and sadness over the one that you lost. There's excitement about what's to come, and trepidation about what each day may bring. There's the hope that comes with another chance, and despair that it all may be in vain. And that's just for starters. Even when you finally give birth to a healthy baby, you will very likely find that tears of sorrow are intermingled with those of joy.

I experienced all of these feelings and others from the very beginning of my subsequent pregnancy. Even though I was overwhelmed with happiness and gratitude, I couldn't help but feel sad and even resentful over my loss. I looked forward to each passing month because it would bring me closer to the day when I might bring home a healthy baby. And yet I feared every minute because I knew that this new life might slip away, too. I tried to maintain a positive attitude and believe with all my heart that, this time, everything would be all right, and yet many times I could not help but worry that the worst would happen again. If I didn't know better, I would have thought I was the only woman ever to have had these thoughts during pregnancy. But because I had talked to many others who had been through a subsequent pregnancy, I knew that all my feelings were perfectly normal.

In the next several chapters, we'll explore the wide range of feelings that you will likely experience in your own pregnancy. We'll discuss the various issues that may be of concern to you in each trimester and offer some tips on how to ease your anxiety. We'll also examine what you can expect at your prenatal visits. Yes, you've been there and done that. But this pregnancy is not going to be anything like your last one. You'll be viewing everything from a different perspective, and, as with the other topics discussed so far, it may be a little easier if you know what to expect.

Common Concerns

Sharing the News

Pregnancy is not something that you can keep secret for very long. Sooner or later, you will have to share the news with family and friends. But will it be sooner or later? That's not always an easy question to answer. In a first pregnancy, couples either tell right away or wait until somewhere close to the end of the first trimester, when they believe that they are "out of the woods." Usually they have little concern about how family and friends may react to the news, because unless there are extenuating circumstances, they know that everyone will be happy and supportive. All they need to decide is whom to tell first.

In a pregnancy following a loss, the issues are not nearly as clear-cut. There are many reasons why couples don't feel comfortable telling others that they are pregnant again when they first find out, such as the fear of another loss or the worry that the baby who died may be forgotten in all the excitement over the next pregnancy. Couples may also be reluctant to open themselves up to all the advice, questions and concerns that are sure to follow their announcement. As for waiting until being "out of the woods" to spread the news, couples know that that day may not come until after the baby's birth. If a couple decides to tell right away, it may not be as much from wanting to share good news as from wanting to solicit prayer and support. They may even find themselves using words like "hopefully" and "if all goes well" in talking about the baby. And unlike the responses to the previous pregnancy, reactions this time can run the gamut, from happiness and joy to outright shock and disapproval.

Just as there was no right or wrong amount of time to wait before trying to conceive again, there is no ideal time for sharing the news of a subsequent pregnancy. Your decision will be based on your particular circumstances and the feelings of you and your partner. But there are some things you might want to consider before making your decision. Let's turn now to reasons for waiting, as well as some motivations for sharing the news right away.

Reasons to Wait

There will be many reasons why you may prefer to keep the news of your pregnancy to yourself, at least for the first several weeks. If you have had multiple losses, or believe that there is a good chance that you could miscarry again, you may be reluctant to tell people for fear that you will have to tell them bad news at some point in the future. Even if your actual chances for a successful pregnancy are pretty good, you may still not be able to shake the feeling that something could go wrong. That's how Phyllis felt throughout most of her subsequent pregnancy:

I remember that it was April, just two months before the baby was born, and I was still walking around in my big winter coat because I wanted to hide my stomach. My husband said, "People are going to think you're crazy." But I didn't want anyone in my apartment building asking me or knowing anything about my pregnancy. I just kept thinking that if they know I'm pregnant then I'll have to tell them if the baby dies. But in a way, I was cheated out of the whole process—letting everyone know about the baby, sharing the excitement, and watching my body go through all the changes. Instead, I was hiding it.

Perhaps you fear that the baby may have the same problem that caused your last pregnancy to end in a loss. In that case, you may want to wait to tell others until prenatal tests confirm that history will not repeat itself. Glenda held off announcing her subsequent pregnancy until after she had an echocardiogram to see if her baby had the same heart condition that caused her son to die. "We didn't tell anybody outside of the immediate family because we didn't know what we were going to do if the results were bad, and we didn't want anybody's opinion," she says.

Your own health may be another reason for not telling others right away. Women who have chronic medical problems sometimes fear the negative reaction that they could receive from others, and not sharing the news is their way of avoiding hurtful comments, at least for a while. Maybe your motivation for not talking about the pregnancy is altruistic; that is, you want to spare your family and friends from worrying. Sharon, who had a serious kidney disease that doctors feared would be aggravated by pregnancy, recalls her reaction when her pregnancy test came back positive.

I knew there would be a lot of opposition to my pregnancy just out of worry for me. And I felt a lot of responsibility for that because they were all put through the mill when my baby died. They were all there. They held her, they cried for her, they buried her. So a lot of people just did not want me to go through another pregnancy, and I can't say that I blame them. I wanted to spare them that worry as long as possible.

Although Sharon's intentions were good, there really is no way to keep friends and relatives from worrying—short of hiding the pregnancy from them. Often, concerns arise only after you have shared your news. And although, more often than not, everything turns out to be fine, it can nonetheless lead to many anxious moments. Carla, for example, waited until she was at thirteen weeks gestation before she told her family about her pregnancy because she wanted to get past the high-risk first trimester. But the very day she shared the news, she started bleeding and was put on bed rest for the rest of the pregnancy. She ended up being fine and gave birth to a healthy baby boy at thirty-eight weeks. Yet no one could have been at ease during what was an extremely nerve-wracking pregnancy.

Your reasons for waiting may not have anything to do with your health, but instead may be based on your emotions. For example, if only a short time has passed since your loss, you may be embarrassed to tell people that you're expecting again. You may feel that if people learn about the subsequent pregnancy, they will assume that you are no longer grieving, even if that couldn't be further from the truth. Or you may want people's focus to remain on the baby who died rather than on the pregnancy and the next baby. That was the feeling that Kim had when she got pregnant only three months after her loss: "I kind of felt like everybody in the world just wanted me to forget about Grace and go on with my life, and I couldn't do that. I thought about her all the time, and was still grieving very intensely. So I didn't tell anybody I was pregnant again for four or five months. I waited until I had to start wearing maternity clothes."

If no one knows you are pregnant, you won't have to explain yourself or listen to advice. It will also help you avoid the attention that naturally falls on every pregnant woman, and that will probably focus all the more on you, given your circumstances. By not telling people right away, you can buy some extra time that may even make the nine months seem shorter.

Depending on how long you wait to tell, you may notice that some people are stealing glances at your bulging stomach. But usually no one will have the courage to ask you if you're pregnant. If they do, you might want to tell the truth so that you don't have to explain later. That happened to me when I was only about ten weeks pregnant with my second baby. We invited some close friends over for dinner and about half way through the meal one of them said, "You're pregnant.

I can tell." Of course, since he was right, I felt like I had no choice but to confirm his suspicions. Fortunately, he kept his promise not to tell anyone.

Even if you decide not to tell family and friends, don't be surprised if you find yourself telling strangers about your pregnancy. Laura's husband was so excited about her pregnancy that he wanted to tell everyone right away. When she asked him to wait for a few weeks, he blew off steam by telling strangers on airplanes and in convenience stores. "Keeping it a secret was driving my husband crazy, so he told people that he didn't even know. He just needed to do that," she says. Another compromise might be to tell a few close friends or family members who you know will be supportive. You can then gradually share the news over time—first with close family and friends and later with those outside your inner circle.

That was the approach I used in telling people about my subsequent pregnancy. Aside from my husband, my grief counselor and the friend who guessed that I was pregnant, no one else knew I was expecting until well into my second trimester. I remember finally making my announcement on New Year's Day, just four and a half months before my delivery. At that point, all I had to do was take off the apron I was wearing to hide my stomach and say, "Guess what?" Based on the reaction, I could tell that we had done a pretty good job of concealing the pregnancy. I even went so far as to keep the pregnancy a secret from my out-of-town relatives until after the baby was actually born. It was easy enough not to tell because, aside from my brother, my entire family lives in Italy. Obviously, with everyone that far away, there was no danger that I would unexpectedly run into someone who hadn't heard the news.

Actually, I might not have remained silent quite that long if there hadn't been a precedent in my own family. More than thirty years earlier, when my mother found out she was pregnant with me, she didn't tell anyone in Italy until after I was born. Her reasons for waiting were different. I was a so-called surprise baby, born six years after my brother, and my mother was a little embarrassed to let her family know she was expecting again. So she opted to write them all letters on hospital stationery shortly after my birth. I figured if she could do it that way, so could I. Only I would use the telephone to spread the news.

One of my biggest motivations for waiting so long to tell was that I was simply afraid that people, in their eagerness to focus on the positive news of my subsequent pregnancy, would forget about the baby who died. Not only was I a little embarrassed to be pregnant again just four months after Patrick's death, I felt it was somehow disrespectful. I knew that I would keep grieving the loss through my pregnancy, but I wasn't sure anyone else would. And although I know that others meant well, it bothered me that so many people thought that another pregnancy would somehow fix everything. That seemed to diminish the magnitude of what had happened. When I finally shared my news with those closest to me, seven months had passed since my loss, which seemed a more appropriate time to start looking ahead to the new baby's arrival while still holding on to Patrick's memory.

There were some advantages to calling relatives overseas with the wonderful news of my baby's birth, as opposed to alerting the chronic worriers in my family that I was pregnant again. This way, no one had to be concerned about me. I didn't have to listen to any unsolicited advice. And it all served to make my subsequent pregnancy feel different from the last one, which is something I was trying to do every step of the way. Fortunately, my husband was willing to go along with whatever I wanted and managed to keep the news a secret until I gave him permission to tell. Although the secretive approach worked well for me, many would argue that there are good reasons for sharing the news right away. Let's explore some of those reasons now.

Reasons to Tell Right Away

One of the main reasons that some people decide not to share the news of their pregnancy is the fear that they might suffer another loss. But that may be the very reason to *want* others to know. You may feel that the support of family and friends will be essential should the worst happen again. This was Lynn's feeling, after she found out she had a genetic problem that made her next baby's chances of survival only fifty-fifty. "My philosophy was that I was going to want my friends to support me if I ended up miscarrying, so I didn't see the need to keep it to myself and tell them after the fact." Cynthia, who had suffered four pregnancy losses, had done it both ways—telling right away in some cases and waiting until after the first trimester in others. But when she got pregnant for what she believed would be the last time, Cynthia felt she needed the prayers and support from her family and friends:

> There was a pregnancy when I didn't tell people until I was sixteen weeks along. We didn't even tell our son until fourteen weeks, so we were very guarded. But it didn't make any difference because a few weeks later we had to tell those same people that we weren't pregnant. So this time, we figured let's tell everybody up front. That way, there will be more people across the United States praying for us. My husband and I thought maybe there's force in numbers. Maybe God will listen if a whole bunch of people are praying for us.

Sheila felt that by telling everyone early she would receive the positive feedback that she needed on a daily basis to stay positive herself. "I told everybody I was pregnant from the beginning—my boss, my coworkers, my friends—so everybody was behind me, and I knew that if I miscarried they would all be there to help me, too."

Another good reason for sharing the news of your pregnancy may be that you are happy and want others to share your joy. For Nancy, who had battled infertility, the pregnancy itself was a victory: "I was excited about it and wanted to be happy and celebrate every minute of it. If something bad happened, then I wanted people close to me to know why I was upset rather than going back and telling them, 'Well, I was pregnant, but now I'm not.' As long as I had reason to be hopeful, I wanted to be positive and rejoice."

Some reasons for sharing the news right away may be more practical. Perhaps your pregnancy is obvious to others because of morning sickness or bed rest. Katie was a flight attendant and quit her job when she found out she was expecting again. As a result, she was forced to tell her family and friends when she was just five weeks pregnant. Martha says she told people because they would have figured it out for themselves if she hadn't. "I had really bad morning sickness, so people knew something was up when I was eating crackers all the time. I hadn't really wanted to tell people because I didn't want to have to give a lot of explanations if I lost the baby, but I went ahead and told them anyway."

Like most women, Sydney felt both approaches had pros and cons, especially when her subsequent pregnancy ended in her second miscarriage. "Not telling is a little bit lonely because you're dealing with the fears all alone while you're pregnant. But on the other hand, there weren't all the people to tell when I miscarried. I got tired of delivering bad news."

How to Share the News

When the time comes to share the news about the pregnancy, most of us choose to tell people either in person or over the phone. But because the reactions to a subsequent pregnancy can be so complicated, you might opt for a third alternative—a letter. Several women I interviewed decided to write to relatives and friends so they could explain that there was a lot more to their pregnancy than just excitement about the new baby.

Katie, whose first baby had died at term, wrote in her letter that she and her husband were expecting their second child, and that the next baby could never replace the one who died. She also stressed that she didn't want congratulations at that point because she felt too vulnerable. However, she told everyone that she would welcome prayers and encouragement. She sent the letters to her parents and in-laws a day early so that they got the news before everyone else. After all the letters were received, Katie was pleasantly surprised by the reactions:

I got a lot of phone calls and a lot of letters back, and the letters were so unbelievable. People said they were praying for me. In fact, my brother said he put the letter on his refrigerator and said a prayer for the baby every day. Other people called and said the letter finally helped them understand how I felt.

Cynthia used a letter to inform only those friends and relatives who lived out of town or whom she saw infrequently. Cynthia had two reasons for writing the letter. She knew that many people would be shocked to learn that she and her husband were trying to have another baby since she had already suffered multiple losses. The letter gave her the opportunity to fully explain her motivations so that many of those who might have opposed her pregnancy could understand why she was going through it again. Cynthia also had a much more practical reason for using a letter to share her news. She knew that her high-risk pregnancy was going to cost a small fortune in medical expenses, and stamps were a whole lot less expensive than long-distance phone calls. Today, you could also use e-mail to share your news, but keep in mind that most people consider this much less personal than a hand-written note.

The Reaction of Others

In most cases, people's feelings about your pregnancy will reflect your own. If you are happy, they will probably be happy for you. Similarly, if you have doubts, you will convey those feelings to them, and they in turn are likely to feel the same way. But you should also be prepared for the unexpected. There will always be someone who voices disapproval or, even without meaning to, says the wrong thing.

Couples who already have other children often find that people have trouble understanding why they would put themselves through the pain of another pregnancy. If you are putting your own health at risk to bear a child, you may discover that people are angry, especially those closest to you. "Your own parents especially might be horrified that you would put your own life at risk for a child that they don't know," says Candace Hurley, executive director of Sidelines National Support Network for women experiencing high-risk pregnancies. That was the case with Brenda, whose pregnancy endangered both her life and that of her baby:

We didn't tell very many people at the beginning because we knew their opinions were not going to be very supportive. So we waited until I was about four months along to tell them. Just as we expected, their reactions were mostly all negative. It was very hurtful. Looking back on it, I can understand. But we were excited even though we were high-risk because we felt it was going to work out this time. They all thought we would be having another funeral.

Not every case is as extreme as Brenda's. Her pregnancy was exceptionally high risk. But even when the subsequent pregnancy is only at slightly greater risk of ending in a loss, telling people can still be difficult. Rita worried that her family and friends would be upset at the news of her pregnancy because her infant daughter, who later died, was still fighting for her life in the neonatal intensive care unit at the time. It turned out she was right. No one seemed to care that Rita's pregnancy was unplanned and more difficult for her and her husband than for everyone else:

My husband's parents were very upset because they couldn't understand why on earth we would go through this again. They were very angry about it. His brother also was a little upset because he and his wife were going through everything with us daily and couldn't believe we were getting ourselves into something that was iffy at best.

At times, the reaction of others may surprise you. Suzanne went back to law school after her baby had died in the hope that staying busy would make it easier for her to cope with her loss. When she got pregnant again a few months later, she never dreamed that her mother would be angry at her for having a baby before finishing school. "My mother was furious. And I said. 'How can you be mad at me for getting pregnant?' She said, 'We're just concerned because you're not going to pass the bar.' And I said, 'Mom, the bar exam is irrelevant to me. I just want a baby.' "

Lynn, who had had several miscarriages, also did not get the reaction she expected when she first shared the news of a pregnancy that later resulted in the birth of a healthy baby boy: "When I told my mother that I was pregnant again, she said something like 'already' or 'again?' It wasn't 'congratulations,' but rather 'here we go again,' which was kind of my reaction too. But you want others to be a little more excited."

Cynthia, who suffered multiple losses before giving birth to twins, had a similar experience when she told her sister that she was pregnant again:

She said, "I support you 100 percent, but if it was me, there's no way I'd be doing it." And I said, "That's not very supportive. That's telling me that you think what I'm doing is nuts or that I'm making a mistake." And then she said, "I just hope it's worth all the agony." Well, wouldn't it be worth all the agony? I mean, if they told me I had to swing from a chandelier five times a day in order to have a baby, I'd do it.

Sometimes you may get no reaction at all, which can often be worse than hearing negative comments. Allison's mother registered silent disapproval when she heard about the pregnancy.

This is the Catholic mother who used to leave information for us on natural family planning, and I know she blamed most of my pregnancy problems on the birth control pills that I had been taking for about eight years. So when she wasn't excited, I thought, "What's wrong with you? You've wanted this for so long, and I am trying."

Other pregnant women are pleasantly surprised when the reaction is better than what they expected. Leslie's family was visibly excited and happy about the news, even though she had already suffered two losses and almost died herself in her previous pregnancy. "I don't think anybody that wasn't there that saw how sick I was had any clue that's what we went through, so I think most people were pretty happy for us. Maybe I'm naive, but I didn't think it was possible for me to lose three babies, and I think that's what other people thought."

Occasionally, though, others can be too happy for your liking. It may especially pain you to be congratulated given that you know the long road that lies ahead of you. As one woman said, "Being pregnant is nothing to congratulate me for. Save your congratulations for when I have a healthy baby." It bothered Martha when her mother-in-law gave her an outfit for the new baby shortly after hearing the news that she was expecting again. "I was thinking that I could lose this one too and then what would I do with the present? She was trying to be kind, but I didn't like it. I felt like it was insensitive of her."

I was especially bothered when people at an office where I worked as a freelance journalist simply gushed over the news of my subsequent pregnancy. I wondered why those same people could not find the words to console me when I first returned to the office after my loss. Yes, they had sent a card, and even made a donation to a children's hospital in my baby's name, and I sincerely appreciated that. But I hated that it was business as usual once I returned to work. I wanted someone to ask me how I was doing, or look me in the eye and tell me they were sorry about what happened. With time, I came to understand that most people don't know what to say to someone who has experienced any type of loss, much less a pregnancy loss. They are also afraid of stirring up fresh emotions, which would make everyone feel uncomfortable.

In fact, it was only after my next baby was born that I realized how wrong I had been to think that everyone had forgotten about my loss. Somehow it was easier for people to share their feelings about what had happened once they knew that I had given birth to a healthy child. There was one woman in particular who told me that she had a baby many years before who suffered from PKU (phenylketonuria), a genetic disorder that, if left untreated, can lead to mental retardation. Today, babies are routinely tested for this metabolic disorder before being released from the hospital, and, if necessary, given treatment to prevent abnormal brain development. But back when my coworker had given birth, testing was available but not yet widespread. As a result, her son, who is now in his thirties, is mentally disabled. What made her story even sadder to me was that she never had another baby. She and her husband were terrified that the same thing could happen to their next child. So although my colleague had suffered a loss of a different kind, she knew all too well how hard it was for me when my baby died. Unfortunately, it took many months and much resentment on my part before I was finally able to understand that.

Although my subsequent pregnancy opened the lines of communication with certain people, I also noticed that a few friends dropped out of touch in the months following my loss and during my subsequent pregnancy. If the same thing happens to you, you might think as I did that they are just too busy to call. But if you dig a little deeper, you may discover that certain people are avoiding you for fear of saying or doing the wrong thing. Or perhaps they feel helpless because they have no idea what they can do for you. You can ease the situation by letting them know how you feel and how they can help. Nancy did this in a letter that she sent to friends and coworkers after her loss:

> I sent all of them a letter and said, "This is what I believe, and this is what I do not want to hear. I don't want to hear things like, it's God's will, or you can always have another baby. I don't believe God wills for babies to be taken from their parents, so if you want to say something helpful to me say, 'I'm happy for what you had and sad for what you lost.' " It really helped me to write that because I didn't want to go back and be bombarded with things I didn't believe.

Beth made it a point to let her friends and family know that it was okay to talk about the baby who died, and not just focus all of their attention on the pregnancy: "I think once I gave them permission to talk about Eric, we all were a lot more open about discussing our feelings. It also made it easier for me to talk about my pregnancy because I didn't feel like I had to be positive all the time. They knew that even though I was excited about the new baby, I was still grieving."

Telling Your Other Children about the Pregnancy

If you have other children, they must also be told about the pregnancy. But considering that they have already spent months awaiting the arrival of a little brother or sister only to be disappointed, it may be difficult to find the right way to share the news. You may also have trouble deciding when to tell them. If you tell them too early, the nine months can feel like an eternity, especially for very young children. On the other hand, by waiting too long, you run the risk that they might overhear a conversation or find out from someone else that you're expecting again. As you try to decide on the best approach for you, you might want to take into account the ages of your children, how far along you were when you suffered your loss and how they reacted to the news. All of those factors will influence when and how you tell them about a subsequent pregnancy.

As with so many aspects of the subsequent pregnancy, it can also help to know how other couples have handled the same situation. Kim, for example, chose to tread very carefully in sharing the news of her pregnancy with her five-year-old son, since he had had a particularly hard time dealing with the death of his baby sister several months before.

> He was in the room with us when the doctor told us that he couldn't find the baby's heartbeat. So in the weeks after the baby died, he was really worried about me because he had heard people say that my heart was broken. He thought I was going to die, too. He also had nightmares that he was going to die, and he would wake up crying almost every night. I explained to him that what happened to his sister happened to little babies sometimes, but not to older kids.

Given the turmoil that her son was experiencing, Kim waited as long as possible to tell him about the subsequent pregnancy for fear that the news would only add to his anxiety. As it turns out, waiting did not make things any easier. She recalls:

When I told him that I was pregnant again, he didn't think another pregnancy was such a good idea. He didn't want another baby. He didn't think there was room in the family, he said, for another baby. There was just him and mom and dad and that was just fine. I couldn't really blame him for feeling that way. I mean, look at what happened the last time I was pregnant. As it got closer to the time when the new baby was going to be born, he got very vocal about it. He talked at one point about getting a knife and putting it in the baby's crib so she could kill herself. So he was very positive that there shouldn't be another baby and we should just forget all of this.

Fortunately, her son's attitude changed once the baby was born. Proud to be a big brother, Brian was very protective of his little sister and liked to show her off to his friends. Despite his tough talk during the pregnancy, he never showed any signs that he might want to hurt the baby.

If your own child has a bad reaction to the news of your pregnancy, you might want to consider seeking family counseling. If you're not sure who to see, you can ask your pediatrician for referrals. This may be an especially good idea if, like Kim's son, your child was there when you were told that your baby had died or if there are other extenuating circumstances that have made coping with the loss especially difficult. You should also consider getting counseling if you know that you will be bedridden during the pregnancy, since this can put an additional strain on every member of your family. Another option is to consult with a specialist *before* you share the news of the pregnancy in order to figure out the best way to handle it. That's the approach that Kelly took:

It helped me to discuss the issue with someone who knew more about how kids think than I did, because you have to be careful about what you say.

Like you can't ask, "Are you afraid this baby is going to die, too?" Or else you're giving them an idea to worry about. They ended up taking the news of my pregnancy pretty well, but things were a lot different than the last time. They had been very excited about the baby who died. They knew he was a boy and they knew his name was Joshua, and we talked about him as if he was already here. This time, we just didn't talk about the baby. We tried for it not be such a focal point. We tried to keep our minds on other things.

Although Kelly went out of her way not to put negative thoughts into her children's minds, many parents find that kids do think the worst and that they are often not afraid of saying it. They may ask you whether this baby is also going to die. Or they may make offhand comments that reveal what is going through their heads. When Sydney would go out with her four-year-old son, he would often spot other couples with only one child and say, "Oh look, Mom, their baby must have died too." Coping with these kinds of comments may be easier if you talk openly with your children.

"It is important to be honest with your child. Make sure she understands that the loss was nobody's fault. It was something that just happened, and does sometimes happen," says Andrea Seigerman, a licensed clinical social worker in the high-risk obstetrics clinic at Yale–New Haven Hospital. "But you should explain that now that you're trying again, you and your doctors will do everything you can so that a loss does not happen again—but it still might. There's always that possibility. And if it does happen, we'll be able to deal with it."

Doing Something Wrong

Once you have decided when to tell people about your pregnancy and how to deal with their reactions, your focus may turn inward to yourself and the baby you are expecting. As anyone who has been through a subsequent pregnancy will tell you, the next nine months will be a time of high anxiety. You may have found yourself worrying about the baby's well-being almost from the moment you discovered you were pregnant again. It may seem at times as though the list of things that could harm the baby is virtually endless. Although some of your thoughts may make you feel crazy, it probably helps to know that you are not alone. Chances are, others have had even crazier fears than you have. One study of subsequent pregnancies quotes a woman who became so compulsive about substances she feared might cause birth defects that she avoided putting bleach in the wash because of the fumes. She described herself as "neurotic about fumes." Later, when she found out she had a hole in her muffler, she cried about it for days.

Although fears about the baby's well-being are normal, you have to guard against stressing out too much, or the stress itself could create complications in your pregnancy. The research is far from conclusive, but some evidence exists that chronic stress can increase the risk of preterm birth. The jury is still out on why stress is harmful. One theory contends that persistent stress can indirectly trigger a preterm birth, since women who are under stress often eat poorly and are less inclined to take care of themselves. Another theory holds that stress increases the production of certain hormones that can interfere with blood flow to the placenta and may be involved in the early onset of labor. Whatever the effect of stress, you should try to avoid too much of it, both for your sake and the baby's.

Seeing Other People's Babies

In the days or weeks since you discovered that you were expecting, you have probably already realized that being pregnant again does not magically erase all of the turmoil you have been experiencing since your loss. Your grief certainly has not gone away, and probably neither have a lot of other feelings that have become commonplace. One lingering sentiment that may even surprise you, given that you are pregnant yourself, is the envy you may experience when you encounter others with healthy babies. Although all of us wish only the best for every pregnant woman, it can still be difficult to see mothers enjoying their newborns when we were deprived of the same privilege.

Pam discovered how hard this can be when she held a friend's baby only a few weeks after her pregnancy loss. "My arms ached for days afterwards. It was the most horrible thing I ever did." It can be especially difficult to be around other babies who were born around the same time that your own died, as Brooke found out:

> My sister had a baby a few days after I did, and I remember her coming over to my house just before Christmas and throwing all these pictures of her son on my coffee table. Bless her heart, she was excited. It was her first baby and those were the first pictures that she had taken, but I thought, "How could you possibly do this to me? Don't you know how this makes me feel?" At the same time, I felt sorry for her because I felt like my grief put a damper on what should have been the happiest time of her life. Even my mother said, "I can't be excited for your sister because of what you're going through." In fact, the first time my parents saw my sister's baby was at my son's funeral.

Brooke's feelings typify the contradictions that permeate a subsequent pregnancy. She was happy for her sister and sad for herself, and yet she also felt sorry that her own tragedy had cast a shadow over her sister's joyous experience. In addition to their awkwardness, these situations are often unavoidable. Given your age, many of your friends and siblings will be having babies and, of course, it will be impossible to avoid running into other mothers when you go out. Trisha, who lost a set of triplets in the second trimester, said she had the wind knocked out of her when she turned the corner in a grocery store one day and saw a new mother of three babies. "I had to find a place to sit down because I literally couldn't breathe. Thank God my husband was with me or I'm not sure what I would have done."

I, too, had an especially hard time seeing other people's babies throughout my subsequent pregnancy. In fact, my situation was so bad that I couldn't even look at pregnancy books or baby magazines without bringing all of the raw emotions of my loss to the surface. I remember one day in particular when my doctor was going to use the Doppler for the first time to listen for my baby's heartbeat. Since I was only thirteen weeks along at the time and still not feeling movement, I was terrified that something might have happened to the baby without my knowledge. I could also not shake the horrible memory of the night when I learned that my baby's heart was no longer beating. Although the nurse knew my history, she had no clue what I was feeling that day. So when she saw me crying, she asked me what was wrong. When I told her that I was nervous about what was about to happen, she just grabbed a baby magazine and said, "Here, this will help put you in the mood." She didn't seem to understand that was the last thing I wanted to see.

In my third pregnancy, my aversion to seeing other babies was not quite as strong, since I had actually given birth to a healthy child. But it still seemed that every time I picked up a book or magazine aimed at pregnant women, it would rub me the wrong way. One article I remember began: "In less than nine months, you are going to be eye to eye with the child growing inside you. When you finally see, touch and care for your baby, the challenges of pregnancy will all make sense." True for most people, no doubt, but when *I* read it, all I felt was sadness.

How You May Be Feeling

Happy

No matter how scared and nervous you are about the pregnancy, you are also bound to be happy that you are expecting another baby. If the pregnancy was a surprise, it may take a while for those feelings to surface. But for many of us, the knowledge that we are pregnant again brings a sense of overwhelming joy, even if that feeling is fleeting. "I was totally ecstatic," says Leslie. "I thought my world was wonderful again, and everything was going to be great." Kim felt much the same way. "I was very happy to be pregnant again, and I really didn't have a lot of fear about it working out. I think I had so much trouble believing that it had happened to me the first time, I couldn't conceive that it could happen again." If doctors were able to determine why your last pregnancy ended in a loss, that may also give you some confidence. After Sheila had surgery to correct a malformed uterus, she felt optimistic about her chances for success in her next pregnancy. "I had some nervousness, but I felt my doctors had fixed my problems and were going to take really good care of me."

While there's no question that it feels good to be happy again, you may feel a little guilty that you are not grieving as much as you were. You may also be worried about what others think about your behavior. If you act too happy about this pregnancy, you may fear that everyone will think that you have forgotten all about your loss. That was one of the fears that pervaded my thinking in the early months of my subsequent pregnancy, and it was the main reason why I waited to tell people that I was expecting again. It didn't take long for me to realize that it was useless to worry about what others might think about my behavior. No one else could really understand how my husband and I felt about losing our child, so it really didn't matter what they thought now that we were expecting again. We still felt so much sadness that I could not begrudge myself for feeling some happiness, too.

Mixed Emotions

Like me, you may also have mixed emotions during your pregnancy. Although you are happy about your new baby, you are still sorrowful over your pregnancy loss. You probably have good days and bad days, with the bad days made even worse by hormonal changes. Kelly's thoughts sum up how many women feel during the subsequent pregnancy. "Part of me was very excited, but I also felt very sad. It was immediate hope and immediate fear." Depending on how much time has passed since your loss, you may still be crying every day or sinking back into depression whenever someone you know has a baby or you come face to face with a child around the same age that yours would have been. Sharon, who suffered a second trimester loss, says she felt grateful to be pregnant again, but continued to be haunted by memories of the baby who died. Although many women report having vivid, and sometimes bizarre, dreams during their pregnancies, Sharon's dreams revolved around her daughter and were extremely disturbing:

> *The dreams were really weird. I remember one when I was in a forest and could hear her calling me, and even though I was close I couldn't get to her. Real haunting things like that. So even though I was looking forward to the new baby, I just could not seem to let go of the "what ifs" and "might have beens."*

Despite my happiness about my pregnancy, I, too, had setbacks on a nearly daily basis. Even the most routine thing could trigger painful memories. Once I visited a sick friend who was at the hospital where I had delivered Patrick, and just as I was walking in, another woman was leaving with her new baby. Seeing her reminded me of how horrible it had been to leave the hospital empty handed and made me feel utterly despondent. On another occasion, I was having lunch with some friends and was unexpectedly seated at a table with a woman who had had a baby two weeks before me. It was almost unbearable for me to sit through the meal as everyone fussed over the new baby. I tried my best to act normal and avoid looking at the baby so that I wouldn't cause a scene. I guess my act came off pretty well, because about halfway through the meal, a friend said, "You seem to be okay with this." I nodded my head in agreement, but it was all I could do to make it to the bathroom before I burst out crying. For weeks afterwards, I cried every time I thought about that day. It did not matter that I was pregnant again. I wanted my Patrick back.

Anxious

The first trimester can also be a time of high anxiety because you cannot yet feel the baby moving and may sometimes worry that the worst has happened again. You may find yourself going to the bathroom just to check if you are spotting. Any abdominal pain, no matter how slight, may send you into a panic. Even if your chances of a successful pregnancy are good, you may not feel reassured. Since you have already experienced something that was supposed to be rare, you can easily imagine it happening again. Statistics are meaningless at a time like this. After all, as Sharon describes, you've already been a statistic: "We have all these statistics that say the chances of what happened before happening again is really nil. But someone made a comment that has really stuck with me. She said, 'What are the chances of you being struck by lightning? Not very high. But those people who have been struck by lightning and have lived to tell about it probably still get very nervous everytime it storms.' "

If at any time you find your anxiety overwhelming, call the doctor's office and ask if you can go in for a checkup. It can be very reassuring to see or hear the baby's heartbeat and get a clean bill of health from your physician. Some of your anxiety may ease once you are past the first trimester and know that your risk of miscarriage is significantly diminished. It can also be reassuring to feel the baby move. But it will be difficult to ever recapture the untarnished bliss that you may have experienced in your pregnancies before the loss. Now you are all too aware that there are no guarantees that a pregnancy will end with the birth of a healthy child. Says Diane:

Really, throughout my pregnancy, I never for once thought that everything was fine. There was never a day that I felt like I could relax. I had level-two sonograms every two weeks, and, at the end of my pregnancy, every week. We could literally see every body part on the baby. But even with all that, I still could not allow myself to think that everything was fine because I knew there were a lot of things that could happen.

Sometimes you may experience problems that you don't even associate with your pregnancy loss. Glenda, for example, had panic attacks for the first year after her baby died. It was only months later that she realized that the panic attacks were directly related to her grief. If you have other living children, the anxiety you feel during this pregnancy may be in sharp contrast to how you felt before. Jennifer describes the differences in her two pregnancies:

*In my first pregnancy I was twenty-eight, and I'd never known anyone who
had lost a baby—ever. So my main concerns were things like, "Will I live
through the labor?" and "Will I be a good mother?" Occasionally I
thought, "I hope everything will be okay with the baby." But that was just
a vague anxiety that all pregnant women get. After my miscarriage, I lost
my innocence. I lost the ability to be happy about the pregnancy.*

Your biggest fear may be that the same thing could happen again.
But even after you pass the critical period without incident, you may
start to worry about something totally unrelated. If your loss was late
in pregnancy, like mine, there may never be a time when you stop
worrying that the same thing might happen again. "Even though a
woman may be very happy to be pregnant again, she's still always
waiting for the other shoe to drop," says Maureen Doolan Boyle, executive director of MOST (Mothers of Supertwins).

Some books on pregnancy loss recount stories of women who were
so fearful in the subsequent pregnancy that they considered aborting
the baby rather than enduring the pain. If at any point in your pregnancy you feel the same way, think hard before making a decision
that you may regret later. Seek counseling to get through what undoubtedly is one of the most difficult periods you are ever likely to
experience in your life.

Pessimistic

Some women deal with their fear during a subsequent pregnancy
by imagining the worst that could happen and how they would deal
with it. The first time you suffered a pregnancy loss you were probably
completely shocked, and you may feel like you need to look at things
differently this time. Dr. Peggy Morton, an adjunct associate professor
of social work at New York University who conducted a research study
on subsequent pregnancies, describes the approach that many women
take. "To protect themselves, many women think if they tell themselves that they're not going to have this baby, then they're not going

to be upset if they lose it, which is crazy because they're going to be upset no matter what." This kind of psychological detachment is known as anticipatory grief.

If you have had multiple losses, you may become more and more convinced that you will never get the chance to mother a child. Katie says that for her it wasn't a question of *if* the next baby would die, but rather *when*. It bothered her when others expressed the optimism that this time everything would be all right. "Sometimes I'd just say, 'Don't count your chickens. Didn't you feel like everything would be all right the last time, and look what happened?' I know that was mean, but that's the way I felt." Even women who consider themselves optimists sometimes can't seem to avoid negative thoughts during the subsequent pregnancy. Brooke says that both she and her husband, who in the past had always been upbeat, often imagined what it would be like if they were to experience the death of a second baby:

The sad part about it was when my husband and I went to look for a coming-home outfit for the baby, we kept saying, "Will this look okay in a casket if he dies?" I just knew he was going to die. I just knew he was. I said I've got to find something for him to come home in, but if he dies, it has to look good in the casket, too.

Unlike Brooke, I had decided early in my pregnancy that I was going to think and speak only positive things. There was no way that I was going to even speak the words "death" or "funeral" in the same sentence as "my baby." I just tried to convince myself over and over that this baby would be fine. But still, pessimism would get the better of me rather frequently. I remember one day when I was only about six weeks pregnant, I happened to stumble on a great sale of maternity clothes. Even though I figured they would come in handy in just a few weeks, I couldn't even bring myself to try anything on, much less buy something. Somehow, I couldn't allow myself to act on my optimism. If you feel the same way sometimes, try not to worry about it. What you are feeling is not unlike post-traumatic stress disorder, in which you relive a painful experience in your mind long after life has returned to normal. With time, those types of episodes will very likely diminish but may never completely go away.

Angry

It also is very normal to experience feelings of anger during the subsequent pregnancy. You may be angry that you are having to go through another pregnancy when you should have been spending this time with your baby. If you are experiencing morning sickness, you may even find yourself blaming either the new baby or the one who died for making you feel so bad. You may also be angered at the comments that other pregnant women make. I would occasionally hear patients at the doctor's office complain about how tired they were of being pregnant, and think to myself "if you only knew." Katie, who suffered a pregnancy loss at term, was furious about how long she had to wait for a baby. She compared herself to a whale, some of which have a sixteen-month gestation period. You may also be angry that you have lost the innocence that you experienced in your previous pregnancies. Sharon recalls:

> I loved every aspect of being pregnant with my daughter. It was twenty-four weeks of absolute bliss. This time, I'm trying to be more grounded and not think that everything is going to be fine. At the same time, I don't want the pregnancy to be over and have a beautiful healthy baby but feel like I cheated myself over the last hurrah of being pregnant because it's such a gift. So I'm trying to find that balance of enjoying the miracle and yet at the same time not wanting to have the rug pulled out from under me again.

Since many people will see your new pregnancy as a solution to all your problems, you may be angry that only a select few understand what you are truly feeling. You may also resent that it seems so easy for others to have babies while you have to struggle so hard. Phyllis saw herself as a victim. "Sometimes I just thought 'Why me? How come everyone else can have this normal, blessed event happen to them while I have to suffer this way?' " If you are around other people with children, it may irritate you to see them lose their patience. Mary, who worked as a flight attendant, would sometimes tell frustrated parents on board the plane about her baby's death and urge them to treasure their children. "I'm not sure that they appreciated my comments, but there was a period when I just couldn't bite my tongue and say nothing." Allison would get upset when she heard her co-worker talking about her newborn baby who had colic. "She always complained about her baby and it really pissed me off, so I tried to avoid her."

Talking with someone who understands your feelings and can lend a sympathetic ear may help you deal with your anger. Katie found that it helped to talk to her sister, who had given birth to a baby with Down syndrome four years earlier. Although Katie was dealing with the death of her baby, her sister had a loss of a different kind—the loss of a normal baby:

> *Both of our babies were born on the same day, January 15, and for both of us it was the worst day of our lives. Even though our situations were different, we both had to deal with a lot of anger. She could understand how I felt, and I could talk to her in a way that I couldn't talk to all my friends who had healthy babies. It was a lifesaver for me.*

Confused

Unless you learn to expect the unexpected, you may find yourself feeling confused by your behavior during your pregnancy. For example, you may have planned to share the news about your pregnancy only after you were past the first trimester, but then ended up telling everyone right away. Or maybe you decided that you would quit your job to take care of yourself, but quickly concluded that staying home would drive you crazy. Perhaps you started out being fanatical about your health, steering clear of anything that could possibly harm your baby, including junk food and caffeine. Then out of the blue you found yourself gorging on french fries or chocolate.

Your feelings may also confuse you. If it took you a long time to conceive, you may be relieved that you are finally pregnant again and yet have trouble believing that it is true. You may resent that you are suffering from morning sickness again, yet worry at the first sign that you are feeling better for fear that something has happened to the baby. The only thing that makes sense during this tumultuous period is that many things about this pregnancy will not meet your expectations. Try to be patient with yourself and realize that there is nothing wrong with your feelings, or, within reason, your behavior. As long as you are doing your best to protect your unborn child from harm, it is okay for you to act irrationally at times. All of us who have been through a subsequent pregnancy have done the same thing. Since you are not going through a so-called normal pregnancy, very little about the experience is likely to be within the guidelines of what's considered normal.

Overwhelmed

Pregnancy is both an enormous risk and a tremendous responsibility, and all the more so after you have suffered a loss. You may be overwhelmed that you are very much responsible for your baby's wellbeing, although so many things are beyond your control. At the same time, you may no longer worry about whatever bothered you previously. In the past, you may have wondered whether you were ready to care for a child, or whether you could afford it, or how the baby would affect your family life. Now your overwhelming worry may be whether the baby will be born alive. Phyllis, who had suffered two miscarriages before giving birth to two healthy children, remembers: "It was a very tense and scary time. I just felt a tremendous burden on me the entire nine months. I'm much happier having the children than being pregnant with them. My pregnancies were all about just waiting for the end. I just wanted them to be over."

Overwhelming feelings often take many different forms. They may make you depressed, irritable or simply nervous. They may also make you even more tired than you would normally be. Although just about everyone is tired during the first trimester of pregnancy, your fatigue may be even worse if you are worried about your prospects for a healthy baby and are still feeling sad about your loss. If possible, take more naps and go to sleep earlier. Your outlook may improve once you feel more rested.

Tips for Easing Anxiety

Pray

If I had to name the one thing that helped ease my anxiety the most during my subsequent pregnancy, it would be prayer. Although at first I was angry at God for allowing my baby to die, I soon found that I could not go on without prayer. I prayed about when to get pregnant again. I prayed as we tried to conceive. And I prayed incessantly once I knew that I was expecting another baby. Many times, I got a feeling of peace that this time my baby would be all right, and that's what sustained me during my darker moments when I feared the worst. Occasionally, I asked myself how I could pray so much when all the prayers I had said in my last pregnancy had seemingly gone unanswered. But as I reflected on it, I had to concede that I would never understand why my baby died. In that way, I was no different than all of the other good people in this world who have had bad things happen to them. But I still had faith that God would protect both me and my baby.

During times of uncertainty, it helped that I was surrounded by people who had very strong faith, such as the counselor I was seeing who prayed with me every time we met and often gave me encouraging Bible verses to read. I also had several friends who put me on prayer lists and prayed with me whenever they got the chance. As fate would have it, I even got a new boss at the news agency where I worked who turned out to be one of the most spiritual people I have ever met. She had already heard about my loss before she arrived, so the first time we got together, she prayed for God's protection over me and my baby. With so many people praying for me so often, I truly felt like I had a sort of protective shield around me.

Of course, there were many times when my faith wavered, and doubts creeped into my mind. In talking with other women, I realized that many of them struggled with their faith at first, but found that it tended to grow stronger over time. Pam, whose twins were stillborn, recalls:

> *I haven't had a very easy life, so when I met this wonderful man and married him, I thought my life had changed and now I was on the good side and only good things were going to happen. And, of course, losing the twins was the most horrible thing that had ever happened to me, so that just crushed the whole belief system that I had constructed. I blamed everybody at first, and God was just one of them. I can't say that my faith just suddenly came back one day, but gradually it did.*

Even those who considered themselves to have strong faith had moments when they, too, were unsure. Sharon, for example, sometimes had trouble praying because she wondered whether God even wanted her to have another baby.

> *I almost felt like I was being greedy because God had given me one beautiful healthy child and she's the sunshine of our lives. And I thought maybe by asking for more, I wasn't being appreciative. But my minister pointed out that God wants what you want if it's good for you, and how can wanting a child be bad? I think that's what got me back on my spiritual path.*

You will have to find your own spiritual path during this pregnancy. Pray or meditate alone if that helps. If you cannot seem to pray for yourself, ask others to pray for you or turn to the Book of Psalms for inspiration. "The Psalmist has put your pain into words, and sometimes into better words than you can. So when you don't have your own words for prayer and you need to talk personally to God, that's a place to turn," says Rabbi Stephanie Dickstein, a chaplain and educator. "It reminds you that you are not isolated and gives you permission to be angry at God because you will see that others have also felt angry and betrayed. And when the time comes to rejoice, the Psalms can also give you the words." You can also attend religious services, or look to a minister, rabbi or other member of the clergy for answers that you cannot come up with on your own. It really doesn't matter what spiritual path you take as long as it brings you a sense of peace and well-being.

Keep a Journal

Keeping a journal is another great way to ease anxiety. Many women I interviewed said that it helped them tremendously to start writing in a journal as soon as they knew they were pregnant again. It was a lifesaver for me as well. You can use a journal to vent all of the feelings we have been discussing, as well as to express the hopes and dreams you have for your new child. Putting your emotions into words can be a way to work through your grief or release negative energy. It can also enable you to better understand your feelings. Sometimes to get a different perspective on a problem, you need to see it on paper. You don't have to write in your journal every day. Just do it when you want to. When you review the entries from weeks and months before, it will help you see how far you have come. And once your pregnancy is over, the journal will be a precious keepsake of your baby's start in life. Carla credits her journal writing with helping her keep her sanity during her high-risk pregnancy.

I talked to the baby all the time. I'd write things like, "Here's what's happening today," or "I believe in you. I know you're going to make it." Even though I didn't necessarily totally believe what I was writing all the time, it was my way of trying to believe it. Now I read my journal every once in a while and I think, "Wow, what a time I had." It's a reminder of all that I went through.

You'll notice that Carla says she talked to her baby all the time. That's a journaling technique that Joann O'Leary recommends to women who are in her Pregnancy after a Loss program at Abbott Northwestern Hospital. But O'Leary says women often find it easier to begin the journal by writing to the baby who died rather than to the one they are expecting. "Sometimes they can journal to the baby who has died about the baby who is coming because they know the baby who has died better. That can be a way to help people start journaling," she says. "Gradually, over the course of the pregnancy, they can begin to journal more to the baby who is coming."

O'Leary's advice is based on the theory that the baby who died is still very much a part of the family and central in the parents' minds. It is important for couples to validate the parenting experience they had and find a place in their family for the baby who died. "People want you to forget about the baby who died, so we label grief as parenting rather than as grief," she says. "People assume that you have to get over your grief, but you don't have to get over your parenting."

Take Care of Yourself

If you got in shape and started to live a healthy life even before you got pregnant, it will probably come naturally to do the same now. But if you're a slow starter, you now have more incentive than ever to do what you didn't do before. A life is growing inside you that depends on you for its well-being, which should be reason enough to go the extra mile to take care of yourself. What you'll find is that you will benefit as well. It is reassuring to know you are doing everything possible for your baby. It's a provider role you will be playing to some extent for the rest of your life, and certainly for the next eighteen years, so it makes sense to start now.

Being healthy means eating a balanced diet of protein, vegetables, fruits, complex carbohydrates and foods that are rich in calcium. As a rule, you should take in between three hundred and five hundred more calories each day than you normally consume. You also should talk with your doctor about ensuring that you have an adequate intake of calcium, iron, folic acid and other essential vitamins and minerals. It is also a good idea to get moderate exercise three times a week. Generally safe choices include swimming, walking, stationary cycling and exercise programs specifically designed for pregnant women. Again, it is essential to check with your doctor before starting any exercise program. Of course, you should avoid potentially harmful substances like cigarettes and alcohol and any drugs that have not been prescribed or recommended by your doctor.

All of this again raises the thorny issue of what you did for your health the last time you were pregnant. You no doubt did everything to safeguard your baby's well-being, yet still it wasn't enough. But when you consider it rationally, you know that you have no other choice this time either, despite that there are no guarantees that everything will turn out all right. In some rare instances, there may even be choices you can make to improve this baby's chances of being born healthy. Virginia, for example, suffered a pregnancy loss at twenty-four weeks when she contracted an infection that was fatal to her baby. Although Virginia was not to blame for what happened, the experience nonetheless made her more cautious during her next pregnancy.

> I was a little bit more careful, but mostly with the things that were directly related to the nature of my loss. If somebody called in the winter and said, "I know we were scheduled to get together, but my son has X-Y-Z," I'd say, "Well, no thank you. I'm not even going to risk it." I wouldn't even send my children to a playgroup if a mother called and said, "So-and-so has a cough." I would say, "I'm sorry I don't want anyone in my family getting infected, which would in turn infect me."

In your own case, maybe you had a few drinks or smoked some cigarettes when you were pregnant the last time, and now find that you don't want to do anything that could even remotely harm your baby. As Bridget recalls, "I tried to do everything perfectly because if anything bad happened this time, I didn't want to feel any guilt whatsoever." But taking care of yourself means more than just looking out for your physical well-being. It means taking care of your mental health as well. Pamper yourself. Take a nap, read a good book, go to a movie, get a massage or a facial. All of these things can make you feel happier and more relaxed. More important, they will help you take your mind off your pregnancy—at least for a while. This means you can reduce your stress level, which will ultimately benefit both you and your baby.

Get Your Partner Involved in Your Pregnancy

Nearly everything about your pregnancy will be easier if you don't have to do it alone. If you are fortunate enough to have a supportive partner, be sure to get him involved. This may mean sharing your hopes and fears and telling him how you feel physically. You should also consider asking him to come with you for doctor appointments. Even if you are normally the type who prefers to do such things on your own, you may find that you benefit by having your partner with you. That's mainly because this time you are likely to feel tense during what others would consider to be routine procedures. Whether the doctor is checking the baby's heartbeat or doing a sonogram, it may make you very nervous. It will be good if you have shoulder to cry on or a hand to hold, should you need it. It will also help if your partner stays apprised of everything that is happening in your pregnancy so that if any important medical decisions need to be made down the road, you can make them together.

Heather learned the importance of having her husband with her at each prenatal appointment early in her pregnancy:

The first time my doctor used the Doppler to listen to the baby's heartbeat, he couldn't find it. He said, "We're not going to panic, we're going to go and do a sonogram." But of course, I panicked right away and I was thinking, "here we go again." My husband was not there during all of this, even though he was supposed to be. He had some meeting and was running late. He did get there by the time they started the sonogram, and I remember looking at him and saying, "You realize you have to be here for absolutely every appointment from now on. You are not going to miss another appointment." And he never did.

Since my doctor's office was across town and I had frequent appointments, I didn't see a need for my husband to come with me every single time. But he was there for what I considered important procedures, such as sonograms and amniocentesis. Fortunately, he was able to come with me whenever I wanted him to since he is in business for himself and can set his own schedule. If your partner does not have that kind of flexibility, arrange to reach him by phone as soon as your appointment is over. Also, be sure to have a plan to get in touch with him should an emergency arise. It is important to know that you can count on your partner's support since research has shown that pregnant women with supportive partners have fewer problems overall.

Attend a Support Group

Depending on where you live, you may be able to find a support group for couples who are expecting again after a loss. These groups are an excellent place to share your thoughts and feelings with others who understand exactly what you are going through. I was fortunate enough to attend a Pregnant Again group near my home once a month throughout my pregnancy, and found that it was a wonderful place to release pent-up emotions that I couldn't necessarily discuss with my family or friends. I grew close to the other women in the group and was thrilled when all of us were making great progress. On those nights when someone unexpectedly missed a meeting, I worried that something might be wrong. Fortunately, during the time that I attended, no one had another pregnancy loss. If someone in the group had suffered a loss, I think it would have been a big setback for me as well.

Another drawback to attending was that I heard many new stories of what could go wrong in a pregnancy. Whenever someone new attended my group, she would share what happened with her pregnancy loss. I'm sure all of us in the room later thought about her experience and wondered if the same thing might happen to us. Heather, who attended the same support group that I did, recounts how she felt about it:

I definitely believe in support groups, but it can be a panicky thing to hear about everything else that can go wrong. Ignorance can sometimes be a little bit more blissful. After you have one pregnancy that doesn't work out, you start finding out that these things really do happen, and they do happen to us.

On the positive side, I was encouraged by seeing other women who were further along in their pregnancies than I was. It made me realize that if they could make it this far, so could I. Lynn, another support group member, says that was one of the main reasons that she continued attending even toward the end of her pregnancy.

I got a lot of emotional support from women who were far along when I was only nine or ten weeks. Now that I'm in my third trimester, I feel like I am giving back what I got. I know that for the other people who are there, it helps to talk with someone who's been there and made it through.

If you cannot find a subsequent pregnancy support group in your area, consider contacting one of the national organizations on pregnancy loss such as SHARE or Bereavement Services/RTS or the Parent Education Department at Abbott Northwestern Hospital. They can either help you find a group or tell you how you can start one yourself. You will find their phone numbers in the back of this book. An alternative is to consider whether you want to continue attending a support group for bereaved parents. But this too can have its drawbacks. Pam remembers:

It got to the point where the support group was making me feel worse because I'm a really empathetic person, and to sit there and hear people struggling with newer losses was very difficult for me. It brought up my own feelings over and over. For a while, I think that's important because until you can really deal with those feelings, you do need to bring them up. But there's a point where that ceases to be a good thing anymore.

Abby, who continued going to her regular support group, worried about what other couples would think once she started showing:

I felt very awkward about going at first because I didn't know if it was going to hurt anybody else to see me there pregnant. But I had one woman come up to me and say she was so glad that I was there and I was pregnant because it made her feel hopeful that someday she would be strong enough to go through it. After that, I quit worrying about it.

Newsletters specifically designed for couples going through a subsequent pregnancy can be another source of support. *PAILS of Hope* newsletter provides information, suggestions and encouragement regarding all facets of pregnancy after a loss. It is produced by Pen-Parents, a non-profit organization that provides a support network for bereaved parents. If you have access to the Internet, you can also communicate with other parents on-line through SPALS, which stands for Subsequent Pregnancy After a Loss Support. You can find their Web site at www.inforamp.net/~bfo/spals.

Continue to See a Counselor

If you started seeing a counselor after your loss, it may help to continue doing so throughout your pregnancy. Contrary to what others may believe, being pregnant again does not mean that all your pain and grief will suddenly vanish. Although you are well aware of that, you nevertheless may be under the mistaken impression that you no longer need professional help even when you do. "Sometimes you've had a good day, and you will want to move on, but in most cases you need to keep going for that emotional support," says Fran Rybarik, executive director of the national pregnancy loss organization, Bereavement Services/RTS.

I know that from first-hand experience, because that was a mistake I made. I'm grateful that my counselor urged me to schedule appointments despite my feeling that I was sometimes wasting her time. Some days I spent most of my time talking about the joy of being pregnant again, but far more often we discussed my unresolved grief and my overwhelming fears. She was a calming influence in my life at a time when I really needed it. I credit her with helping me make it through the pregnancy with as much emotional stability as I had.

In my case, my counselor was someone whom I had been seeing since the pregnancy loss itself. But some women realize only after they are pregnant again that they need professional help. Donna, who suffered a second-trimester miscarriage, handled her grief relatively well at the time. She had another child to take care of and focused much of her attention on when she could try to conceive again. But once she became pregnant again, the many feelings she was repressing started to surface. She found herself crying every day and was unable to sleep or carry out her normal activities. Things got so bad that she actually contemplated suicide, and that was the point when she finally realized she needed help. She recalls:

> It just didn't seem right that I was alive and fine, and my baby was gone. I really hit rock bottom when I saw a bottle of pills that my husband had been taking, and I actually wondered how many I would have to take to not wake up. I could not see that I would ever get beyond where I was. Even the fact that I was pregnant didn't seem to give me the will to live. The counselor helped me in so many ways. She was my reality check when my thoughts would run away from me.

You don't have to have suicidal feelings to be a candidate for counseling. Perhaps you are having anxiety attacks or are not getting along with others. Or maybe you're depressed. There can be many reasons why you might benefit from the help of a professional. If you feel as though you need help, ask your physician for a referral.

Lean on a Friend

We all need someone to talk to, especially when we're feeling anxious or scared. As we've discussed, your partner will play an important role in giving you that much-needed support, but friends can fit the bill as well. There may be certain things that you just can't talk to your partner about, or maybe his patience will only stretch so far and every once in a while you find yourself needing to speak to a new set of ears. Friends can be a great source of support in both good times and bad, and this is one of those times when you will depend on them more than ever. Sometimes, though, the people who you least expect to be supportive will be there for you, as Diane discovered during her subsequent pregnancy:

> All of my friends tried in their own way to be supportive and helpful, but most of them didn't know what to do or say. But I had two or three friends—and it was not the people I expected—who would specifically say, "I want to help you but I don't know what to do." That was better than people who would try to manufacture some way to help me. So I was able to cry with them, and they would cry with me, and I would just say, "I'm having a hard time" and they would say, "Oh Diane, I'm so sorry." They didn't have a lot of words of wisdom. They were just there.

Other times, you may find that those who are farthest away geographically are the ones who are closest to your heart. Nancy says that encouraging words came from all over the nation. "I received a lot of cards and telephone calls from friends who said, 'We want you to know we're thinking of you,' or 'I'm in a prayer group, and we're going to be praying for you and your baby.' " Whether your friends are near or far, you will want to talk to someone who will listen in a non-judgmental way to what you have to say. Although your friends won't necessarily understand everything that you are going through, a sympathetic ear is really all you need. And if those closest to you have been fortunate enough to have had babies themselves, they will serve as a reminder that most pregnancies do result in the birth of a healthy baby

Find Success Stories

It also helps to talk to women who have made it through a pregnancy after a loss. They are living proof that it is possible for someone with your history to have a healthy baby, even though, at times, you may have a hard time believing that you will be so fortunate. Although I was jealous of every pregnant woman I saw in the months immediately following my pregnancy loss, I had completely different feelings when I met women who had had successful pregnancies after a loss. I remember going into the home of the very first woman I interviewed for this book and being so uplifted when I saw pictures of her children. It seemed like a dream that these two beautiful babies could have been born to someone who had experienced the same horrible thing that I had. That gave me hope.

If you don't personally know anyone who has made it through a subsequent pregnancy, there are several ways to go about finding someone. You can start by asking the leader of a support group for bereaved parents, if there is one in your area. You also can ask your doctor or friends if they can put you in touch with anyone. While it may take time to find the right person, it will be well worth your effort. As Perry-Lynn Moffitt, coauthor of *A Silent Sorrow: Pregnancy Loss* points out, women who have experienced a subsequent pregnancy will be in a unique position to help you. "People who haven't been there— as much as they love you and as much as they want to support you— don't really understand what you are going through," she says. "Someone who has been through a loss and a subsequent pregnancy will also have the patience to listen."

I hope this book will serve as another source of encouragement, since, as I told you back in chapter 1, every woman quoted ultimately gave birth to a healthy baby after experiencing the pain of miscarriage, stillbirth or infant death. None of us will tell you that a pregnancy after a loss was easy. But it was worth all the pain and anxiety we had to go through to reach our goal.

Treasure Every Moment You Can

All of us who have suffered a pregnancy loss know that life is too short not to treasure every precious moment, no matter how brief. You no doubt have special memories that you cherish from your last pregnancy, and those memories keep your baby alive in your heart. The baby that you are carrying now deserves its own special memories, too. Today, right at this moment, this baby is alive, and that is cause for celebration. Each time you hear your baby's heartbeat or feel a kick, celebrate the moment. No matter what the outcome of your pregnancy will be, you will want to hold on to these special memories. In fact, they will be all the more important if the worst happens and you are unable to share your life with your child. You will never be able to recapture these moments if you let them pass unnoticed. So, today, resolve to be grateful for what you have while you have it.

Remember, too, that it probably wasn't too long ago that you wondered whether you would ever be pregnant again. Maybe you didn't even dare hope that you would have another child. Now, you have a baby growing inside of you and that is much for which to be thankful. So rather than seeing the pregnancy as a task whose only purpose is producing a healthy baby, if possible, try to enjoy some of the aspects of being pregnant.

Prenatal Visits

When Visits Are No Longer Routine

We've been focusing on the many things you can do to ease your anxiety during your pregnancy. But something that we've touched on only briefly, which can do wonders for your peace of mind, is scheduling many prenatal visits with your doctor. Every time you have an appointment, you will learn everything is progressing as it should be. You will also be reassured that if any signs of trouble arise, your doctor will have the opportunity to identify them. If you're wise, you did your homework before you got pregnant again and selected a physician who is competent, compassionate and willing to accommodate your special needs. If not, it is definitely not too late to find someone new. By asking your doctor questions and bringing up any concerns that you may have, you will gain a sense of control that will enable you to be your number-one advocate.

Be forewarned, however, that your prenatal visits themselves will cause anxiety. In your last pregnancy, most of your appointments consisted of weighing in, getting your blood pressure checked, giving a urine sample, having your tummy measured and checking the baby's heartbeat. Although all this may have seemed rather routine in the past, it will be anything but routine this time. You may have anxiety attacks before every visit for fear that the doctor may diagnose a problem, and then leave with a sense of elation once you and the baby receive a clean bill of health. Cynthia, who had suffered multiple losses, went to see her doctor weekly from the very beginning of her pregnancy, since her pregnancy was considered extremely high risk. She says the frequent visits were a mixed blessing. "The day of the appointment, I would become a nervous wreck because I was never sure what he was going to find. But then I'd get a rush of relief every time he told me that everything looked fine."

Prenatal visits are typically scheduled once a month in the first and second trimesters. Then, beginning at twenty-eight weeks, they are scheduled every two weeks and, in the last four weeks of the pregnancy, weekly. Given your history, your doctor will probably want to see you more often. In my case, I don't think there was ever a time when a whole month elapsed between visits to the doctor. During the last trimester, when I was the most nervous about the baby, I visited my doctor as often as two to three times a week. Some women even go in every day just to have the baby's heartbeat checked. Talk to your doctor about the schedule of prenatal visits that best meets your needs.

Also, keep in mind that your first visit will include a number of procedures that will not be repeated at later visits. Generally, your doctor will want to do a physical, including a pelvic exam and a Pap smear. You will also have your blood tested to check for such conditions and diseases as anemia, rubella, hepatitis B, HIV and venereal diseases.

Checking the Heartbeat

As you may already suspect, one thing that is likely to provoke the most anxiety at your prenatal visits is checking the baby's heartbeat. This is especially true if, like me, you discovered your pregnancy loss when the doctor could no longer detect the baby's pulse. Assuming your first prenatal visit is six weeks into your pregnancy, the doctor will probably not even check the baby's heartbeat until your second visit, or when you are about ten weeks pregnant. But because there is a chance that a hand-held Doppler cannot pick up a pulse that early in your pregnancy, you can avoid unnecessary anxiety by asking to wait until you are at least twelve weeks along before checking. At that point, the chances of hearing the heartbeat with the Doppler are extremely good. If either you or your doctor do not want to wait that long, you can ask whether it would be possible for you to have a vaginal sonogram done immediately if, for whatever reason, the doctor has trouble locating the heartbeat with the Doppler.

Planning ahead this way will help you avoid what Jessica experienced in her subsequent pregnancy when she had her first prenatal visit. She was ten weeks along at the time, and her doctor routinely reached for the Doppler to hear the baby's heartbeat. But after trying for several minutes to locate it, he finally gave up. Although he reassured Jessica that most likely everything was fine, he scheduled her for a vaginal sonogram just to be sure. Since her doctor did not have an ultrasound machine in his office, Jessica could not have a sonogram right away. She had to wait from Friday until the following Monday morning for an appointment at a local hospital. That the doctor was not overly concerned might have comforted most women, but, given her history, Jessica was inconsolable. All she could think about was what had happened in her previous pregnancy when the doctor couldn't find her baby's heartbeat. She and her husband spent an agonizing weekend fearing the worst, before learning on Monday that everything was indeed just fine.

Doctors accustomed to dealing with women who have suffered a loss will often do a vaginal sonogram on the first visit to avoid that kind of unnecessary anxiety. But even then there is no guarantee that the heartbeat will be detectable. Jennifer, for example, went in for a vaginal sonogram at six weeks since she had a history of early miscarriages. Everything about the experience turned out to be nerve-wracking.

They had warned us that it might be too early to see the heartbeat, and I was furious at my husband because he wanted to take a videotape with us. I had a big fit and said, "You want to go and videotape it, and it's going to show our baby's dead." Finally I just stuck the tape in my purse, but I didn't give it to the technician. As it turned out, I did the right thing because the doctor came in and said things looked good, but he couldn't detect a heartbeat, so he said we would have to wait until the next time. During the two weeks that I had to wait, I cried and prayed a lot. Fortunately, my son was in the first grade so I had to get up in the morning and get him to school. That whole period was so stressful that I've blanked out a lot of the details. When we went back in at eight weeks, we saw the heartbeat, and that was the first time I actually thought, "We're seeing some progress here. Maybe everything's going to be all right after all."

The date when the heartbeat can be detected will vary from pregnancy to pregnancy. I was fortunate enough to have a vaginal sonogram at six weeks that showed the heartbeat. My doctor then waited until thirteen weeks to listen to the heartbeat with the Doppler. This ensured that there was very little chance that I would have to endure the anxiety of thinking that something bad had happened when in reality everything was just fine.

Good Communication

The importance of good communication with your doctor is something else to remember as you embark on your next round of prenatal visits. Whether you have concerns about prenatal testing or how often you will be going in for visits, it is important to speak to your doctor clearly and succinctly. Don't worry about asking stupid questions or asking the same thing more than once. Asking questions—no matter how dumb you think they are—is a sign that you are smart enough to take a proactive role in your own health care. It can help to write down your questions beforehand. And if you don't understand the answers, ask for clarification, especially if your doctor tends to use medical jargon. Don't be embarrassed to ask your doctor to explain in plain and simple terms.

Good communication is even more important when it comes to conveying physical symptoms that may be concerning you. If anything happening to you does not feel right, call your doctor and explain it as clearly as possible (and graphically, if necessary) to ensure that there is no misunderstanding. You do not have to use medical terminology, just straightforward language. In most cases, that will be enough. But do not be afraid to trust your instincts if you feel that something is wrong and your doctor is taking your concerns too lightly. Be persistent, request a visit and, if necessary, go to the nearest emergency room. The old adage "it's better to be safe than sorry" is definitely applicable in this case.

Nancy learned this lesson the hard way when her water broke about midway through her pregnancy, resulting in the death of her twin boys. Despite her best efforts at communicating her symptoms, Nancy's concerns were downplayed by the nurse that she talked to:

I tried not to diagnose myself, but just to be very specific. I said I'm leaking enough to soak a panty shield. I didn't know—and she didn't realize—that it was my water and I was leaking amniotic fluid. She attributed it to urine and told me about doing Kegel exercises.

There were no guarantees that Nancy's doctor would have been able to save her babies through early intervention, but she will never know for sure. In her next pregnancy, she was a much stronger advocate for herself and insisted on being seen by the doctor whenever she had a valid concern.

Don't hesitate to discuss your anxieties with your doctor either, even if you get the feeling that everyone would rather be focusing on the future instead of the past. It's normal for you to be afraid and nervous at times. But remember, your doctor cannot read your mind, so if you are worried about something, say so. You may find out that your fears are completely unfounded.

Prenatal Tests of the First Trimester

There are a number of tests that you can have throughout your pregnancy to check on the baby's well-being. These range from vaginal sonograms early in the pregnancy to amniocentesis close to the midpoint and non-stress tests at the end. As you discuss with your doctor which tests are right for you, keep in mind that some tests can result in false positives. That means that the baby and pregnancy may be perfectly healthy even though the results indicate there may be cause for concern. We'll talk more about the roller coaster of prenatal testing in the next chapter, but, for now, let's look at the limited testing options that you have during the first trimester.

Vaginal Sonograms

As we've already discussed, many doctors perform vaginal sonograms during the first trimester to ensure that everything is progressing well in the pregnancy. In the procedure, a transducer is inserted into the vagina, thereby providing a view of the uterus. A heartbeat can usually be detected as early as five to six weeks of gestation. In cases in which the heartbeat is not visible by eight weeks, the pregnancy may have been dated incorrectly or the baby is simply developing at a slightly slower-than-average rate. It does not necessarily mean that anything is wrong with the baby.

A sonogram is a noninvasive procedure that can provide a lot of valuable information. And in over three decades of use, it has never been found to be harmful to pregnant women or their babies. We'll talk more about how sonograms are used later in pregnancy in the next chapter.

hCG Levels

The level of the human chorionic gonadotropin hormone (hCG) in your body is another indication of the viability of your pregnancy. This hormone is produced by the developing placenta and is present in both your urine and blood. In fact, home pregnancy tests work by reacting to the hCG in your urine. If at some point in the first trimester, your physician has any concerns about your pregnancy, your hCG levels can be checked with a blood test. You will most likely have more than one test to determine whether the levels are rising rapidly from one exam to the next, as they should be. Keep in mind, though, that hCG levels can vary from one pregnancy to another, so the hormone tests are only one way of detecting a potential problem. If the results are inconclusive, your doctor may recommend a vaginal sonogram to check for the baby's heartbeat.

Chorionic Villus Sampling

Chorionic villus sampling (CVS) is a controversial procedure that, like amniocentesis, can detect certain genetic problems in a baby. It is generally performed between the tenth and twelfth weeks of pregnancy. In the procedure, a needle is inserted through the abdomen into the uterus to obtain a small number of cells from the chorionic villi, tiny pieces of tissue that eventually form the placenta that carry the same genes as the baby. Another method for obtaining this fetal tissue is by inserting a catheter through the vagina and cervix and into the uterus. The tissue is then sent to a laboratory, where the chromosomes are analyzed.

The type of information provided by CVS is similar to that provided by amniocentesis. That means it can identify certain chromosomal problems, such as Down syndrome. The analysis also can detect a host of other abnormalities, such as anencephaly, skeletal diseases and certain metabolic problems. Babies can be born with many other abnormalities, however, that cannot be identified by either CVS or amniocentesis.

The advantage that CVS has over amniocentesis is that it can provide some answers in the first trimester when termination of the pregnancy is medically easier and, in some cases, less traumatic for the woman. This may be especially important if you had to terminate your pregnancy in the second trimester last time because of problems detected with the amniocentesis. CVS also requires a shorter waiting time between sampling and diagnosis than amniocentesis. Preliminary CVS results are generally available within forty-eight hours, with complete results taking about a week.

CVS is considered controversial by many doctors since some evidence suggests that women who have a CVS have a higher incidence of giving birth to a baby with limb defects. The concerns first surfaced in the early 1990s when a panel of experts convened by the Centers for Disease Control and Prevention (CDC) concluded that the risk of having a baby with missing or undeveloped fingers or toes was six times greater for mothers who underwent CVS, although the percentage of children who had such abnormalities was still a minuscule 0.03 percent. But a later study of more than one hundred thirty thousand CVS procedures reported to the World Health Organization between 1992 and 1994 found that there was no increased risk of limb defects after CVS. Given the conflicting reports, some doctors have chosen not to offer the procedure at all. Other genetic counselors and obstetricians suggest that a woman be informed of the research so that she can make her own decision about CVS.

Home Monitoring of Your Pregnancy

Why Home Monitoring Is Important

It is important for you to be proactive during this pregnancy and to be aware of signs of potential problems. You can do this through home monitoring. People may tell you not to be paranoid, but, in your case, a lack of paranoia could mean that you start ignoring critical symptoms. By being informed, you will learn the difference between the normal aches and pains of pregnancy and life-threatening developments. Being anxious and vigilant is valuable only if it leads you to intervene at the first sign of trouble.

Another advantage to being well informed is that it will help you deal with all the advice that you are likely to receive from both friends and strangers throughout your pregnancy. Although some of the advice will be well worth following, much of it should be ignored. A good way for you to make the distinction between good advice and bad is to arm yourself with plenty of information. If you understand the inherent risks of your subsequent pregnancy, you can respond better to those who offer unsolicited comments.

More important, by being well informed you will be better equipped to ensure that your next pregnancy ends with the birth of a healthy baby. Knowing the signs and symptoms of preterm labor, for example, will enable you to quickly identify it should it happen and to take steps to prevent a premature delivery. If you are up to date on all the latest prenatal testing and monitoring, you can make better decisions about which procedures are right for you. And even though you will undoubtedly trust your doctor to determine your best course of treatment, the more informed you are, the better able you will be to take a proactive role in your prenatal care.

Potential Danger Signs

In the first trimester of your pregnancy, the most important things for you to know are the signs of an impending miscarriage. Call your doctor immediately if you notice any of the symptoms listed below. But try not to panic. None of these danger signs alone necessarily means that you are miscarrying. For example, about half of all women who bleed do not have miscarriages. And remember, if you detect a potential problem early enough, you have a better chance of successfully treating it.

Signs of a Possible Miscarriage

Bleeding or spotting with or without cramping and pain. Bleeding can result from implantation of the fertilized egg or the aftermath of intercourse. But bleeding can also be a sign of a miscarriage or ectopic pregnancy. Be prepared to explain when the bleeding began, how heavy and what color it is, and whether you have pain or cramping. The longer the bleeding occurs and the more pain you feel, the more likely it is to be a miscarriage. **Call your doctor right away if you experience any bleeding or spotting.**

Any loss of fluid from the vagina. Amniotic fluid is the watery liquid that surrounds the baby, providing vital protection throughout pregnancy. Occasionally, the fluid can escape either as a gush or a slight leak. **Check with your doctor immediately if you suspect that you are losing any amount of amniotic fluid.**

A feeling of not being pregnant anymore. Sometimes a sudden feeling of not being pregnant anymore can be an indication that a miscarriage has occurred. Perhaps your breasts are no longer tender, or your nausea suddenly disappears. Keep in mind that these feelings tend to decline anyway around the end of the first trimester, so there is no need to panic. But call the doctor to be sure.

Other Signs of Trouble

Although the symptoms listed above are the most common signs of an impending miscarriage, other symptoms that are not normal in the first trimester can be signs of trouble. In the book *How to Prevent Miscarriage and Other Crises of Pregnancy*, Dr. Stefan Semchyshyn describes a dozen other symptoms that you should watch out for during the first trimester and report to your doctor:

Backache (a nagging lower backache or pain). Although a backache could just be a sign that you strained your back, it could also indicate a serious problem, such as a backward-tilted uterus. It is not normal to have chronic back pain throughout pregnancy, and you should call your doctor if the problem persists for more than a day. Call the doctor immediately if it's accompanied by other symptoms on this list.

Sudden swelling of your hands, feet or legs or puffiness in the eye. This could indicate a number of serious conditions, such as hypertension or edema (fluid retention). Call your doctor immediately.

Weight gain of more than two pounds per week. This could simply be a sign that you're overeating, or it could be a symptom of a more serious problem, such as excess fluid retention or diabetes. Report the weight gain to your doctor to find out more.

Frequent faintness, feelings of dizziness, headaches, blurred

vision. Some dizziness and faintness are normal in early pregnancy. Fainting or constant dizziness are not. Neither are painful
headaches or blurred vision. They could indicate serious problems, such as blood pressure changes, an infection or ectopic
pregnancy. Call your doctor immediately.

Continuous or intermittent abdominal pain. This could be a
sign of ectopic pregnancy or fibroid tumors. Call your doctor right
away.

**Burning sensation on urination, cloudy urine or blood in
urine.** This could indicate a urinary tract infection, which can
be easily managed by antibiotics. Left untreated, however, the
infection could spread and ultimately be life-threatening to both
you and your baby. Report your symptoms to your doctor.

Severe nausea or vomiting. While some vomiting and nausea
is normal, they could be dangerous if you are unable to eat or
keep down fluids. They could also be signs of other problems,
such as a kidney infection, flu, molar pregnancy or even food
poisoning. Let your doctor know if the problem persists for more
than a day.

Rash of unknown origin. This could simply be the result of an
allergic reaction to a particular food, or it could be a sign of a
potentially harmful illness such as German measles, chicken pox
or Lyme disease. Have it checked out by your doctor.

Chills, fever or shakes. A fever of 101 degrees or more with
or without chills or shakes could be a sign of infection or an
ectopic pregnancy and should not be left untreated. Do not let
it go unattended, or it could jeopardize your pregnancy.

Unusual vaginal discharge. It is normal to have a thicker vaginal discharge during pregnancy. But it should not be mucous,
which could be a sign of an incompetent or weakened cervix,
nor foul-smelling, which could be a sign of vaginal infection.

You will need to be examined by your doctor to determine the cause and possible treatment.

Chronic exhaustion, depression. We've already mentioned that you might sometimes feel depressed or exhausted, but very severe symptoms may be a sign of anemia or other nutritional problems. Talk it over with your doctor.

Diarrhea, constant urge to move bowels. Diarrhea could be a sign of food poisoning or a viral infection, particularly if you also feel achy and feverish. Feeling the urge to move your bowels and not being able to do so, however, could indicate a problem with a tilted uterus. Be specific in describing your symptoms to your doctor so that they can be correctly assessed.

chapter five

Pregnant Again: The Second Trimester

ONE DAY, EARLY in the second trimester of my subsequent pregnancy, I was in my car when I suddenly began experiencing all of the classic symptoms of a panic attack: shortness of breath, heart palpitations, shaky hands, cold sweats. I wondered what could have triggered that kind of reaction. Possibly, it was because I was reaching the point in my pregnancy when I would soon start feeling the baby move. Typically, feeling movement is one of the most joyful moments of pregnancy; but mine, as you know, was no typical pregnancy. The idea of feeling the baby move terrified me because I was sure there was no way that I would endure the times when the baby did not move. They would remind me too much of the last day that I was pregnant with Patrick, the day when I had lain on my bed waiting and waiting for a kick that never came, fearing the worst but trying to convince myself that everything was all right. There was also the long ride to the hospital when I kept telling my husband that I wasn't feeling the baby, yet denying to myself that anything could be wrong right up until the moment when the doctor told me the baby's heart was no longer beating. No, there was simply no way I could have survived all the weeks that lay ahead of me without losing my mind. I was sure of it.

But it turned out that I was wrong. Once I started feeling the baby move somewhere between sixteen and seventeen weeks, it was very reassuring. Sure, there were moments of absolute panic. There were times in the middle of the night when I woke up and felt nothing; mornings when I could not get out of bed until I felt a kick; and busy days when I didn't take the time to really monitor what the baby was doing until I broke out in a sweat at the thought that I hadn't stopped to check on him in a few hours. But all of those scary times were far outnumbered by the times when I was reassured because I could actually feel that my baby was still alive. Usually, all I had to do was lie down and wait a few minutes. And sure enough, it wasn't long before I'd start feeling those flutters and nudges.

If your pregnancy loss occurred before you ever had the chance to feel your baby move, you will soon be getting the first taste of the wonder of it all. For the rest of you whose losses came later in pregnancy or shortly after birth, the baby's movements will be a reassuring—albeit sometimes nerve-wracking—sign when you need it most. As we consider the concerns and feelings that you are likely to have during the second trimester, we'll examine what you may experience once your own baby starts moving. We'll also discuss other concerns that may come up at this point in your pregnancy, such as how to answer all those awkward questions about your baby, how to decide whether to have the battery of prenatal tests that will be made available to you and how you may feel if you find out whether you are expecting a boy or a girl.

In some ways, the second trimester will be the best time of your pregnancy. You'll know you have safely made it past the point where most women miscarry. You'll probably be feeling your best physically, since any morning sickness has usually gone away by this time. This will also be the time when your child makes the transition from a tiny baby that could not possibly survive outside the womb to a baby who, if for some reason had to be delivered at the end of this trimester, would have a fairly good chance of survival. Only two decades ago, a baby had to be born at twenty-eight weeks gestation to have any hope of surviving. Today, babies are routinely saved as early as twenty-four weeks, although the goal still remains to bring them into this world full-term and healthy. Despite the progress you will be making during this trimester, this period of your pregnancy will by no means be easy, especially if your loss occurred around this time. You will have to get through all the painful reminders of what happened before, knowing as you've known all along that there are no guarantees this time, either.

Common Concerns

Answering Awkward Questions

Since you may be showing by this point, you will begin facing the inevitable questions that go along with any pregnancy. Is this your first baby? How many children do you have? Do you want a boy or a girl? These seemingly innocuous questions may be difficult for you to answer. Barbara, who suffered a loss in her first pregnancy, says she felt guilty when she told people that she didn't have any children, but couldn't seem to come up with a better answer. "I could say, 'none living,' but then they may wonder how many are dead," she says. Answering these types of questions can be even more awkward if you have one or more babies who are surviving multiples. Says René: "Everyone keeps referring to my two surviving children as twins, and they're not. They're triplets, even though one of their brothers is in heaven. Now that I'm pregnant again, it's even more complicated to try to explain things. I try to avoid the subject altogether."

It helps to know how other women have coped with these same issues and then plan ahead should they happen to you. The best thing is to prepare a simple answer that you are comfortable with so that you will be ready when the time comes. It really doesn't matter what that answer is, as long as it feels right to you. What you may find is that there are no good answers to certain questions. Whether you tell people about your pregnancy loss or choose to avoid it, it will probably be difficult.

Most of us who have suffered a loss in our first pregnancy learn to tailor our answers to the situation. If it's the television repairman or a stranger in the elevator asking a question about our subsequent pregnancy, we might just say we're expecting our first child and then whisper a silent prayer letting our babies know they are not forgotten. If it's someone we are likely to see again or strike up a friendship with, we might choose to tell them the whole story. Beth, whose first baby died shortly after birth, said she was grateful whenever she had the opportunity to acknowledge her son's brief life.

> *There are times when you know that the people you are around just don't want to listen, or if they're pregnant, you don't want to bring it up. But most of the time, I do say something about our first baby because although he only lived four days, he was still our child and we loved him very much. I'll just explain that I had a little boy a year before and he died of trisomy syndrome. Some people say, "I'm sorry" and I go on my way and I feel better. Others say, "What's that?" and then I explain. If I can educate somebody about it, then I will.*

No matter how many times you tell the story, it can still be difficult, if not always for you, then for those you tell. Allison, a dental hygienist whose baby died at term, had to answer awkward questions repeatedly as patients returned for their six-month checkups. She recalls: "I almost feel more sorry for my patients at this point because I'm used to it and I can talk about it without crying, but they feel really bad after they've asked."

Heather also had gotten used to answering awkward questions during her last pregnancy when she was carrying a baby she knew had anencephaly and would die shortly after birth. "People would ask if I was having a girl—which I was—and since I already had a little boy they would say, 'Now you'll have a boy and a girl and you can stop. You'll have the perfect family.'" Of course, Heather knew all too well that the outcome would be far less than perfect. Now that she has three living children, Heather has found an answer that is right for her when people ask how many children she has: "I say, 'I have three surviving children.' And if I say three children without saying 'surviving,' the kids will correct me."

If you also have surviving children, you can avoid the numbers game altogether by simply stating the ages of your kids. Nicole found that worked well for her. "Whenever someone asked if it was my first pregnancy, I would just say, 'I have a three-year-old and a five-year-old at home.' If that person turns out to be someone I want to know better, I can always tell them the full story later." I, too, found that that approach worked best once I had given birth to Andrew and was expecting my third child. To this day, I avoid answering the question of how many children I have and usually just tell people the ages of those who are still living.

The only approach that I ever found that backfired was if I told people about Patrick without specifically letting them know that he had died. The first time I did that, I was shopping for some new outfits when the saleslady started making small talk with me. I told her it was the first time that I had shopped for clothes since having a baby a few months before. She asked me whether I had a boy or a girl. I told her I had a boy, but didn't elaborate. She responded, "Lucky you." As you can imagine, I was wishing that conversation had never taken place.

A few months later I was at a furniture store and a lady started asking the usual questions about my pregnancy. When I told her I was expecting my second child, she asked, "Oh, what did you have before?" I said, "A boy." She continued, "Is this one a boy or a girl?" I said, "It's another boy." And she said, "They'll be great buddies." Up until that point, I had been so focused on what my husband and I had lost, that I really hadn't given much though to the fact that the baby I was expecting now had been deprived of a brother. After that episode, I learned not to mention Patrick unless I also explained that he was no longer with us.

Finding Out the Baby's Sex

In some cases, a sonogram will show whether you are expecting a boy or a girl. If you have an amniocentesis to check for chromosomal abnormalities in the baby, you also will have the option of finding out the gender. Most couples have very definite ideas on this subject. Some are certain they want to know the sex of the baby before it is born, while others prefer to do it the old-fashioned way and get the news in the delivery room. Some of those who want to know in advance say they don't need any more surprises. "The surprise for us will be if the baby is born alive," says one mother who had suffered a pregnancy loss. Others say that knowing the sex of the child helps them think of the baby in more concrete terms. "I'm having a hard enough time acknowledging this pregnancy to begin with," says Camille. "Not knowing whether it's a boy or a girl just makes it that much harder."

Joann O'Leary says most of the couples who participate in the Pregnancy after a Loss program that she helps run at Abbott Northwestern Hospital want to know the sex of the subsequent baby. "Most couples are desperate to know because that helps them individualize the next baby, and that is very important," she says. "In our program we spend a tremendous amount of time trying to help couples separate the babies in their minds."

Whether you and your partner opt to find out your baby's sex before or after birth, be prepared for an onslaught of emotions. Although it goes without saying that the only thing any of us really wants is a healthy baby, it's unusual not to have some feelings one way or another about the sex of the next child.

Many of the women I talked to felt that they wanted to have a baby that was the same sex as the one who died. Kim, who had given birth to a healthy son five years before losing a baby girl, said she was very glad when a sonogram showed she was expecting another girl. "From the time we lost Grace, I knew I wanted a girl because I have always wanted a girl. I didn't want to have my only chance for a girl taken away from me. Not that another baby would ever replace Grace, but I still wanted a girl."

If you feel the same way, and it turns out that your baby is a different sex, it may be a major disappointment. Suzanne, whose baby boy died near term, tried to convince herself that the sex of the next child did not matter. But deep down, she could not help feeling that having another boy would somehow make the loss easier to bear. Still, she was not prepared for the overwhelming grief and denial she felt when she found out she was expecting a girl. She recalls:

The sonogram clearly showed that it was a girl, but I just kept looking at the video and thinking that the doctor had made a mistake. It took a while for it to finally sink in. And when it did, I sobbed like I had never sobbed before, not even when we lost Jeffrey. I knew that this was a different baby, and it had a different soul. But I guess I still had not had any kind of closure after the loss. That, to me, was the hardest part.

Others are just as certain that they do *not* want to have a baby that is the same sex as the one that they lost. Glenda already had one girl when she gave birth to a son who died within a few hours. Neither she nor her husband wanted another boy in the subsequent pregnancy. She recalls how they felt when they found out they were expecting a girl:

We were really glad because we felt everyone would think that if we had a subsequent child that was a boy that he would replace Nicholas. We didn't want anyone to think that, much less say it. So if we had had a boy and he had been healthy, we would have been thrilled, but we were hoping we wouldn't have another boy.

Another common feeling among those who want a baby of a different sex is the desire to have everything different in the subsequent pregnancy. That's how Heather felt after her newborn daughter died. "I did not want to get the babies mixed up. I didn't want to get the names mixed up. I wanted the delivery to be totally different. I wanted it to be a happy occasion if it could be, so I wanted everything to be different." Heather got her wish in her first subsequent pregnancy and gave birth to a boy. But when she got pregnant again, she found out she was expecting a girl. "I cried hysterically when they told me because I felt like I was doomed to lose every girl," she says. "Besides, I felt like I already had my girl in heaven and she was more perfect than any other."

Still others are not sure what they want. Here's how Brooke describes her feelings about the sex of her next child. "I don't want it to be a boy because I don't want it to be the same sex, and yet I want it to be a boy because we lost our first boy and we already have two girls. I don't know what I want. I'm like, 'I'm going to cry if it's a boy and I'm going to cry if it's a girl.' "

Regardless of which category you fall into, you might want to consider finding out the sex of your baby ahead of time so that you can get used to the idea and perhaps even have an easier time bonding with the child. As one mother told me, "I felt like I needed to have time to come to terms with the news if it was a boy or a girl, either one. There was going to be a period of acceptance when I had to accept that this baby was not the one who died." If you do find out the sex once the baby is born, be prepared for the possibility that you may have some feelings of grief despite your joy at the birth of a healthy child.

Occasionally, women and their partners do not agree on whether they should find out the sex of the child before birth. In that case, you can compromise and ask that the information be given to you in a sealed envelope and the person who wants to know can open it later in privacy.

My husband and I agreed that we wanted to know the sex of our subsequent baby in advance because it would make him or her more real to us. If it turned out that we only had a limited amount of time with this child, too, we wanted to be able to think of the baby as our son or daughter from the very first possible moment. I suppose I felt so strongly about the issue because I was so grateful that I had known beforehand that Patrick was a boy. That gave me twenty weeks to appreciate him as my son before he died.

I also had some definite ideas about the sex of the next baby. Although I had always imagined myself having girls, that changed after our son's death. Now I wanted as many boys as possible because

I felt like each baby brother who was born would give me a glimpse of what Patrick might have been like. Needless to say, I was overjoyed when I found out I was having another boy. When I got pregnant again the third time, I felt like I had even more reason to want a boy; I didn't want Andrew to grow up with his only brother in heaven. When I found out that my third one was a boy, I was thrilled again.

Whether You're Having More Than One Baby

If your pregnancy loss involved twins or triplets or even more babies, your first concern may not be so much the sex of the next child, but whether you are expecting multiples again. "A lot of times, couples really hope to have multiples again," says Janet Bleyl, founder and president of The Triplet Connection, an organization for multiple birth families. "They were so looking forward to having those babies that they lost, that they would really like another chance." But if you do find out you are pregnant with more than one baby, it can sometimes be a mixed blessing. You may be scared about being placed in the high-risk pregnancy category again. Depending on how many children you are expecting this time, your physician may even pressure you to consider selective reduction, where one or more babies are aborted in an effort to give the others a better chance of survival. We'll address these complicated issues on high-risk pregnancies in chapter 7.

If you're not expecting multiples this time, you may be disappointed that your unique opportunity to raise two or more children together has been taken away from you. You may find that it takes time to get used to the idea that you are carrying only one child this time. Hillary says her first thought was of the twins when she heard the news that she was expecting one baby girl. "When I found out that I was having only one baby, I thought, 'Which of my twins will be the guardian angel for this baby?' And then I decided, 'They both will be.' " While other mothers sometimes get the names of their children mixed up, you may find yourself mixing up the number of babies. Pam remembers:

Sometimes I find myself referring to this baby as "the babies," and that was really hard at first because I felt guilty. But I finally have gotten to the point where it doesn't bother me so much. My mother-in-law and I were talking on the phone the other day and she made the same mistake, and I could tell it really upset her, but it didn't really bother me. I thought people who have children who are actually alive get them confused sometimes so what's wrong with doing that while I'm pregnant? It's okay that it happens.

In addition to dealing with the idea that you are having only one child, you will also have to cope with the ambivalence you are likely to have about the sex of the next baby. If you lost both a boy and a girl, for example, you may lament that you can have one gender but not both this time. Pam, who had lost a twin boy and girl in the second trimester of her pregnancy, was glad to hear that she was expecting a girl but sad that she was not having a boy. "I still look at the little boy clothes that I had bought for Andrew and know I will always miss that."

Trisha was disappointed to see that her subsequent pregnancy was not greeted with the same kind of excitement as her pregnancy with triplets. "A singleton pregnancy is wonderful, but there's a difference in the way you're treated which adds to the grief factor. When you're expecting multiples, you're a celebrity. When you're only expecting one baby, it's no big deal."

Delivering Too Early

If your baby died because of problems due to prematurity, your biggest fear in this pregnancy may be that you will deliver too early again. We discussed earlier that it is during the second trimester that your child will make the transition from a tiny baby with no hope of survival outside the womb to a baby who, if for some reason had to be delivered early, would have a fairly good chance of living. In fact, statistics show that babies born after the twenty-eighth week of pregnancy have a better than 90 percent chance of survival (although some have serious complications). But the prognosis for any baby born before twenty-four weeks gestation is grim, as you know all too well if you previously delivered before that point.

Pam, who had given birth at twenty-two weeks gestation to twins who did not survive, was constantly in fear that she might go into early labor again in her subsequent pregnancy: "Until I reached twenty-eight weeks, I was more afraid of delivering early than I was excited about the pregnancy. But once I got past the second trimester, it just started to sink in that maybe everything was going to be okay."

Depending on the reason for your preterm delivery last time, your subsequent pregnancy may be considered high risk. We'll talk at length about the treatments available for women at risk for preterm labor in chapter 7.

Working Too Hard

Although a lucky few women manage to make it through a subsequent pregnancy without worrying too much, most of us are concerned about things that other pregnant women usually don't think twice about. Work is a perfect example. The American College of Obstetricians and Gynecologists (ACOG) estimates that more than one million working women become pregnant every year. Many of them stay on the job until a short time before delivery and return to work within six weeks of giving birth. Research generally shows that women who work during pregnancy do not have any significantly increased risk of adverse outcomes. An exception to this rule would be any job that requires strenuous activity, especially long hours of standing and walking, since these may increase the risk of preterm delivery. But as long as your job is no more strenuous than everyday life, you probably have nothing to fear.

Having said that, though, several factors could prompt your doctor to recommend that you either cut back on your hours or stop working altogether. Your physician may advise that you curtail your activities if there is a risk that the problems you had in your last pregnancy might repeat themselves. You may also have to change your routine if you have already developed complications in this pregnancy or if you have problems with your own health. Pam, who worked as a computer programmer, had an incompetent cervix that caused the premature delivery of her twins. Her obstetrician urged her not to work in the subsequent pregnancy unless she could arrange it from home. When her company frowned on the idea of telecommuting, Pam decided to take a leave of absence. Financially, it was not a problem since she was legally entitled to disability pay. But she is still unsure whether it was the right decision personally:

> *I don't know if it would have been better or worse to keep working because my job is kind of stressful, so I know I would have worried that that might have hurt something. But I had been working there four and a half years, so it was really hard to give it up. There were so many times when I thought, "God, if I could just have some work to take my mind off my pregnancy."*

Even if your pregnancy is not considered high risk, you may find that making changes in your work habits will help you deal with normal discomforts such as morning sickness and fatigue. You may want to negotiate to work fewer hours per week or arrange to work the same number of hours on a flexible schedule. Another alternative is to switch temporarily to a less stressful position. Katie, a flight attendant, arranged to do office work at the airline until after she delivered her baby. Nancy, who worked as a school teacher, decided to do only substitute work during her high-risk pregnancy.

By law, employers cannot discriminate against you because you are pregnant. Any medical condition that results from your pregnancy must be treated the same as any other temporary disability. In practice, however, some companies will be more accommodating to your needs than others. It will help if you have a sympathetic boss who knows your history and realizes how important it is for you to take care of yourself during this pregnancy. If your superiors are not very understanding, you may consider talking to your doctor about what—if any—changes in your work routine you are medically required to make.

I had made no changes in my work routine during my first pregnancy but decided to try to lighten my load considerably in my subsequent pregnancy. I was worried because the freelance work I did for a news agency kept me running from one assignment to the next, covering everything from courthouse shootings to national press conferences. I felt I needed to be more careful and avoid those kinds of high-stress situations. I briefly considered giving up journalism altogether and focusing instead on writing this book. But just as many women find they cannot go to support group meetings and hear pregnancy loss stories, I felt as though I could not work on this book while I was pregnant. So I talked to my boss about limiting my work to articles that could be written based on telephone interviews and suggested that someone else be sent out to cover the breaking stories. Since I worked for someone who was well aware of my history, she understood and shared my concerns. That made it easy to reach a compromise that made us both happy.

Women who are not fortunate enough to have a sympathetic employer sometimes choose to take medical leave during their pregnancy, as Pam did. Others may quit altogether, especially if they have already decided to give up working once the baby is born. "We had struggled so long and so hard to get to this point that I decided I shouldn't take any chances whatsoever," says Lynn, who gave up her high-stress job midway through her pregnancy. "It was hard at first because my job was really active and I traveled all the time, and then all of a sudden I was at home. But now that I have my son at home with me, I wouldn't trade it for the world."

Since Terri's baby had died of SIDS while under the care of a babysitter, she felt she could never work again once she had another baby. "There was no way that I was going to leave another baby in day care, so I just went ahead and quit as soon as I found out I was pregnant." For others, quitting is not an option. Says Marcia, an advertising executive: "I thought, what if I quit and then I lose this baby, too? Then I'd have nothing."

If you decide to stay on the job and plan on returning to work after the baby is born, now is the time to begin thinking about how much time off you would like. Depending on where you work and how long you have been in the job, you may be able to take up to twelve weeks unpaid leave under the Family and Medical Leave Act in addition to your regular maternity leave. Consider whether you can afford to take this unpaid leave to spend some well-deserved time with your baby or whether you will only take the paid maternity leave offered by your employer. Then talk to your boss about it when the time is right.

Be aware, however, that since pregnancy is so unpredictable, even the best-laid plans are subject to change. You may plan to work until the end only to find yourself put on bed rest three months before delivery. Or you may try cutting back and then discover you have too much time on your hands. And there's really no way to know for sure how you'll feel once your baby finally arrives, so give yourself permission to change your mind.

Exercising during Pregnancy

If you've always been a couch potato, now is not the best time to begin a rigorous exercise program. But if you are accustomed to physical activity, you may want to continue exercising regularly throughout your pregnancy. Exercise will help you maintain muscle tone and better manage all the extra weight you will be carrying around. It can also improve both your energy level and your mood. "I find that exercise is so good for relieving stress," says one mother in the midst of a pregnancy after a loss. "It's good for your head and it's good for your body." Research also shows that exercise can reduce pregnancy-associated discomforts.

Despite these advantages, you may worry about the possibility of doing too much and somehow harming your baby. There are some cases when exercising will probably not be allowed, for instance, if you have a history of recurrent miscarriages or preterm labor or if you have been diagnosed with placenta previa, an incompetent cervix or cardiac problems. Exercise will also be discouraged if you are expecting more than one baby. If you have certain other conditions, such as high blood pressure or bleeding during pregnancy, you may be advised to avoid vigorous exercise and work out only under the strict supervision of your doctor. Those of you who are allowed to exercise should be sure to follow the following ACOG guidelines. Discuss them with your doctor so that you can evaluate your exercise program together.

- Base your exercise program on your fitness level before pregnancy, but avoid competitive exercise and any activities that require jumping or rapid changes in direction or deep stretches.

- Do not exercise on your back once you are past the first trimester of pregnancy, since this could interfere with the blood flow to your uterus.

- Some ideal forms of exercise for pregnant women include swimming, stationary cycling and modified forms of dance and calisthenics.

- Before you begin any vigorous activity, warm up for at least five minutes. Then limit strenuous exercise to fifteen minutes or less.

- Be sure that your heart rate does not exceed 140 beats per minute, and stays about 25 to 30 percent lower than when you are not pregnant.

- If you are doing any floor exercises, get up gradually to avoid sudden drops in blood pressure.

- Drink plenty of fluids and avoid exercising in hot, humid weather so that you do not get dehydrated.

- Try to exercise regularly if you can. It is much better to work out at least three times per week, than to only exercise irregularly.

- If at any time you experience any of the following warning signs, stop exercising immediately and contact your doctor: back pain, bleeding, difficulty walking, dizziness, faintness, pain, palpitations, pubic pain, rapid heart rate or shortness of breath.

Your Relationship with Your Partner

Now that your morning sickness has (presumably) gone away and you are feeling more energetic, you may finally find yourself thinking about something besides being pregnant. And that may mean you start focusing again—maybe for the first time in months—on your relationship with your partner. The pregnancy loss has no doubt been stressful on both you and him as individuals, and may have even strained your relationship with each other at times. It probably hasn't helped matters that sex was likely the last thing on your mind once you conceived again and started feeling nauseated and tired.

But for many women, the second trimester of the pregnancy is different. They are not only interested in romance, they're interested in sex again, and that can definitely be good for your relationship. Unfortunately, it can also be one more thing to worry about. Some women fear that having sexual intercourse can harm the baby or put an already tenuous pregnancy at higher risk. While there are some cases when having sex can be a problem, in general, sexual intercourse does not increase the risk of miscarriage. It can, however, be dangerous for some women who are already at high risk due to complications such as placenta previa or incompetent cervix. Your obstetrician may also advise abstinence if you have a history of preterm labor since orgasms can cause uterine contractions. Another reason to abstain is if either you or your partner has a sexually transmitted disease, since bacteria can enter the vagina and cervix and harm the baby. It's always a good idea to talk with your physician about what is best in your particular case.

If you are not among those women who take a renewed interest in sex during the second trimester, don't worry about it too much. Your lack of interest may stem from grieving your loss and feeling guilty about doing anything that gives you pleasure. Or the reason could be much simpler. Maybe you just don't find sex pleasurable when your tummy is bulging and you are packing on the pounds everywhere else. Whether you are abstaining from sex by choice or on doctor's orders, there are still plenty of things you and your partner can do together to keep romance alive. You can start exploring the possibilities by going out on a date at least once a week, especially if you don't have any children at home. Once your baby is born, not only will you find that you want to spend more time at home, you may not have any other choice if you cannot find a trusted sitter. So enjoy your freedom while you can. If you are confined to bed rest during this pregnancy, you may already have lost that freedom, which is something we'll examine in chapter 7.

Common Feelings

Reassurance—and Panic—by the Baby's Movements

Sometime between sixteen and twenty weeks gestation, you will begin to feel the baby move. At first the movements will be little more than flutters, and days may pass when you feel nothing at all. But over time, the baby's movement will become more regular and strong, eventually turning into outright punches. By twenty-eight weeks, you should be able to detect a regular pattern of movement on a daily basis. Try not to be too alarmed if you do not feel the baby move by the twentieth week in your pregnancy. Any number of reasons could cause that. Maybe your dates are slightly off or the baby is positioned in such a way that you don't feel the kicks. Before you panic, talk to your doctor. You can then have a sonogram or other tests to determine whether or not there is a problem.

As much as you would like it, no one can give you any hard and fast rules about how often your baby should move, especially this early in your pregnancy. Each baby's activity level is different and can range from as few as fifty kicks per day to as many as one thousand kicks. But most doctors agree that "normal" movement is what is normal for your baby. If your baby typically kicks up a storm all day long and is then suddenly quiet, that could be cause for concern. But if you usually do not feel a whole lot of movement, that may be normal for your baby. In the next chapter, we'll talk about using kick charts to keep tabs of your baby's movements. During this trimester of your pregnancy, it's enough to always be aware of what your baby is doing and to call your doctor at any sign of a noticeable slowdown.

It's important to point out that all babies have periods when they sleep, and if you are really in tune with your baby, you may eventually be able to detect a regular pattern of sleep and wakeful periods. But given your history, it will not be unusual for you to panic any time you feel that too much time has passed since the baby last moved. That's a feeling that all of us who have been through a subsequent pregnancy have had at some point. One of the best things to do is to drink some orange juice or eat something sweet and then lie down and wait for something to happen. If that doesn't work, call your doctor. Chances are, everything is just fine. But occasionally babies slow down because there is a problem that—if caught in time—can mean the difference between life and death. It is much better to check things out than to wonder whether you could have done more and didn't.

Even the most active babies can have days when they do not move as much. The only way to know whether there's a problem or not is to call your doctor. That's what Glenda did when she realized that her normally active baby had been exceptionally quiet one day. She recalls:

I told my husband, I don't mean to sound paranoid, but the baby hasn't been moving today and it really makes me nervous. Normally, she would kick so much that we would joke that she was going to grow up to be a soccer player. So when it got to be about nine o'clock at night, I called my OB and he told me to go to the hospital immediately. The whole drive down there, my husband and I were very quiet. Both of us were so worried. Un-

beknownst to us, our OB had called the hospital and said, "Put a fetal monitor on her right away and let her hear the heartbeat if it's there. Let's reassure her before we do anything else." Well, the nurses did that as soon as I walked in and sure enough there was a heartbeat, but there was still no movement. So they gave me some orange juice and then the baby was kicking up a storm.

Sometimes not even orange juice will do the trick, as Sharon discovered one night when she was worried about her baby's movement. Like Glenda, Sharon had to go to the hospital to be checked out because it was after regular office hours. But since her six-year-old daughter had already gone to sleep for the night, she decided to go alone. She explains:

We either would have had to take Samantha to a friend or drag someone out of bed at midnight. And I just wanted to do it by myself because I thought, "If I am being neurotic, there's no sense in getting everyone worked up," although, of course, my husband was worked up anyway. So I drove myself to the hospital and when they strapped me to the monitor, they couldn't find the baby's heartbeat. So they brought an ultrasound in and we saw him. The way he was curled up it was just hard to get to his little heart. I was actually pretty calm while they were doing everything, but after we saw the heartbeat, I got the shakes. I called my husband right away and we let him hear the heartbeat over the phone, and then I just sat there for literally forty-five minutes and listened to the baby's heart.

It is not unusual for babies to start moving again just as their mothers are walking into the doctor's office or the hospital. Allison's baby gave her a swift kick as the nurse was strapping on the fetal monitor. She called the experience her "$600 panic attack." It *can* be very expensive to make an emergency trip to the hospital. But because you know that these stories do not always end happily, you can't afford to ignore your concerns. And even though your behavior may make you feel neurotic at times, try to keep in mind that all of us who have been through a subsequent pregnancy have felt the same way at some point. In my first pregnancy, it didn't even enter my mind that the baby could die. In my second and third pregnancies, that was always my first thought whenever the babies didn't move. I was relieved each time they kicked again and I knew that I had been spared the agony of another loss.

Reluctance to Bond with the Baby

For many women, the period when their baby begins to move also marks the time when they really begin to bond with their child. If you reached that point in your last pregnancy, you probably remember what that was like. Maybe you started dreaming about what the baby would look like or began making plans for the future. Depending on how far along you were when you suffered your loss, you may have "nested" or prepared for the baby's homecoming. These are all signs that you were becoming attached to the baby long before birth. As Kathi, who had a pregnancy loss in her second pregnancy, explains, "To me it always felt like it was worse to lose a second child because with Lauren I knew exactly what it would be like, and so my thoughts and dreams and plans for her were so much more detailed."

Given the tragic outcome of your last pregnancy, you may find that you behave much differently this time around. Maybe you try not to think about this baby in concrete terms for fear that something could go wrong again. You may choose to keep your emotional distance until the results of the amniocentesis or other tests are available. You may even feel that you will never be able to love this baby as much as the one that you lost. I think I was well into the second trimester before I could stop thinking, "This is not the baby I really want. I want Patrick back." Julie, another bereaved mother, also had trouble bonding. "I called it a pregnancy of denial," she says. "I didn't even want to acknowledge that there was a pregnancy."

Perhaps your feelings are fluctuating from one day to the next. You may dream about the baby when everything is going well and then put up your guard at the first sign of trouble. Brooke's comments illustrate just how confusing feelings about the subsequent baby can be: "Everytime the baby would kick, I'd say, 'Stop kicking. I don't want to feel you. I don't want to bond with you.' And then when he wouldn't kick, I'd say, 'Kick! I want to know you're there.' It was just a roller coaster. It was horrible."

If some of these feelings sound familiar, it may help to know that you are not alone. Studies document that women who go through a pregnancy after a loss often find it difficult to bond and plan a future with their babies. As one mother says, "It's hard to dream about a child that you're not even sure is going to be born alive." And while many pregnant women like to talk to their unborn baby or stroke their stomachs, you may be reluctant to do so, sometimes without even being consciously aware of it. Pam, who suffered a pregnancy loss in the second trimester, says, "I don't talk to this baby as much as I used to talk to the twins. I remember when I was driving to work, I used to sing to the twins, but I don't do that so much with her. At first it bothered me, but I think I can only let myself get involved up to a certain point."

The fact that women who have suffered a loss often have trouble bonding with their unborn babies is well documented. What is not so clear is whether this does any harm to the mother-child relationship after birth or even to the health and well-being of the child itself. Certainly, that's something all of us have worried about in the subsequent pregnancy. There are some studies that suggest a mother's attitude during her pregnancy does have an effect on the baby inside her womb. In *The Secret Life of the Unborn Child*, Thomas Verny writes that more studies are showing that prenatal bonding "to a great extent determines the future of the mother-child relationship." There is also evidence that babies can hear sounds from the outside world by about six months' gestation, leading some to theorize that negative and angry sounds might upset the baby. But prenatal psychology is far from an exact science. Although evidence exists that maternal anxiety can affect the unborn baby, the consequences of that influence are not as clear.

I worried a lot about how my behavior during pregnancy would affect my baby, but I ultimately chose to focus more on anecdotal evidence than scientific studies. I have yet to meet a woman who sensed that her unhappiness or reluctance to bond during her subsequent pregnancy rubbed off on the baby after birth. Diane's comments are typical of what I heard from most of the women that I interviewed:

> In pregnancy I could not get excited. I did wonder sometimes if this baby was going to feel that I was not connected. But when she was born, it was so great. I never felt a distance from her at all from birth. I think my lack of excitement must have been a mechanism I had to have in order to keep my sanity during pregnancy. I don't think there's anything wrong with that now, but at the time I felt guilty about it.

If anything, most of the women I talked to said they felt closer to their babies after birth because of all the hardships they had to go through to get them into this world. Now that I have made it through two subsequent pregnancies, I share that belief. I believe I am a better parent than I would have been if I had not suffered a pregnancy loss because I treasure my children so much more. And from the looks of my happy, healthy boys, I don't believe for a minute that they are feeling any of the effects of my anxiety, sadness or rejection during pregnancy. We'll further discuss parenting and the subsequent child in chapter 9. Like so many things that follow pregnancy loss, there are no easy formulas for predicting what you can expect.

If you are worried about the scientific evidence that supports the importance of bonding with your unborn child, keep in mind that taking care of yourself physically is also a sign that you are bonding with the baby. "Just by complying with her physician's recommendations and by being even more cautious than what the doctor advises, she really is bonding with her baby even though she may tell herself that she isn't," says Maureen Doolan Boyle, executive director of MOST (Mothers with Supertwins).

If that is not enough to reassure you, consider doing other things to nurture your relationship with your baby. Avoid negative thoughts and emotions. Tell yourself that your baby is healthy, happy and beautiful and picture it in your mind if you can. Talk and sing to your baby whenever you get the chance. Make plans for your baby's arrival and dare to dream about a wonderful future together. Other pregnant women do these kinds of things all the time. Maybe you can, too.

Anxiety over Getting Past the Critical Week

If your loss occurred before you reached full-term, you may find it easier to bond with your baby once you get past the point in your pregnancy when the baby died. Somehow, there's something almost magical about getting past that critical week. It may be the first time in the entire pregnancy that you actually breathe a sigh of relief. This is especially true if the baby you lost was your first. You know that once you get past the point of your loss, this pregnancy will become a whole new experience. As one mother says, "I can feel it now when a little foot moves, and that's something I never got to experience before. I really like that." Laura, who suffered a pregnancy loss at twenty-three weeks, says getting past that point has made it easier for her to focus on the baby she is expecting rather than the one who died: "We've never been to this point before, so this is a whole new ball game for us. I was doing so much comparing before and carrying all the old baggage. Now there is nothing to compare it to. It's just this baby's pregnancy. I feel a little more joy, not just fear."

For Sheila, making it further in the pregnancy than she ever had before gave her the confidence to start making preparations for the baby's homecoming. "For the first few months that I was pregnant, we didn't do anything at all. But when I got past the five-month mark where I had miscarried the last time, both my husband I felt like now we're ready." Stephanie, who had given birth at twenty-one weeks gestation, was heartened to reach the point where she knew her baby had a chance of surviving outside of the womb:

I knew that at twenty-one weeks she would not survive. But I would celebrate when she got to the next level because I knew at twenty-four weeks she could survive, but she would have a lot of complications. And then when I got to twenty-eight weeks I thought, "This is a lot better." So from about twenty-one weeks to thirty-one weeks, I went through and read what would happen if my baby was born right now.

As much as you look forward to making it past the point where you suffered your loss, living through this period can be difficult. Pam was not prepared for how nervous she would feel when she reached twenty-two weeks gestation, the same point when her twins had died. "I was on the phone to my doctor a lot more around twenty-two weeks. I also kept thinking, 'Is next week as far as I can make it?' Since I had never made it any further in a pregnancy, I wasn't sure that I could." Although you will definitely feel relieved once you pass this particular hurdle in the pregnancy, the relief may be only temporary. Don't be surprised if some of those old anxieties and fears come creeping back a few days or a few weeks later.

Maybe in your case the critical week in your pregnancy is not the point when your loss occurred, but the anniversary date. Sharon, for example, was anxious to get past what would have been her daughter's first birthday. "I feel like once we get through that terrible week in September, then maybe it will be time to concentrate on the joy." Living through the anniversary period may remind you about the loss more than you expected but then give you a sense of closure that enables you to face the future with more confidence.

Superstition

Nearly all of us have been subjected to an old wives' tale or two during pregnancy. Maybe you've been warned not to reach too far with your arms because it could put a knot in the umbilical cord. Or you may have been told that the shape of your tummy is a sign of whether you're expecting a boy or a girl. Neither of these statements is true, of course. The only reason not to reach when you're pregnant is that you might lose your balance and fall. And as for the shape of your tummy, that's determined by your anatomy, not by the sex of the child.

If you're carrying out front, it's probably because you have a short torso so the baby has nowhere to go but out. But if your tummy is wide, it may simply be an indication that your torso is long or your baby is in a sideways position.

Even those of us who consider ourselves too smart to believe old wives' tales can find that superstitions get the better of us during our subsequent pregnancies. You may have convinced yourself, for example, that if you are too optimistic about this baby and make plans for its arrival, the worst will happen again. Or you may feel just the opposite and fear that thinking bad things will make them a reality. Some women tell themselves that if only they do everything differently in the subsequent pregnancy, the baby will be all right. Julie is one example:

> *There was no way I could have the same doctor or the same hospital or the same anything or else this baby would die, too. I even threw out all my maternity clothes. I didn't want to see them again. Everything had to be different. It was like bad luck to use anything again. I think my doctor felt bad that I was not going to go back to him, but I didn't care if I had the best doctor in the world, I knew I had to find someone else.*

When we think about it in logical terms, we know that nothing we think or say can hurt our babies. And, assuming we are doing our best to take care of ourselves and seeing our doctors regularly, nothing we do, within reason, will hurt our babies, either. Certainly, wearing the same maternity clothes or returning to the same hospital will not put a jinx on us or our babies—at least that's what logic tells us. But logic does not always prevail in a subsequent pregnancy.

When you find your thoughts running away from you, stop for a minute and consider whether they really make sense. Keep reminding yourself that thinking bad things will not make them so, and being hopeful will not bring a curse down on you. And if you have superstitions that are harmless to both you and your baby, go ahead and indulge yourself. Anything that makes you feel better during this pregnancy is worth doing as long as it does not hurt. You may look back and laugh at yourself later, but at least you will be doing something to make your life easier when it really matters.

What kinds of harmless superstitions am I talking about? They could be anything from not driving the same route to your doctor's office to putting off all baby showers until after the baby is born. Margo, whose first baby was stillborn, recalls her obsession with working on things for the baby:

Even before I knew what I was having, I went and got a Christmas stocking for a little girl and started needle-pointing it. When I finished that, I started working on a baby blanket. I guess I really thought that if I did that, the baby would survive. As long as I kept working on things, the baby would stay alive. I never did that for my first baby.

Your superstition may involve not doing something that you regretted doing last time. Allison decided that if she did not find out the sex of the baby she was carrying, it would make up for the bad reaction she had during her pregnancy that ended in a loss. She says:

My husband and I both really wanted a boy, so when we went for the sonogram and they told us we were having a girl, I cried. I felt so guilty for doing that and I still do. I think sometimes that I caused [the pregnancy loss] to happen because I wanted a boy. So this time I decided I am not going to find out what we're having because I don't want to worry about how I'll react.

The kind of superstition that Allison had is especially common for women who were never given a reason for their baby's death. Rather than acknowledging how completely helpless they are to prevent certain things, they try to regain a sense of control by telling themselves that if they do things differently this time, they can keep their babies safe.

Whatever your superstitions, they might sound as silly to others as old wives' tales sound to you. But again, the thing to remember is that if it helps you feel better and it does no harm, then you should probably go ahead and do it.

Fear

All of the feelings that I have mentioned until now have their roots in the fear that pervades subsequent pregnancies. And that fear can be exhausting, as one bereaved mother points out:

> *I am so tired of being afraid all the time. I wish I could just go to sleep and wake up seven months from now with a live healthy baby in my arms. Even my children expect the worst. If they don't see my car in the driveway when they come home from school, they automatically assume I must be at the hospital because I've had a miscarriage.*

You may find that your fears take the pleasure out of doing simple things that other pregnant women take for granted. Things like picking a name or preparing a nursery. Melanie, who had miscarried in her first pregnancy, could not bring herself to buy maternity clothes until she could no longer fit into anything that was in her closet. "To me, buying those clothes was a sign of commitment, and I didn't want them if I was going to lose the baby."

There is no easy way to stop being afraid, short of delivering a healthy baby. But there are some things you can do to ease your fears. One good practice is to try to avoid worrying about things that have not happened yet. In other words, if you can't stop worrying altogether, resolve to worry only about the problems you actually have, not ones that don't yet exist. Your current worries should keep you busy enough. It can also help to be as informed as possible about any problems that you are actually facing, especially if those problems are medical. Often our imaginations are far worse than reality. So ask your doctor to explain things thoroughly and in plain English. If you find it helpful, do your own research, too. The more you know, the less you will have to fear the unknown. Another good idea is to try to counter every negative thought with a positive one. We'll talk more about how to do that a little later in this chapter.

Hopefulness

Underneath all the fear, anxiety and worry is the hope that motivated you to get pregnant in the first place. As I said in chapter 1, every woman quoted in this book gave birth to a healthy baby after going through the pain of pregnancy loss, and if you did not think the same thing was possible for you, you probably never would have contemplated another pregnancy. Hang on to that hope when times are tough. Remember that many of us have felt exactly as you feel right now, wondering whether we would ever have the joy of holding a live baby in our arms. Our dreams eventually came true and we hope that yours will, too.

Tips for Easing Anxiety

Think Positive (If at All Possible)

We have all heard about the power of positive thinking, but not very many of us have mastered it, especially when it comes to our subsequent pregnancies. What exactly does thinking positive mean? It means expecting the best rather than imagining the worst. It means not conjuring up scenarios of all the bad things that could possibly happen but looking forward to the good things that the future holds. It means affirming over and over that everything will be all right. The theory behind this is that your mind controls your body, and thoughts can either help or hurt you. But as we've already discussed, this can be very difficult to do in a subsequent pregnancy. One resource that many people have found invaluable through the years is Norman Vincent Peale's classic, *The Power of Positive Thinking*. In the book, Peale blends modern psychiatry with biblical teachings to illustrate how to counter negative thoughts with positive ones. Sheila, who had suffered a loss in her first pregnancy, credits that book with changing her outlook on life.

I started reading that book every day and decided to adopt that way of thinking. It just helped me think about why good things happen, and that really sustained me when I would start to get nervous about something. Even as they were giving me the epidural I was practicing the positive thinking.

If Peale's Christian teachings are not part of your belief system, you can consult plenty of other books and tapes on positive thinking as well. Go to your local book store or library and browse through the self-help or religion section. You will find something that works for you.

Something else that helped me was to focus on there never being a better time to have a baby. In the last several decades, a number of medical breakthroughs in treating pregnancy complications have been discovered that in the past might have been fatal. The therapy for autoimmune problems discussed in chapter 1 is just one example. Tremendous progress has also been made in the treatment of premature babies. Infants who just a few years ago would have died are now not only surviving but thriving. Even if you feel like the medical profession let you down somehow in your last pregnancy, keep in mind that women are receiving better prenatal care today than ever before.

Despite all your reasons to be positive about the future, it is important not to let that optimism get in the way of recognizing symptoms or conditions that need immediate medical attention. Martha learned that lesson the hard way. She developed a serious condition in her subsequent pregnancy known as HELLP syndrome, which stands for hemolysis, elevated liver enzymes, and a low platelet count. Although Martha had many of the classic HELLP symptoms, her doctor did not immediately diagnose her condition. She remembers:

I was always trying to remind myself of everything that was positive and good about my pregnancy, like my amnio results. Once I got the news that

the baby had no chromosomal problems, I just kept thinking about that
and telling myself that everything would be fine in this pregnancy. But I
think that I over-reassured myself so that when I started having health
problems, I didn't really convey the seriousness of my condition to my doc-
tor. A lot of it is my fault. I didn't communicate very well. I wanted to be
positive when I was at my appointments, so I really didn't tell my doctor
in strong enough terms how I was feeling.

Fortunately, Martha's mother recognized the symptoms that her
daughter was having and intervened. She insisted on taking Martha
to the hospital, where she described in detail what had been happening. When doctors were finally alerted to the seriousness of Martha's
symptoms, they were able to act in time to save both her and her baby.

Being positive does not mean that you will not have problems during your pregnancy. But it does mean that you can face them with a
sense of confidence that you will overcome them before they overcome
you.

Keep Busy

Many women find that if they keep busy during their pregnancy, it
leaves them less time to feel anxious. The second trimester is when
you will be feeling your best, so take advantage of your extra energy
to take on new projects or complete unfinished ones. If you work
outside the home, focus as much attention as possible on your job. If
you have other living children and are a stay-at-home mom, you will
have no problem keeping busy. As Virginia, who had two children at
home, says: "There were a lot of other distractions, so I couldn't just
stare at my navel and think about being pregnant."

Some women find that they need to do something new to keep them
from dwelling too much on their pregnancy. Kathy decided to go back
to school for an advanced degree. It wasn't a cure-all, but it helped.
"I had to study a lot, so that was good," she says. "But there were a
lot of times when I would be sitting in class and thinking about the
baby." Kelly, on the other hand, found it helpful to keep her focus

on others. "I was much better about sending birthday cards or calling friends—anything that would shift the focus off of myself and onto somebody else." Those of you who are put on bed rest during the pregnancy will find it more challenging than ever to keep busy. We'll examine some of the things you can do while restricted to bed rest in chapter 7.

Try Not to Make Comparisons

Any doctor will tell you that no two pregnancies are alike. So do your best not to dwell on comparisons between this pregnancy and the last one. If problems crop up that are similar to what you experienced before, don't panic until you have had time to discuss the situation with your doctor. It may be a false alarm or the same problem may be taking a different course in this pregnancy. Laura, for example, panicked when she stepped on the scale at one of her regular prenatal visits and discovered that she had gained more weight than usual. She immediately concluded that she was retaining fluid, a problem that preceded her pregnancy loss last time. She recalls: "I was sure there was something wrong. There just had to be some dark ugly thing that was causing me to gain too much weight. But it turned out that I had just eaten more than I should have."

Although it is now easy for me to tell you not to make comparisons, I wasn't always able to follow that advice myself during my own subsequent pregnancy. One time when my blood pressure was slightly elevated during a prenatal checkup, I immediately concluded that I was having the same problem with high blood pressure that I had experienced in my first pregnancy. I talked to my doctor about it, and he cautioned me that it was premature to draw any conclusions. He also gave me advice that I am now passing on to you: don't compare pregnancies.

At the time, it didn't matter to me what he said. I thought I knew better and was inconsolable. I told him, "I can see the pattern. I'm sure that the same thing is happening all over again." But I was wrong. My blood pressure was lower at my next visit and continued to be low throughout the rest of my pregnancy. If I had listened to my doctor and stopped myself from making comparisons and drawing conclusions, I could have avoided the anxiety-filled days that I spent convincing myself that all kinds of bad things were going to happen.

Some complications do recur in pregnancies. But your obstetrician is well aware of this and can take steps to treat any condition that you already have or are at risk for developing. In many cases, if your doctor has prior knowledge of potential problems, he can make the treatment even more effective. Leave the comparisons to your doctor.

Take a Proactive Role in Your Care

Whatever medical condition or complication you may face in the subsequent pregnancy, it is a good idea to be as informed as possible about it. Even though you may trust your doctor implicitly, you are only one of literally hundreds of patients being cared for at any given time. The better informed you are, the more you will be able to ensure that nothing about your case gets overlooked. When you are knowledgeable about the medical aspects of your pregnancy, you can also better discuss treatment options and outcomes with your doctor. You can ask questions and challenge anything that does not sound quite right. You will know when it's time to seek a second opinion. And perhaps most important, you can more readily recognize symptoms that require immediate medical attention. Being informed does not mean that you will be charting the course of your own care, only that you will be actively monitoring it.

Sydney, who suffered a second-trimester loss, explains how she played this role in her subsequent pregnancy:

> I learned to research and I learned to question my doctor—not just accept everything he said at face value. Doctors are authority figures, and we've been taught to listen to authority figures. But I realize that my doctor is going to go on and live his own life no matter what happens in this pregnancy, while I have to live with the consequences. So I want to be sure that I am playing as active a role as he is in deciding what's best.

As you can imagine, I also made it my responsibility to stay informed during my subsequent pregnancies and talk to my doctor about anything that I considered important. I did that mainly because I bitterly regretted not being more proactive during my first pregnancy. Rather than blindly trusting my doctor about when to induce labor (he had decided to induce the day after my due date), I wish that I had questioned his decision since I had a family history of big babies. I now know that my baby, who weighed over eleven pounds at birth, could have been safely delivered at least two weeks before my due date and still have been considered full-term. If I had raised that possibility with my doctor, the outcome may likely have been very different.

In my second and third pregnancies, I was determined that things definitely *would* be different. I became my own advocate on all matters related to my medical care. So although my obstetrician told me early on that his policy was to deliver no earlier than thirty-eight weeks gestation unless there were complications, I made it a point to talk to him extensively about this. I think he considered what I had to say and took it into account when he ultimately decided to deliver the babies at thirty-seven weeks gestation. Both boys weighed around eight and a half pounds at birth and were so hefty that the deliveries themselves were difficult, which to me proves that the doctor made the right decision to deliver even earlier than he normally would.

Your medical concerns may not be as straightforward as mine were. The complications that you face may be very difficult for you to understand. But with the power of the Internet, medical information is now as close as your fingertips. You can access medical databases and read up on the latest research on virtually any topic. You also can use e-mail and chat rooms to communicate with other women who have been in similar situations. All of these avenues will help you better understand your case. It is important, however, not to use that information to self-diagnose. Simply use it as a springboard to open a discussion with your doctor. If you are not satisfied with the answers you get, go to someone else for a second opinion.

As Candace Hurley, executive director of Sidelines National Support Network for women experiencing high-risk pregnancies, puts it, "I believe you should become as educated as possible about everything—what happened the last time and what you can do this time to ensure it does not happen again. Most women feel like they put their head in the sand the first time and they want to be as involved as possible in their subsequent pregnancy."

If too much information makes you nervous or you do not feel comfortable conducting your own research, consider asking your partner to do it for you. He can accompany you to your prenatal visits and ask all the questions.

Avoid Other Women's Horror Stories

Pregnancy can bring out the worst in women who get a kick out of relating how horrible their own pregnancies were. They may want to talk about every complication they ever had or give you details about their excruciating labor. If you come across someone who also has had a pregnancy loss, she might want to tell you all about it, right down to the details. Listen only to as much or as little as you feel comfortable hearing. If the conversation starts to make you nervous, cut off the discussion in a polite way or even walk away if you must. You have already lived through your own horror story; you do not need to hear anybody else's.

You should take the same approach with any unsolicited advice that comes your way. Listen to anything that sounds useful; ignore anything that does not apply to you. Tell the other person that you have a doctor who is giving you the best possible care and that you are confident in him. There is no sense in getting angry with people when they mean well. But there is also no point in subjecting yourself to advice that you don't need to hear. "It is important to have a little bit of humor where advice is concerned; don't take things so seriously," suggests Fran Rybarik, executive director of the national pregnancy loss organization Bereavement Services/RTS. "Just realize you are doing what's best for you."

Take One Day at a Time

As you live through each day of the subsequent pregnancy, you no doubt have your eye on the prize. All you really want is to reach the end and deliver a healthy baby. But counting the days until your due date can be overwhelming, since imagining the next hundred or so days is sometimes more difficult than living through them. Instead, try whenever possible to focus on the day at hand. Kelly says her motto in her subsequent pregnancy was simply "live for today." She says, " 'Live for today' sounds so awful, but I think you can get so caught up in what's down the line that you don't enjoy today." Trisha told herself over and over again, "today, I am pregnant." She recalls, "That was as far as I could go. I couldn't think about tomorrow. Then once I got past the point where I had suffered my loss, I started telling myself, " 'Today, I am more pregnant than I ever have been.' "

The one-day-at-a-time approach might be a sharp contrast to the way you handled your previous pregnancies. Kelly, for example, says that in each of her three other pregnancies she had made a ritual of marking the days off her calendar as her due date approached. After her loss, she never did that again. "I just tried to do the best job I could that day. I didn't look to tomorrow. If someone asked me how much more time to my due date, I was like, 'I don't know.' I didn't want to think of the fifty-five more days to go. I did not mark it on the calendar at all."

Many times in life you will count the days in anticipation of some exciting event. But your subsequent pregnancy should not be one of them. You will already be feeling like your pregnancy lasts forever. Counting the number of days left to go will probably just make it seem longer. Instead of using a calendar to count the days until the end of your pregnancy, consider getting a *pregnancy calendar* instead. It will describe how your baby is developing in utero each week of the pregnancy and can help you focus on the baby being alive and well *today*.

Feel Free to Continue to Grieve

No matter how much time has passed since your loss, you are bound to still be grieving to some extent. It is important to continue working through those feelings even while you are pregnant again. It is only by experiencing the pain of your loss and working through it that you can eventually come to terms with what happened to your baby. If you feel like crying, do it. If it makes you feel better to visit the baby's grave site, go. Do whatever you need to do to mourn your baby.

Melissa Swanson, editor of the *PAILS of Hope* newsletter for parents going through a pregnancy after a loss, has this advice: "You have to allow yourself to continue to grieve and to continue to feel and to continue to cry. You're crying not only for the baby or the babies who died, you're crying for the unknown and the fear in this pregnancy. And letting that out is so much healthier than keeping it in."

You may worry about the effect that all these emotions will have on the baby you are expecting, especially in light of the studies that we discussed in the last chapter, which indicate that stress could increase the risk of preterm birth. But as I pointed out, the research is far from conclusive. The best advice might be for you to avoid too much stress by finding a balance between grieving for the baby who died and looking forward to the one that is on the way.

Put Yourself First

In the previous chapter we discussed taking care of yourself, including indulging in some healthy pleasures such as facials and massages. This trimester, you should try to take that idea one step further and, whenever possible, put your needs above those of everyone else's. That's not to say that you would always want to live your life that way, but this is a unique period when your needs really should come first for your own sake and that of the baby's. This means that if the holidays are approaching and you are dreading the inevitable battery of questions from well-meaning family members, bow out if you want. Simply tell everyone that you need a break this year and plan to do something else with your partner. If you have friends who want you to do things that make you uncomfortable—whether it's attending a baby shower or going to lunch with someone who has a child about the age that yours would have been—politely decline. And if you feel pressured at any point to do more than you feel comfortable doing, either at work or at home, just say no.

But also do positive things for yourself. If your doctor says it's okay to travel, go somewhere you have always wanted to visit. The second trimester is typically the best time in your pregnancy to take a trip because your body has adjusted to being pregnant and you may have more energy. The rate of complications is also lowest in the second trimester. If you don't feel like leaving town, do things that you've always wanted to do in your area. Go to the art museum, look for bargains at a flea market or take a good friend to a restaurant you've been waiting to try. All of us need to find the right balance between work and play, but taking care of yourself is more important than ever right now.

Prenatal Visits

Frequency

Now that you are in the second trimester of your pregnancy, your prenatal visits will probably become more frequent. Instead of seeing your doctor once a month, you may start going in as often as every two or three weeks. Most of the time, the visits will be brief, consisting of blood pressure and weight checks, urinalysis and measurements of your tummy. Your obstetrician will also be checking the baby's heartbeat and asking you about any complications that you may be experiencing.

Usually, you will be in and out of the office in fifteen minutes, not including the time you spend waiting for the doctor. (You may have to hang around a while longer when you're having prenatal tests or on the day you undergo a glucose tolerance test to screen for gestational diabetes.) But if at any time you feel like your physician is not spending enough time with you, remind the staff that you need an extended appointment. You may ask to be scheduled late in the day or first thing in the morning when the doctor has more time to sit down with you. Do not be afraid to ask for what you want. That's what your doctor is there for.

Visits with the Perinatologist

Sometime in your second trimester, you may also begin seeing a perinatologist. These visits will be in addition to your prenatal visits with your obstetrician. You may see the perinatologist for special diagnostic procedures, such as a level-two ultrasound or an amniocentesis. If you are required to have any special treatment, such as a cerclage for an incompetent cervix, you will probably see the specialist right before and then again right after the procedure.

Since you will be so closely monitored, there may be times when the specialist becomes concerned about a problem that corrects itself over time. It may be something that you otherwise would never have known about. That is one of the drawbacks to having frequent checkups. On the other hand, by being monitored closely, your doctors can detect potentially serious problems before they become life-threatening.

Prenatal Tests of the Second Trimester

To Test or Not to Test?

At some time during the second trimester, you will need to make some hard decisions about prenatal testing. Your first decision will be whether to have a maternal alpha-fetoprotein test, a blood test that shows if you are at higher risk of having a baby with Down syndrome or a neural tube defect. Depending on the results of that test, you will then decide whether to have a level-two ultrasound, possibly followed by an amniocentesis.

As you contemplate which prenatal tests are right for you, it is important to keep in mind that while the tests that are currently available can *detect* certain problems in the baby, they usually cannot *correct* them or determine the degree of impairment. In some cases the baby can have corrective surgery while still in the womb, but that is the exception rather than the rule. Whether surgery can be done after birth will depend on the diagnosis. There also are a wide range of problems that neither sonograms nor amniocentesis can detect. So while you may be able to rule out certain problems if your test results are favorable, you must guard against getting a false sense of security that nothing could go wrong. Many things can and do go wrong, even after prenatal test results come back normal. There also is a risk—albeit small—associated with amniocentesis, which we'll discuss later in the chapter.

Something else to consider as you make decisions about prenatal testing is what you will do with the information once you get it. Will you terminate the pregnancy if the tests show that there is a problem? Will you carry to term knowing that the outcome will be less than perfect? Or are you not sure what you would do? If you are having trouble making a decision, a genetic counselor can answer questions you might have about prenatal testing as well as give you details about your particular risk for birth defects. A counselor can also talk about what options you would have should your diagnosis be bad. "By seeing a genetic counselor, a couple can be provided with information about their situation and what it means for a subsequent pregnancy. Then they can make a decision about their next step," says Donna Jeane Pappas, a licensed professional counselor in the Department of Obstetrics and Gynecology at the University of North Carolina at Chapel Hill.

As is the case with every difficult decision in the subsequent pregnancy, it might help to read about some of the reasons that other women have decided to have prenatal testing and what they planned to do with the information.

To Avoid Giving Birth to a Child with Special Needs

By far, the main reason that women opt to have prenatal testing is because they fear giving birth to a child with special needs. By finding out ahead of time whether the baby has chromosomal abnormalities or other problems, they know they will then have the option of terminating the pregnancy. "I was pretty certain that I would have aborted," says one bereaved mother. "I didn't feel like I could deal with a disabled child." You may feel the same way. Perhaps you believe that you have had your share of pain and are unable to handle any more. You may be especially concerned if you are over the age of thirty-five and are therefore at higher risk of giving birth to a baby with chromosomal problems. Of course, terminating a pregnancy will not be without its own pain. But it is ultimately a decision that only you and your partner can make. Either way, you are the ones who will have to live with the consequences.

To Prevent History from Repeating Itself

Maybe your reason for having prenatal testing is that you have already experienced the pain of having a baby with a birth defect and do not want to risk having the same thing happen again. Brooke, whose third child died as a result of chromosomal problems, says she wanted to spare the next baby the kind of pain that her son had endured:

> I knew that for the ten hours my son was alive he was in pain the whole time. That's why we couldn't touch him, because every time the nurse did anything to him, you could tell just the way he reacted that it bothered him. So because of that, I knew that if another baby were to be diagnosed with the same thing, we would terminate the pregnancy. We wouldn't have any choice because I would not put another baby through that.

Even if you have not given birth to a baby with genetic problems, you may opt to have prenatal testing if you have a family history of birth defects or you have a genetic disorder that puts you at higher risk of giving birth to a child with problems.

To Minimize the Risk of Unhappy Surprises

If you did not know that your baby had a problem until the actual delivery, you may want to do everything possible to ensure you never get another unhappy surprise. Having the prenatal tests does not necessarily mean that you would terminate the pregnancy this time, only that you want to know one way or another so that you are not caught unaware. Kelly explains her reasoning along those lines:

> I had an amnio because I was thirty-nine years old and I thought it was wise. I didn't know what I would have done if it turned out that there was a problem, but I wanted to be aware, whatever the situation was. I didn't want to know about it on the delivery table. I'd already gotten one shock in the delivery room, so I wanted to reduce as many shock factors as possible.

If testing does reveal a problem and you decide to continue the pregnancy, you will then have the option of preparing for the birth by planning to deliver the baby at a hospital equipped to deal with whatever condition was diagnosed.

To Gain a Sense of Control

When your pregnancy ended in a loss, it probably dawned on you just how helpless you were to do anything to change the outcome. Although you could take care of yourself and follow doctor's orders, there was simply no way to prevent your baby from dying. Given that so many things are out of our hands during pregnancy, prenatal testing can give you a much-needed sense of control over the situation. As one mother says, "Even though all the tests scared me, I also felt like they would give me a sort of control and give me the ability to know my baby more."

Andrea Seigerman, a licensed clinical social worker in the high-risk obstetrics clinic at Yale–New Haven Hospital, says it is common for women to want to control everything they can in the subsequent pregnancy. "Since they did not have control over what happened to their body and their baby when their pregnancy ended in a loss, the next time around women may strive to have control over as many things as they can," she says. "It is important to remember though that many aspects of the pregnancy will remain beyond your control, with or without prenatal testing."

For Peace of Mind

Your reason for wanting prenatal testing may simply be that you yearn for any information that can give you peace of mind during the pregnancy. This may be especially true if your loss came at term or shortly after birth, as Glenda's did.

> When you have a miscarriage or you lose a baby at seven months and you get past that point in your next pregnancy, you start feeling better mentally, but I had gone full term and everything was wonderful, so I didn't have a point I could get past and start feeing better about the pregnancy. For me, testing was the only thing that would give me some peace of mind.

Strangely enough, what you thought would bring you peace of mind sometimes does just the opposite, as Kathi discovered in the pregnancy that followed her baby's death. "Anytime we did any kind of test and the results came back normal, I would come home and be very, very depressed. Part of me was happy that my baby was doing well and another part of me felt, 'Why couldn't it have been this way for Lauren?'"

What these experiences show is that women deal with a lot of unknowns during subsequent pregnancies. Prenatal testing can minimize some of those unknowns but sometimes helps create others. The important thing is to make a well-thought-out decision. Don't have tests simply because your doctor says you should. Think about whether or not you really need or want the kind of information these tests provide. And ask yourself what you would do with that information once you had it. Also consider whether the tests pose risks and whether you are willing to take them. By knowing more about the tests themselves, you will be able to make more informed decisions.

Maternal Alpha-Fetoprotein Test

Between fifteen and eighteen weeks gestation, your doctor can check the alpha-fetoprotein, or AFP, levels in your blood to see if your baby is at higher risk for neural tube defects or Down syndrome. AFP is a protein produced by the baby's liver. Levels are higher than usual when the baby has a neural tube defect and are lower than normal when the baby has Down syndrome or some other chromosomal abnormality. In many cases, the AFP is tested in combination with two other substances in what is known as the triple or multiple marker screen. Levels of the hormone hCG are also tested, since they can be elevated if the baby has chromosomal abnormalities. A recent study also found that elevated levels of hCG can be indicative of a higher risk of pregnancy complications, such as pre-term birth, low birthweight, and preeclampsia. The third screen is for estriol, a by-product of the hormone estrogen, which is found at lower levels if the baby has chromosomal problems.

If any of these three screening tests comes back positive, which means that the results are either above or below normal levels, it does not necessarily mean that your baby has a problem, only that he or she may be at higher risk for one. In most cases, nothing is wrong. Often, the problem is that either the pregnancy has been dated incorrectly or the woman is carrying more than one baby. To verify the results, the doctor usually does the test a second time. If the results still come back positive, your doctor will probably recommend a level-two sonogram and possibly an amniocentesis.

Since both the AFP test and the triple screen produce a lot of false positives, it is important not to jump to any conclusions until you receive all the facts. This will help you avoid the kind of pain that Shelly experienced in her subsequent pregnancy:

I went through a major depression when my AFP results came out bad. My doctor told me there were a lot of false postives, but he still suggested that I come in and have an amnio right away. He had us in his office doing an amnio that very same day. He also sent us to get a level-two sonogram because he felt like we needed to see our baby. But during the time that we had to wait for the results of the amnio, I was almost suicidal. I was scaring my family because I thought I was going to lose another baby. During that time, I'd go to work, and I'd come home, and I wouldn't cry at work, but I would cry the entire time I was home, and I would cry myself to sleep. My husband called my doctor and said this is a major clinical depression, so the doctor said he would put a rush on the amnio results and we got them back about two days later. My depression lifted once I got the results because I really felt confident that the test was accurate.

Discuss the pros and cons of the test with your doctor and then consider your own feelings and that of your partner before undergoing the test.

Sonogram

Many women who have never had a pregnancy loss think of a sonogram simply as a way of catching a glimpse of their unborn child and perhaps finding out if they are expecting a boy or a girl. But those of us who are in the midst of a subsequent pregnancy tend to focus more on its being a valuable tool in prenatal diagnosis of certain detectable birth defects. By using high frequency sound waves to produce a picture of the baby on a monitor, ultrasound enables doctors to check for a wide range of problems, including abnormalities of the spine and of major organs, such as the brain, heart and kidneys. In some cases, Down syndrome is also detectable through sonography, although most of the time, it is not.

Ultrasound can reveal other potential problems in the pregnancy as well. For example, a sonogram will show if the placenta is positioned correctly and whether the cord insertion is normal. It can also enable the doctor to check that the baby's growth and movement are good and that an adequate amount of amniotic fluid is present—all signs of fetal well-being. In most cases, obstetricians schedule this type of high-level ultrasound sometime between the eighteenth and twentieth week of pregnancy, since that is the best time to check for structural abnormalities in the baby. Some doctors will continue to do ultrasounds throughout the pregnancy to check on the baby's progress and to give you peace of mind.

But as reassuring as sonograms can be, they are by no means offered routinely by all doctors. In fact, the American College of Obstetricians and Gynecologists does not recommend the use of prenatal ultrasound unless there is a specific reason, such as unexplained bleeding or uncertainty about the date of conception. Most obstetricians, however, will perform at least one sonogram during the course of a subsequent pregnancy to confirm the due date and rule out the possibility of a multiple pregnancy. A sonogram is also routinely scheduled if results of the AFP or triple screen come back abnormal or if there is some other reason to suspect that a woman is at higher risk of giving birth to a baby with birth defects.

Although ultrasound can detect actual and potential problems and rule out others, many problems cannot be detected with a sonogram, chromosomal abnormalities usually being among them. In many respects, the scan is also only as good as the person performing it. Sonographers are not required to be accredited, but you might want to ask whether your sonographer has gone through the rigorous accreditation process administered by the American Institute of Ultrasound in Medicine.

Since having an ultrasound can sometimes be a nerve-wracking experience, you may ask the person performing the sonogram to talk you through the procedure to point out such anatomical structures as the baby's head, heart and other major organs. The sonographer might be more willing to do this if you explain your history of pregnancy loss. But even then, there are no guarantees that your needs will be met.

I remember one ultrasound in my subsequent pregnancy when I specifically told the sonographer that I was nervous and wanted to know as much as I could about what was taking place. She assured me that she understood and did a fairly good job of explaining things as she went along. But at one point, she inexplicably left the room after telling me to "get comfortable." Although it seemed like an hour—I think she was actually gone only about twenty minutes—and you can imagine everything that was racing through my head during that time. And I'm not sure how she expected me to get comfortable with ice-cold jelly smeared all over my exposed midriff. When she finally returned, I breathlessly asked her if there was a problem with my baby. She casually said, "No, not at all." She just needed to consult the doctor about another patient—so much for being sensitive to my needs.

In addition to being nervous during the procedure itself, you might also worry during the time leading up to the sonogram. As Katie recalls, "I could hardly sleep the night before my sonogram. I remember lying in bed, thinking there's going to be something wrong with the baby." Even when your doctor performs frequent ultrasounds, the experience can still be nerve-wracking. Laura, who saw a perinatologist throughout her high-risk pregnancy, describes the roller coaster of emotions that she felt before every ultrasound:

Usually a couple of days before the doctor's visit I start to notice that I have more thoughts of what he is going to see and whether everything is going to be okay. Then when we get a good report, I feel like I'm on cloud nine for the rest of the day. I call my mom, and my husband calls his parents, and we tell them we saw the baby. But then before my next appointment, I start getting nervous all over again.

Despite the anxiety a sonogram can provoke, you might feel, as these women did, that the reassurance provided by the procedure far outweighs any nervousness you feel beforehand.

Amniocentesis

Amniocentesis is another sophisticated tool for prenatal diagnosis. In the procedure, which is typically performed between the fifteenth and eighteenth week of pregnancy, the doctor inserts a needle through the abdominal wall and into the uterus and withdraws a small amount of amniotic fluid. Fetal cells obtained from this fluid are then grown in a tissue culture, and the chromosomes are studied. This type of analysis can detect chromosomal problems as well as a host of biochemical problems. It usually takes about two weeks to get the results, which can feel like an extraordinarily long time. "I wasn't scared about doing the procedure itself," says Lynn, who was in the midst of a high-risk pregnancy, "but waiting for the results was real stressful."

An amniocentesis is routinely scheduled if either parent is known to have a genetic defect that can be passed on to the child, or if an ultrasound shows the possibility of a fetal abnormality. It is also generally offered as an option to women who will be thirty-five years old or older when they give birth or to those who have a family history of birth defects. If the amniocentesis shows a problem with the baby, you would have the option of either terminating the pregnancy or preparing yourself for a less-than-perfect outcome.

Since doctors now use ultrasound images to find a pocket of fluid around the baby and guide the needle, amniocentesis is much safer today than it once was. About 1 in 200 women will have a miscarriage after an amniocentesis that they otherwise would not have had. In other cases, women continue to leak amniotic fluid after the procedure. But the rate of complications can vary depending on the experience of the physician performing the procedure. It is a good idea to ask your doctor about the rate of complications wherever you plan to have your amniocentesis performed.

Although the risk of miscarriage after amniocentesis is low, the risk may seem too high for you given your history of pregnancy loss. Laura explains how she felt when her doctor recommended that she have an amniocentesis:

One half of one percent sounds really low to everyone, but to us it sounded really high. When the time came to make the decision I went back and forth a little bit because I figured if it showed something I could prepare myself, but we eventually decided that we just could not take the risk.

Even women who have a history of genetic problems sometimes decide against having an amniocentesis. Beth, for example, had a baby with a rare chromosomal problem who died shortly after birth. Even though her doctor recommended that she have an amniocentesis in her second pregnancy, she decided against it because the risk of miscarrying after the procedure was greater than the risk of having another baby with the same genetic problem.

Even if the results of the amniocentesis come back completely normal, you may find that it is not enough to give you peace of mind. You know all too well that while amniocentesis can rule out certain problems, it cannot rule out everything. As one worried mother put it, "When the amnio results came back that everything was fine, then I thought, 'well it's going to be a cord accident.' I was just convinced that something else would go wrong."

If the results of the amniocentesis are not good, you and your partner will have to deal with the painful issue of what to do next. Deciding to terminate the pregnancy can be heart-wrenching, especially given your history of loss, but so can the idea of giving birth to a child with special needs. Lynn, who was at high risk for having a baby with a chromosomal problem, describes how difficult it was for her to choose between the two options:

My husband had no question that we would abort if the amnio results were bad, and when I thought about it academically, I thought that was the right approach. But because of my religious upbringing, I had a lot of problems. I was raised Catholic with the Catholic stand on abortion, so I wrestled with a lot of moral problems. Looking back, I think we probably would have gone ahead and opted to abort the child if there was a problem. But I don't know if I would have been able to live with that decision.

Fortunately for Lynn, she never had to make that decision because her amniocentesis results were normal in each of her two subsequent pregnancies. But another woman who did opt to terminate her pregnancy after her baby was diagnosed with a severe neural tube defect says she knows it was the right choice for her and her husband. She recalls:

It was the most horrific and difficult decision anyone could make. Before making our decision, we spoke with a lot of doctors, and did quite a bit of reading and talking with our family. Ultimately, we made a decision that was best for us and our baby.

Percutaneous Umbilical Cord Blood Sampling (PUBS)

This relatively new prenatal test is done to check the baby's blood for infections and other problems. The procedure itself is very similar to amniocentesis. The doctor guides a needle through the abdomen and into the uterus, but instead of extracting amniotic fluid, he retrieves a sample of the baby's blood from the umbilical cord vein. Because the risk of miscarriage is about twice as high for PUBS as for an amniocentesis, it is performed only rarely.

Home Monitoring of Your Pregnancy

Home Uterine Monitor

Since prematurity is a leading cause of newborn death, some physicians believe that a home uterine monitor is one of the most useful tools you can have if you are at risk for preterm labor. Your doctor can arrange for you to monitor any contractions you may be having beginning at about twenty weeks gestation. If the monitoring shows that you are going into early labor, your doctor can immediately administer drugs to stop it and give the baby more time to develop. We'll more closely examine how home monitors work in chapter 7.

Doppler

Some hospitals and medical supply companies rent Dopplers that you can use to check the baby's heartbeat at home whenever you are especially anxious. If you feel that you need one for peace of mind, talk to your doctor. Pam, who had suffered a second-trimester loss, found that her Doppler gave her reassurance at times when she needed it most. "It was so helpful to be able to pull out the Doppler and just sit there and listen to the baby's heartbeat," she says.

But as you know from your experience at prenatal checkups, babies can sometimes curl up into positions that make the heartbeat difficult to detect. You may have to spend several panicked moments searching for a pulse before you actually find one. It is also easy to get your own heartbeat mixed up with that of the baby's. Once you begin feeling movement, you may find that you no longer need a Doppler. It may be easier to simply eat or drink something and then lie down and wait for the baby to kick. But if you decide to rent a Doppler only to discover later that it creates too much stress, just stop using it.

Potential Danger Signs

In the last chapter, we discussed the danger signs of an impending miscarriage. Although the risk of miscarriage drops dramatically in the second trimester, there are still some potential danger signs that you should be aware of so that you can immediately report them to your doctor should they occur. In his book *How to Prevent Miscarriage and Other Crises of Pregnancy,* Dr. Stefan Semchyshyn describes a dozen symptoms that are not normal during the second trimester and what they may mean.

Sudden swelling. Sudden swelling in the second trimester can be a sign of preeclampsia. Other symptoms of this serious condition include high blood pressure and protein in the urine. It is important that preeclampsia be treated immediately to avoid serious complications for both you and your baby.

Less than average weight gain—under one pound per week. If you are not gaining enough weight, it could be that you are not eating enough. But it also could be a sign that the baby is not developing properly and has a serious condition known as intrauterine growth retardation, or IUGR. Let your doctor know if you are not gaining enough weight or you suddenly lose weight.

[C]ontractions or stiffening and hardening of the abdomen. Occasional contractions may not be a cause for concern, but if you have more than four contractions in an hour or notice a sudden increase in the number of contractions, call your doctor so that you can be assessed for signs of preterm labor.

Bleeding or spotting. Just as it was in the first trimester, bleeding or spotting is worrisome. In the second trimester, it could be a sign of a serious condition, such as placenta previa or placental abruption. Let your doctor know immediately if you see any sign of blood.

Abdominal pain. Call your doctor if you experience any kind of abdominal pain. It could be a sign of a number of serious conditions.

Gush or trickle of fluid from vagina. If fluid is coming out of your vagina, it could be a sign that you are leaking amniotic fluid. The only way to know for sure is to contact your doctor.

Unusual vaginal discharge. If there is a change in the color, consistency or odor of your vaginal discharge, let your doctor know. It could be a sign of infection or another serious condition.

Menstrual-type cramps. These types of cramps can be a sign of uterine contractions that signal the onset of preterm labor. Have your doctor check it out to be sure.

Pelvic pressure or pain in lower abdomen, back or thighs. These types of sensations could all be signs of preterm labor. Report them to your doctor.

Backache. If you have a backache that you cannot relieve, it could simply be that you strained your back. But it could also be a sign of anything from a kidney infection to premature labor. Begin monitoring for contractions as soon as your back starts to hurt. If you are not having any contractions, chances are your backache is not a sign of labor. But if the pain persists more than twenty-four hours, let your doctor know.

Chills, fever. These could be signs of a simple cold or they could be indicative of a more serious problem. Call your doctor to be sure.

Diarrhea, intestinal cramps. Again, this could be another sign of preterm labor. The only way to know for sure is to contact your doctor.

Dr. Semchyshyn also states that it is important not to discount your intuition. If you have a feeling that something is wrong, let your doctor know. If you are wrong, so much the better. But it is better to be safe than sorry.

chapter six

Pregnant Again: The Third Trimester

By THE TIME I reached the middle of the third trimester of my subsequent pregnancy, I was ready to deliver my baby. No, I wasn't having any complications to speak of, but I was determined not to go to term again. Since my first baby had died on my due date and weighed over eleven pounds, I figured it would be crazy for me to carry this second baby too long. I targeted thirty-two weeks as my delivery date because I knew of three babies, all born at thirty-two weeks gestation, who were now happy, healthy children. It wasn't that I really believed that my doctor would allow me to deliver that early by choice, I just started secretly praying that somehow I would go into labor at that point. Then something happened to change my mind.

One night when I was at the hospital attending a support group for women who were pregnant again after a loss, I was telling my counselor how impatient I was to deliver my baby. She listened to what I had to say and then did something for which I will be forever grateful. She escorted me to the neonatal intensive care unit to look at babies who were born prematurely. What I saw there shocked me. Some newborns there were barely bigger than my hand, and all of them were smaller than any baby I had ever seen. They were hooked up to monitors and had wires and tubes coming out of them. Many were breathing with the help of respirators. I also saw anxious parents huddled over the incubators, most unable to even hold their babies.

I knew right then that I did not want my baby to pay the price for my anxiousness. My baby deserved every chance to be in the best environment for as long as possible, and there was no question that the best place for him right now was in my womb.

Visiting the neonatal intensive care unit that night was one of the best things that I could have done. It made it so much easier for me to endure the next several weeks of my pregnancy. If you are feeling as anxious now as I was then, you might want to consider doing the same thing. Go to an NICU and look at babies who were born too early. I promise that it will have a profound impact on you. It's understandable since you've now reached the third trimester that you may be more eager than ever to get the pregnancy over with so you can hold your baby in your arms. But try not to forget that babies continue to develop during the last few weeks of pregnancy, and you owe it to your unborn child to give him or her the best possible start in life.

In this chapter, we'll look at ways for dealing with impatience at this stage in the pregnancy. Since this is usually the time when you'll decide whether to make preparations for the baby's homecoming, we'll examine the conflicting feelings that you're likely to have toward this. As usual, we'll discuss what you can expect at your prenatal visits and what kind of testing you may undergo. But let's begin by exploring the issue of early delivery a little further, since the most important thing to do for your baby right now is to go full-term or as close to it as possible.

Common Concerns

The Possibility of Early Delivery

In the previous chapter, we explored the fear that some women have of delivering too early, which is usual for anyone who gave birth to a premature baby who died. But there are other women, especially those who suffered a loss near term or shortly after birth, who want their babies to arrive as soon as possible and who may even pressure their doctors to induce labor a few weeks before their due date. "In the third trimester we see a huge increase in parental anxiety because they know the baby could survive outside the womb," says Joann O'Leary, who helps run the Pregnancy After a Loss Program at Abbott Northwestern Hospital. "Their feeling is, 'Get the baby out while it's still alive.' That is very normal."

In most cases, obstetricians will not deliver before thirty-eight weeks gestation unless serious complications are present. Here's why: The baby continues to develop until term. The lungs, in particular, are among the last parts of the baby to mature. That's why preterm infants often develop respiratory distress syndrome, also known as hyaline membrane disease. Basically, this means that their lungs are not yet ready to function on their own.

If you have a good reason for delivering your baby early, such as pregnancy-related complications, your obstetrician can order an amniocentesis to check for lung maturity. That's what my doctor did at thirty-seven weeks gestation, since my baby was measuring much larger than normal and his movement had noticeably slowed down. The test showed that the baby's lungs were ready, and he had absolutely no problems when he was born later that same day. But even that far along in the pregnancy, the lungs can sometimes still be immature.

The birth of my third child is a perfect example of the complications that can result from early delivery. He also was born at thirty-seven weeks gestation because he was measuring big for his gestational age and a sonogram showed that my amniotic fluid was low. But the fluid was so low that it wasn't possible to do an amniocentesis to check for lung maturity. As I've already mentioned, the baby's lungs were immature at birth and he ended up in the NICU for eight days. At nearly eight and one-half pounds, he was the biggest baby in the unit, but he was just as bad off as all the other tiny infants who were hooked up to oxygen. As hard as that experience was for me, I felt fortunate that it happened in my third pregnancy and not my second. This last time, I never prayed for an early delivery because I knew how important it was for him to stay in my womb until he matured. That meant that I didn't feel guilty when fate determined otherwise.

If you are hoping for an early delivery, you may want to talk to your doctor about delivering at thirty-eight weeks gestation, which is considered full-term. This may be an option if, like Melinda, your loss occurred close to term for unknown reasons. "My doctor said it probably wouldn't happen again, but, then again, we didn't know why it had happened the first time. So he said, 'Let's just take the baby early.'" Laura's doctor felt the same way: "At thirty-eight weeks I was slightly dilated, and my doctor induced me the next day. He figured, 'why prolong the agony?'" Your doctor will have to determine whether you are a candidate for early delivery based on the medical aspects of your pregnancy.

Preparations for the Baby

The third trimester is usually when your nesting instinct is at its strongest. You may have already experienced it in one of its many different forms. Maybe you have developed a sudden desire to clean your house or an obsession with completing every unfinished project on your to-do list. But you may be more ambivalent in making preparations for the baby's homecoming. Typically, preparing the nursery is an integral part of the nesting instinct. But in a subsequent pregnancy, that is often not the case. "Many women make no preparations at all for the child," says Dr. Peggy Morton, an adjunct associate professor of social work at NYU who has done a study on subsequent pregnancies. "They might have made preparations in the pregnancy that they lost, but then they don't in the subsequent pregnancy."

Julie is a case in point. She had set up a beautiful nursery when she was pregnant with her baby girl. But after that pregnancy ended in a loss, she refused to have any baby things in the house until after she had a baby to accompany them. "If you had come in the day before I had Timothy, you wouldn't even have known that I was going to have a baby." Phyllis took a similar approach. She says, "I really acted like it was never going to happen. I made absolutely no preparations."

I, too, found that I couldn't face the prospect of setting up the nursery during my subsequent pregnancy. In my first pregnancy, I had everything ready, right down to the matching comforter and sheets and drawers full of baby clothes. With only a few days to go before my due date, I worried that I might have forgotten something and fretted that I simply wouldn't have time to do anything once the baby was born. Of course, as you know, my first baby never came home, and when I finally did, all the baby things had already been packed away. Although I had asked for that to be done while I was still in the hospital, I wasn't prepared for the utter desolation that I would feel when I stepped foot inside the empty room that had once been a nursery. As a result, I was determined that I would not, under any circumstances, take the chance of feeling that way again. When my second son, Andrew, was born, I had not a single thing ready for him at home. Everything was packed away in the attic.

This sounds like a recipe for disaster, but it really wasn't. During the three days that I was in the hospital, friends brought me basic necessities, such as diapers, gowns and a bassinet. I discovered that was all I really needed for the first several weeks. When the baby was about six weeks old, I finally asked my husband to pull everything else down from the attic, and we set up the nursery while my son watched us from the comfort of his infant carrier. For me, that was absolutely the right thing to do, and I did the same thing again the next time I got pregnant. When we received word that my son was about to be released from the NICU, I sent my husband to the store to buy everything I needed.

Other couples, however, prefer to do exactly the opposite. Those couples whose loss occurred before they ever had time to set up a nursery, for example, often look forward to preparing for the baby's homecoming in the subsequent pregnancy. "I wanted to celebrate that I had made it further than I ever had before in the pregnancy," says Lauren, who had suffered a loss at fifteen weeks gestation. "It was finally my time to enjoy things like every other pregnant woman."

Suzanne, who had not prepared a nursery for her baby who died, was also determined to make things different in her subsequent pregnancy. She recalls:

In my last pregnancy, I couldn't bring myself to do a nursery. I just had this strange feeling that something bad was going to happen even though my pregnancy was completely normal. I just had an intuition about it. So in my next pregnancy, I felt like if I did the nursery, maybe everything would be okay.

Suzanne is unusual in that she had a feeling that her pregnancy would end in a loss. Most of us, of course, did not have a clue that our babies would die, and so we made all of our preparations in absolute bliss. If your baby died after coming home from the hospital, you even experienced the joy of seeing your child in the nursery you had so lovingly prepared. Not surprisingly, the experience of setting up a nursery is not quite the same the next time around. "Putting up the nursery was sad. It wasn't the happy occasion it once was," says one bereaved mother. "Every time we pulled something out, I would cry." Heather found that it was easier if she prepared it in stages: "I would have my husband pull down the crib, but I wouldn't let him put it up for a few weeks. Then after a while I asked him to bring down the clothes, but I didn't sort through them for a week or two. Each time I did something, I could go on to the next stage. I just really had to get used to the idea."

Some women find that they cannot do certain things until after the baby is born. Margo, for example, set up the nursery but did not wash any of the baby clothes. She says:

I wanted to do a nursery even though it was very hard to pull everything out again. While I was doing it, I would break down and cry, then I would feel guilty that the baby I was carrying did not really have my love because I was so wrapped up in my other baby. But even though I fixed the nursery, I didn't wash any of the clothes. I think that was my way of holding back.

Kelly felt much the same way. She says, "To this day, I can't buy Ivory Snow anymore because that smell brings back all the memories of packing up Joshua's clothes and putting them in boxes. This time, I got my husband to wash everything while I was still in the hospital."

Some couples don't have to make a decision about setting up a nursery because they never took theirs down to begin with. Allison, whose baby died at term, says, "My mother-in-law offered to take the nursery down, and I said, 'Are you kidding me? It's like a shrine to my daughter.' " Beth had packed away her baby boy's clothes but left the crib and the stuffed animals and other parts of the nursery just as they were. When she found out she was expecting a girl in her subsequent pregnancy, she modified what was already there. "We just put pink bows on everything," she says.

Even though you may use most of the same baby things, you might want to set aside a few special items that remind you of the baby you lost. Says Pam, "We went to Disneyland when I was pregnant with the twins, and we bought these two little outfits for them. My husband doesn't want our next baby to wear those, and I understand that." Although Brooke kept the same decor in the nursery, she felt that certain things belonged to her late son. "I took a shelf that was in the nursery and put it in the hall, and I put all of Dylan's things on it. I thought, at least he will have this."

Martha also found a compromise between using the same baby items and keeping mementos of her son. "My mother had made a quilt for Luke, and I wanted to use it because I really loved it, so I said let's put Luke's initials on one side and Mark's on the other and that really made me feel good. So Luke has a place in Mark's room."

Occasionally, in preparing for the baby's arrival, you might encounter stumbling blocks that you had not anticipated. Sylvia, for example, had surprisingly little trouble setting up the nursery but later found that she simply could not bring herself to buy a car seat to take to the hospital. She recalls:

After my baby died, I went back to the store to return the car seat that I had bought, and the girl was not very nice. She just kept asking me, "Why are you returning it?" and I was trying to avoid answering her, but she just would not give it up. Finally I burst into tears and said, "Because my baby's dead." This time, there was no way I was buying a car seat. If I had to borrow one, I'd do it. I knew we'd figure it out.

It is important for you to do only as little or as much as is comfortable. There are no rules that say you must set up a nursery or buy clothes for the baby. All of this can be done on your own time schedule. On the other hand, if you enjoy doing those things, don't feel guilty about it. You should be doing whatever makes you feel best.

Baby Shower Offers

During your third trimester, you might also start getting offers from friends who want to host a baby shower in your honor. Your reaction to these offers may depend in part on when your loss occurred in your last pregnancy. If you miscarried in the first or second trimester and never got the chance to have a shower, you may be feeling optimistic that you have made it this far in the pregnancy. This may be the first time that you have reached the point where your baby could actually survive outside the womb, which you might view as a cause for celebration. Sharon, who had a second-trimester loss, describes her feelings this way: "In the third trimester, I really seemed to have an attitude adjustment. I was just so tired of being sad all the time. So I completely redid the baby's room and had three baby showers. I really had fun toward the end as long as I could separate myself from the fear."

Virginia, who had two other living children, says that she was more willing to celebrate her baby's impending birth once she made it past the twenty-four-week mark, where she had suffered a loss the last time. "I actually had two showers because my friends knew I was having a boy, and since I only had girls, I didn't have anything for him. Plus, it had been so many years since I had had a baby that I had given everything away."

As much as you appreciate your friends' kind gestures, don't be afraid to tell them if you are uncomfortable with the idea of a shower. It is understandable that you might cringe at anything that focuses so much attention on you and presumes that a healthy baby will be the inevitable result of your pregnancy. If your baby died after birth, you may feel a shower is unnecessary because you already have everything you'll need for the next child. Rather than rejecting their offers altogether, consider suggesting that friends host a "Come See the Baby" party instead, after your child is born. My friends did that for me when Andrew was about two months old, and I thought it was a wonderful idea, especially since I had already had a baby shower in my first pregnancy. In fact, I had so many presents that the hosts asked guests to bring diapers instead of gifts. I went home with a several months' supply of diapers, and my closest friends got to see the baby that they all had been so eagerly anticipating.

Melinda's friends also came up with a way to celebrate the new baby without making her feel awkward.

With Preston, they had given me a shower, and I had gotten all this stuff. After he died, I really didn't know what to do with it. I mean, what do you do, return it? So I had all this stuff, and they were offering to give me another shower, but I declined. Since everybody really wanted to do one, that was hard for me. But they ended up taking a collection and giving me a check at the hospital so that I could buy some new things for the baby.

Occasionally, some people won't take no for an answer. Marie's coworkers, for example, threw her an impromptu baby shower at the office without telling her in advance. "They were happy for me, but I just couldn't share in their happiness. When I got home I just stuffed everything away in the closet. I didn't want to see anything." You can avoid this type of misunderstanding by letting your friends know how you are feeling throughout your pregnancy. Opening the lines of communication can be difficult but is well worth the effort.

Picking a Name

Picking a name is another way to prepare for the baby's arrival. For many couples, naming their baby helps them think of him or her as an individual and to mentally separate this child from the one who died. It can also be a way to bond with the baby before birth. Some couples choose a name based on its meaning, with many selecting one that expresses their gratitude for a healthy child. Others find out later that the name they have chosen has a special meaning. According to Sharon, "We had decided to name our baby boy Zachary, and then we looked it up and found out it meant 'God has remembered.' That sent chills up and down my spine."

As surprising as it may sound, a few people may expect you to give the next baby the same name as the one who died. This practice was more commonplace several decades ago when women were typically encouraged to forget about their loss, particularly once they were pregnant again. Some people, especially those who are older, may expect you to do the same today. Some close family friends of mine assumed that I would name my next baby Patrick. Since I knew that their comments were based on outdated ideas and not spite, I gently explained that these two babies would be brothers and therefore each would have his own name.

Your Other Children

If you are fortunate enough to have other surviving children, they can provide much-needed joy and happiness during your subsequent pregnancy. They will also help distract you so that you can focus your attention on something besides your pregnancy. But there will undoubtedly be times when they will only add to your stress. If they are toddlers and difficult to manage, you may resent that you hardly ever have any time to take care of yourself and the baby that's on the way. You may worry about overexerting yourself, especially if you were initially concerned that your pregnancy loss was caused by something you did.

You may also be more worried than ever about your surviving children's well-being, and this could cause you to become hypervigilant. Take Lynn, for example. When her three-year-old son developed a sudden fever one night, she rushed him to the emergency room without even stopping to think whether it was really necessary. She explains:

Now that I have lost a child, I know how fragile life can be. He probably wasn't sick enough for the emergency room, but it was after office hours, and there was no way I was going to take any chances with his health. So now, instead of just worrying about the baby that I'm expecting, I'm worried about my other son, too.

You may also worry about how your surviving children are coping with the stress of your subsequent pregnancy. Like you, they may be scared about the outcome and worry that something bad could happen again. O'Leary at Abbott Northwestern Hospital says it is helpful to encourage children to talk about their feelings. "Children always pick up on the feelings in the home, and usually they have the same feelings as their parents," she says. "The more open parents are to their children's questions, the more children can express what they are feeling."

Your Weight

Most doctors agree that it is ideal to gain somewhere between twenty-five and thirty-five pounds during pregnancy if your weight was in the normal range at the time of conception. But what if you're like me and have packed on thirty-five pounds or more by the beginning of the third trimester? Like many women who gain a lot of weight during pregnancy, I dreaded stepping on the scale at each prenatal visit and could not imagine why I was gaining so much weight. All told, I gained nearly sixty pounds in each of my three pregnancies and was always subjected to lectures from nurses and doctors. This caused me an incredible amount of worry and stress, mainly because

I felt that I was so powerless to control it. It seemed that no matter what I ate, the pounds kept adding up. This was all the more frustrating because I normally have no problem maintaining an average weight, and, in fact, I easily lose the extra pounds once I am no longer pregnant.

If you are worried about your own weight gain, it is important to remember that you should not diet while you are pregnant. Dieting could prevent the baby from getting the nutrition it needs for proper growth. Instead, cut out sweets and high-fat foods to see if that makes a difference. If you are doing the best you can and still gaining too much weight, talk to your doctor. What you may discover is that although gaining too much weight is frowned upon during pregnancy, it is only of serious concern if it is truly excessive or if it happens very suddenly and therefore might be an indication of a dangerous condition like toxemia.

Aside from excessive or sudden weight gain, you may have cause for concern if you are not gaining enough weight. At this point in your pregnancy, you should be gaining about a pound per week. Researchers have found that women who have inadequate weight gain in the third trimester nearly double the likelihood of delivering preterm. Women who were underweight at conception had a similar risk for early delivery. Therefore, it is important to eat the right combinations of food in adequate amounts. Again, talk to your doctor about what eating plan is best for you.

Common Feelings

Obsession over the Baby's Movements

As the baby's movements become more frequent and regular, you may notice that you are getting obsessed about checking for them. Maybe you wake up in the middle of the night to ensure that the baby is still alive or refuse to get out of bed in the morning until you have felt that first reassuring kick. A strong possibility also exists that you will have the kind of panic attack that I described in the last chapter and end up taking an unexpected trip to the hospital. Like Adriane, many women cannot help fearing the worst anytime the baby has a quiet period, especially once they know that the baby could survive on its own. Adriane describes the experience she had in her third trimester:

When my baby didn't move for a while one day, I was sure he was dead. My doctor asked me to go to the hospital so he could check me out, and I packed phone numbers, thinking I'd have to call everyone from there. I wore an old outfit, expecting it to be a "bad news' outfit that I would want to throw away. And I took one last look at my belly before we left. Then a few hours later we were smiling and looking at sonogram pictures of our beautiful son. He was okay.

If your loss occurred late in your last pregnancy, it is also not unusual to have flashbacks. Suzanne blamed herself for her baby's death at thirty-five weeks gestation. She kept asking herself whether her baby could have been saved if she had followed her intuition and called the doctor when she first suspected that the baby was not moving enough. Since she had replayed that day over and over in her mind, it wasn't surprising that she convinced herself that the same thing was happening in her subsequent pregnancy. She explains:

One day, my baby kicked once and then stopped, and that's what had happened with Jeffrey the day he died. So I called my doctor, and he said, "Try to relax. Eat a candy bar and drink a Coke and lie down for a minute," and almost right away, the baby started going crazy.

Although there's no need to obsess over the baby's movement, it is very important to always be aware of his or her pattern of activity. One of the best ways to do this is to stop what you are doing at least three times a day and monitor the baby's movements. You can then record that information on a kick chart, which we'll describe in more detail later in this chapter. The reason for keeping a chart is simple.

If you don't have a routine for checking on the baby, some days you may get so caught up in life's hustle and bustle that you forget to do it. It will also help you to identify a pattern of normal activity for your baby.

I remember once in my subsequent pregnancy when my day was especially hectic, and I completely lost track of what the baby was doing. I had been busy all morning finishing a writing assignment and then jumped in the car to rush it over to the editor's office, which was more than thirty miles away. The meeting lasted longer then I expected and distracted me enough to get my mind off the baby for a change. It was only after I had finished working and decided to go to the cemetery to visit Patrick's grave that it dawned on me that I couldn't remember how long it had been since I had felt the baby move.

I'll never forget sitting at the grave site begging God not to let this baby die, too. I prodded and poked my stomach, trying to get the baby to move. Unfortunately, he wouldn't cooperate so I had to drive all the way back home, fearing that something horrible might have happened and wondering whether I should rush to the nearest emergency room. Once I got home, ate something, and lay down on my bed, I could finally feel the baby move. But after that experience, I never again forgot to fill in my kick chart.

Worry

If your loss occurred late in your pregnancy, the third trimester may be a time of high anxiety, fearing that lightning may strike twice. As we discussed it's very likely that at some point you will replay in your mind what happened last time and believe that it may happen again. Even if your loss had occurred earlier in your pregnancy or shortly after birth, you may still fear that something could go wrong. Phyllis, who had suffered multiple miscarriages, says she was never able to relax. She recalls:

Once I got through the first trimester, my doctor was really wanting me to be optimistic because I had never made it that far in my pregnancy before. I had also had an amnio and the results were fine, and the sonograms showed the baby was doing well. But at all these milestone points when you think you should have some sense of relief, I could never relax. I would just think things like now I know it's a boy and he's really real and now if I lose him what would I do?

You might also find yourself overwhelmed with all the new information you have acquired about problematic pregnancies. Complications that you might not have even known existed before now seem like a possibility. "I must have read a million problem pregnancy books. I read them over and over again, so I knew everything that could go wrong," says one mother. You may replay in your mind every story you have ever heard about pregnancy loss. Leslie says, "Once you lose a baby, you start talking to other people who have lost babies, and you realize there are a whole lot of different ways it can happen. So I was a lot more aware of the reality of it. I wasn't as naive as I used to be."

Even if you sometimes get a brief respite from your worrying, you may immediately panic for fear that thinking good things will somehow make bad things happen. Adriane describes how that would often happen to her in her subsequent pregnancy:

It was so hard for me to just let go of the worry. I would feel hopeful one minute and that would scare me to get my hopes up, and then I would be sick with worry the next. Sometimes I would just feel sorry for myself. I felt like I had been through hell and now it was time for something—this baby—to go right.

Toward the end of your pregnancy, you may hesitate to do certain things or go certain places for fear that it might jeopardize your baby's health. Now that you have made it this far, you don't want to do anything wrong. That used to happen to me all the time. I would get spurts of energy where I would run errands and clean the house, then

I would panic and think if anything happened to the baby it would be all my fault for having overexerted myself that day. Looking back I realize that my reasoning was faulty since my doctor had assured me that I would continue my normal day-to-day activities. But that didn't stop me from worrying at the time.

The stress may become so overwhelming that you begin to wonder whether you made the wrong decision by even getting pregnant again. One mother says: "Sometimes I wonder if this pregnancy was a mistake. My emotional state has not improved that much, even though I am getting close to the end. It helps me to feel the baby move, but between movements I wonder if the baby has died, and I still miss my other baby very much."

If you feel this way, try to remember that there is no point second-guessing your decision. The fact is you *are* pregnant and there is not a whole lot you can do about it at this point. Besides, once you make it through the next few weeks, it is doubtful that you will ever again regret your decision to get pregnant. Assuming all goes well, you will have a beautiful baby to care for and love, and I have yet to meet anyone who has ever lamented that.

Being Pregnant Forever

The forty weeks of pregnancy feel like a very long time to almost every woman, but pregnancies after a loss tend to really drag on. You may find it hard to remember what it was like not to be pregnant and wonder whether you will ever reach labor and delivery. It will not help matters if toward the end you encounter friends and acquaintances who are surprised to see that you are *still* pregnant. Laura, who had endured a stillbirth followed by a miscarriage, says her subsequent pregnancy was unbearably long. "I've spent most of the last two years pregnant. I really feel like I've been pregnant for a long, long time." You may still be angry, as Katie was, that you are having to go through yet another pregnancy while others you know are enjoying their babies. "I'm resentful that I'm having to be pregnant again. I mean, it seemed like I just went through all this yesterday, and I have no baby to show for it."

You may also feel as though you have had to put your life on hold during your pregnancies. Perhaps you have quit your job, cut back on your hours or jumped off the career track for awhile. You may have given up leisure activities that you love for fear that they may be too dangerous for the baby. You undoubtedly are tired of the frequent appointments with the doctor, and are looking forward to having your old life back. As hard as it may be for you to believe, a day will come when the pregnancy seems like a distant memory, and that day may not be too far in the future. In the meantime, try to enjoy the pregnancy while you can. Even if you only get relief for a short time, it will be well worth the effort.

What are some ways to do this? For starters, consider what a miracle it is to be giving life to another human being. No matter how much you may fear that the worst will happen again, your baby is alive today, and that is reason enough to be happy. If you are being pampered by your partner and others who love you, savor that and take advantage of the excuse to relax for a change. Be grateful for the hope that you have that you will soon be giving birth to a healthy baby. Try to remember how you felt just a few months ago, before you were pregnant, when you weren't even sure whether it would be possible to conceive again. It will be a lot easier to make it through the next several weeks of your pregnancy if you can occasionally appreciate your blessings rather than always focusing on your fears.

Being Misunderstood

If your pregnancy is progressing well, you may find that some people will lose patience with your ongoing anxiety. A few may even warn you that worrying so much will harm the baby. "My mother-in-law kept telling me that my daughter was going to end up having attention deficit disorder because I was so stressed out during my pregnancy," says Trisha. "But you know what? She is a happy, well-adjusted, intelligent little girl." You may also encounter friends or family members who do not understand why you are still grieving instead of acting just like every other mother-to-be.

If your loss involved one or more of multiples, you may find that people have an even harder time understanding how you're feeling. "A lot of our families will lose only one or two of triplets, and the whole world is telling them not to grieve because they still have a baby," says Janet Bleyl, founder and president of The Triplet Connection. This insensitivity can carry over into the subsequent pregnancy, when people may wonder why you are scared that the baby you are expecting will die, too.

While it would be easy to lash out at people who behave so insensitively, it helps to remember that those who have never experienced a loss cannot even begin to imagine what you are going through. It takes a very special person to be able to put him or herself in someone else's shoes. If you have the time and the patience, you could explain for probably the millionth time that although you are happy to be pregnant again, this baby will in no way replace the one who died. Furthermore, you can stress that it is difficult for you to be as optimistic as other pregnant women usually are. For you, pregnancy is difficult and will continue to be until you deliver a healthy baby. And even then you will continue to worry, especially if your baby died after birth.

You may also find it helpful to censor the information that you share with those who tend to be insensitive because, by controlling the flow of information, you can also control the feedback that you receive. Brenda, for example, chose to share only good news with most members of her family:

If my prenatal visits were positive, then I shared the information. If I had any doubts or concerns, then I didn't share that. I just shared all the good news. Sometimes I felt like I was not even pregnant because nobody really wanted to talk about it. No one really wanted to plan a future.

Another option is simply to avoid certain people altogether. According to Trisha, "I had to stay away from people who didn't know what I had been through and didn't understand why I felt the way I did. Otherwise, it just made me even more stressed out." You will have to find the approach that works best for you, but you will have enough stress in your life without needing others to add to it.

Annoyance

Since your pregnancy is by now obvious to the entire world, you may encounter a common problem for pregnant women: unsolicited advice. Other people—and other mothers in particular—will want to tell you what to eat, do, expect and even think. Anyone who has ever been pregnant has been annoyed by these sorts of comments at some time or another, but it is usually even more unbearable when you are in the midst of a subsequent pregnancy. Since many women can't help but feel that they somehow failed when their pregnancy ended in a loss, it can be even harder to reject the advice that others want to give.

It is also not uncommon to feel as though you are constantly being judged. If you're extra careful, for example, you may be afraid that you'll be labeled neurotic. If you act carefree, you may fear that others will think you are foolhardy. If you choose to continue working until you are near term, you may wonder if your coworkers are being critical. You probably already know that it is impossible to please all of the people all of the time. Therefore, the only people you should try to please right now are yourself, your baby, your partner and your doctor—but not necessarily in that order. As for how to handle others, use your doctor as an excuse whenever possible. Simply tell anyone who questions your behavior that your obstetrician has approved you to do certain things and has advised you against others, and that you in turn want to follow doctor's orders. Not many people will want to argue with that.

Excitement

Now that you are getting closer to your delivery date, you may finally start feeling excited about this baby's arrival. Many women find that once they can see the light at the end of the tunnel, they can finally breathe a small sigh of relief. Laura describes how she felt as her due date approached: "I'm getting a lot better at being relaxed about my pregnancy as time goes by. Each time we see the doctor and we get a good report, I breathe a little easier." Sheila, who had suffered a second-trimester loss, says she had a newfound sense of confidence that she decided to act on. As she explains, "I signed up for everything there was—CPR, childbirth preparation and baby care. I just felt like it's finally my turn to enjoy this pregnancy because I had never been this pregnant before."

You might also discover, as Virginia did, that you are gaining a new appreciation for the miracle of pregnancy and childbirth. According to her,

> Before Haley died, I think I just took pregnancy for granted. I had given birth to two children with no complications and just never really thought about it. Now I really understand what a miracle it is, so my awareness of the forty-week process, and how much can go wrong, heightens my sense of gratefulness and appreciation.

As the due date nears, you may even find it easier to bond with the baby. Mary Ann says it was in her third trimester that she finally decided it was time to enjoy her baby:

> I wanted to make sure Madeleine existed even if she never existed outside my womb. We named her and everyone started referring to her by name. She was an individual before she got here. If something had happened, I think we would have had more support than if we had not done that.

Tips for Easing Anxiety

Take a Prepared Childbirth Class

If you didn't take one during your previous pregnancy, a prepared childbirth class can help you face labor and delivery with greater confidence. This can be especially important if you have never been through labor before. A class can teach you how to recognize the different stages of labor and how to manage your pain both through relaxation techniques and the use of medication. But as helpful as these classes can be, there is one important caveat: before you sign up, you must consider whether you would be comfortable attending classes filled with happy, expectant parents who are experiencing their first pregnancy. Nancy, who lost twins in her second trimester, decided that was something she was strong enough to handle. She explains:

> *I decided early in my pregnancy that I wanted to go to the class, and I was prepared for the things that I might feel. And that was the key: being prepared. It was when I was blindsided by something that I didn't expect that I would be crushed. Like when I was in the grocery store one day and I heard a song that I always sang to my twins while I was pregnant. That's the kind of thing that ripped me apart, not seeing other parents in the class.*

Unlike Nancy, Trisha did not anticipate how she might feel seeing other parents when she signed up for a prepared childbirth class. She simply enrolled because she had never had the opportunity to go when she was pregnant with her triplets who died in her second trimester. The experience turned out to be traumatic:

> *It didn't really cross my mind until I saw everyone with their happy faces and little naive stars in their eyes. It just made me burst into tears, I was sobbing. I had to leave the room. I did manage to get myself together enough to go back in there, but when they asked everyone to introduce themselves, I had trouble again. At first I couldn't say anything; I just*

stammered. Then my husband said, "This is our second pregnancy." That's
all we said because we didn't want to wig anybody out.

Joann O'Leary of Abbott Northwestern Hospital says it can be painful for couples who are experiencing a subsequent pregnancy to attend
a childbirth class with people who only know about healthy pregnancies. "It makes you feel crazier at a time when you need to feel val-
idated for who you are," she says. O'Leary's hospital is one of only a
handful in the nation that offers a class called Birth Planning in a
Subsequent Pregnancy after Loss that is especially geared to issues
of concern to couples who have had a loss. The hospital has also
published a manual for other hospitals considering starting a class of
their own.

If you cannot find such a class in your area and are uncomfortable
with the idea of going through regular childbirth lessons, try to arrange
for private instruction. Talk to a support group leader or counselor
about whether there is an instructor who would be uniquely suited to
your special needs. It must be someone who will understand that your
concerns this time go far beyond breathing and relaxation techniques.
You may be every bit as worried about how to handle flashbacks to
your last delivery and how to prepare yourself to expect a happy
outcome rather than a tragic one. The right person will be able to help
you cope with these and many other issues that you will be facing
during labor and delivery.

Write a Birth Plan

Something else to help ensure that the labor and birth process goes
more smoothly is to formulate a birth plan. This is designed to inform
your health care providers of your history and what you expect during
labor and delivery. For example, you may want to request an obstetrical nurse who is aware of your pregnancy loss and understands that
you are not a typical mother-to-be. You can also outline your preferences about the labor process itself. Consider the type of environment you prefer—a room softly lighted, or with music playing, or just

a place of peace and quiet. How much monitoring do you want of the baby and what kind of pain relief do you favor—only natural methods or an epidural? Do you want to walk around during labor or do you prefer to stay in bed? What are your views on an episiotomy? What are your preferences for baby care? Do you want to hold the baby right away and then watch as the baby is weighed and given a bath? The plan can also address issues such as feeding and having the baby stay in the room with you.

Your birth plan will be unique to you, but you can talk to your childbirth educator about the various issues that should be addressed. You should also discuss your plan with your doctor to ensure that your wishes are not at odds with hospital policies or what your physician considers acceptable. Then keep in mind that even the best-laid plans can change, especially if changes must later be made to protect either your health or your baby's.

Consider Getting a Doula

Given that you will be dealing with myriad emotional issues and may need more support than most women during the birth process, now is also the time to consider whether you will want the services of a labor support professional, also known as a doula. These are women who have been specially trained to provide emotional and physical support during labor, birth and the postpartum period. They don't replace the father in the delivery room, but instead provide extra support. For example, a doula can help with massages or other forms of natural pain relief and offer advice on the best positions for labor and birth. In an ideal world, the role of the doula could be carried out by obstetrical nurses, but they are often busy attending to other duties. A doula also can provide assistance during the pregnancy itself by explaining medical procedures, giving suggestions on how to make the pregnancy more comfortable, and helping with the preparation of a birth plan.

If you think you require the services of a labor support professional, you can get more information from the Seattle-based Doulas of North

America (DONA), which has a certification process for doulas. Some doulas are also midwives or obstetrical nurses, but many are simply women who have an interest in assisting at childbirths and have decided to be certified. It is important to interview prospective labor support professionals before making your selection. In your case, you will want to find someone who has experience working with bereaved parents. That way, in addition to being your labor coach, she can give you much-needed support during what is likely to be a very emotional time.

Call the Doctor

If at anytime you suspect that you may have a problem, trust your intuition and call your doctor immediately. Don't worry if it's after office hours or in the middle of the night. Obstetricians are used to being on call, and yours will probably understand why you are more anxious than most expecting mothers. In my first pregnancy, I remember sometimes thinking that I didn't want to bother my doctor with what I considered to be a minor concern. But after my loss, nothing could stop me from picking up the phone if I was worried. I had learned the hard way that seemingly minor problems can be a sign of serious complications.

Occasionally you may not be able to reach the doctor and will have to talk with a nurse instead. Often that will be all the reassurance you need. If there is a simple explanation for your problem, you can be assisted over the phone. But if at any point you feel like a health care professional is trying to downplay concerns that you consider to be serious, forcefully let that person know that you are worried or else you would not be calling. Then insist on talking with your doctor or having your call returned by him as soon as possible. If you feel that time is of the essence, go to the nearest emergency room. It may be a cliché, but it's worth repeating one more time that it really is better to be safe than sorry.

After you have delivered your baby, consider writing a letter to let your doctor and his staff know whether or not your needs were met.

"By letting your doctor know how you feel, it will be one more person that you can educate so that the next woman who experiences a loss will be treated better," suggests Perry-Lynn Moffitt, coauthor of *A Silent Sorrow: Pregnancy Loss.* "But don't just write about what you didn't like; write about the good things that happened, too. The good letters are as important as the critical letters because often doctors and medical staff don't know if they have done something right, either."

Moffitt adds that if you really want to make an impression, you should write to the head hospital administrator or other staff members with power who have a right to know whether a particular doctor or staff member has done an especially good or bad job. That will help ensure that your message gets across to the right people.

Insist on Frequent Monitoring

Even if your pregnancy is not considered high risk, you can insist on frequent prenatal visits for your peace of mind. Don't be embarrassed if you just want to hear the baby's heartbeat or get your blood pressure checked. Your doctor may even consider doing more sonograms or non-stress tests to check on the baby's well-being if you have reason to be concerned. Sheila says her doctor seemed to have a sixth sense about when she really needed to see her baby. "If I looked teary-eyed, he'd say it looks like a sonogram day today," she says. Not every doctor will be as adept at reading minds, so the best thing you can do is make your feelings known.

Of course, since monitoring can be expensive, the number of sonograms you can have may depend in part on your insurance coverage. Some plans will cover only one sonogram unless there are complications that make another one necessary. (Insurers usually don't consider a mother's anxiety to a good enough reason for testing.) My insurance company balked at paying for prenatal monitoring, but I decided not to worry about it. My doctor ordered several sonograms, non-stress tests and biophysical profiles in my subsequent pregnancies, both to check on the baby and to give me peace of mind. To me, they were worth every penny. Many doctors and hospitals will be willing to work out a payment plan for you, so you can slowly pay off the balance over a period of months or even years. It will probably be a lot easier to make those payments once you have your baby and know that you have been given a truly priceless gift.

Have a Glass of Orange Juice

We've already discussed how reassuring it is to feel the baby move. Not surprisingly then, one of the best ways to ease your anxiety during the third trimester of your pregnancy is to stop what you are doing every once in a while and check for movement. You'll generally get more cooperation if you drink a glass of orange juice or eat something sweet and lie down.

I always liked to check on the baby before getting out of bed in the morning. It was my way of making sure that nothing had gone wrong while I slept. If the baby was asleep, I would try not to panic. Instead, I would just push on my belly. He would almost always push right back and it would turn into a little game. I also found it helpful to check for movement before leaving for my doctor appointments. As long as I had already felt my baby kick, I could relax when my obstetrician pulled out his Doppler.

Some women find that they can't even make it through the night without waking up to check on the baby once or twice. "Every so often, my husband would wake up and find me in the kitchen eating something or lying on the couch," admits one mother. "He thought it was strange, but it really had become part of my regular routine. I never could manage to sleep through the night because I always had to make sure that the baby was all right. It turned out to be good training for when my baby was actually born." Be sure to put your hands on your stomach when you're checking on the baby. This will allow you to feel subtle movements that you otherwise might miss.

Eliminate Unnecessary Stress

Subsequent pregnancies can be extremely stressful. They're stressful from the instant you consider whether to try again to the moment the doctor pronounces that you have given birth to a healthy baby boy or girl. And even then, the stress of raising that child is only just beginning. Given these unusually high stress levels, it is crucial to do everything possible to try to eliminate all *unnecessary* stress.

This might mean cutting back on your hours at work or saying no to overtime. It could be declining an invitation to volunteer at your church or bowing out of a dinner party. Anything that adds stress to your life should be off-limits to you right now. Instead, pamper yourself. Take naps during the day. Let the housework go. Read a good book. Do something you really like.

Practice Relaxation Techniques

Relaxation is an art that has been practiced down through the centuries in many different forms. Yoga and meditation are two of the most widely used relaxation techniques. Both involve breathing slowly while clearing your mind of distracting thoughts or worries. This is something you can easily do anytime you feel yourself getting tense or nervous. You also might find it helpful to sit quietly and picture a beautiful place in your mind. Keep your focus on the beauty of the scene and try to imagine it in detail, including colors and sounds. Push away any ugly or frightening thoughts and soon you may find yourself relaxing. Soothing music can also help relax the mind as well as the body. If you want to learn more about relaxation techniques, read one of the many books that describes common relaxation practices. You may also want to consider getting a book on panic attacks or anxiety disorders that describes how relaxation can help you cope with the common symptoms of those conditions.

Keep Your Eye on the Prize

In the third trimester of pregnancy, sometimes it can be hard to feel anything but miserable. Your belly is getting bigger, your clothes are getting tighter and you may have reached a point where you are having trouble moving around. Even getting a good night's sleep can be difficult since you are constantly getting up to go to the bathroom or to check that the baby is still alive. When you combine all these minor annoyances with your fear of another loss, it's easy to see why you may be sick and tired of being pregnant.

When you're feeling your worst, it may help to reflect on why you decided to put yourself through this pregnancy in the first place. The reason is obvious: it's because you wanted a baby and have wanted one for a very long time. As bad as things may be right now, this pregnancy will soon be over and, with any luck, you will have your long-awaited healthy baby. That doesn't mean you will not still miss the baby who died. In some ways, your family will always be incomplete because of your loss. But you will have the joy of giving birth to a baby who may not have been conceived otherwise and raising that child to adulthood. That, and that alone, is the prize that makes everything else worthwhile.

Prenatal Visits

By the beginning of your third trimester, you may be seeing your doctor as often as once a week, and toward the end, at least twice a week. You might start seeing a perinatologist in addition to your regular obstetrician. In the third trimester, the doctor will be closely monitoring the baby's movement and growth as well as the amount of amniotic fluid around your baby. If all three of these are normal, your chances for a good outcome are greatly improved.

Unless you are having complications, the majority of your prenatal visits will continue to be routine. You'll have your weight and blood pressure checked, and a urinalysis will be done to check for sugar or protein in your urine or signs of infection. Your obstetrician will continue to listen to the baby's heartbeat and measure your tummy to be sure your baby is growing normally. As your due date approaches, your physician will start doing pelvic exams to look for changes in your cervix. You might also be undergoing a variety of prenatal tests to check on the baby's well-being. Depending on your particular circumstances, you may have sonograms, non-stress tests or biophysical profiles. We'll examine these tests later in this chapter.

Since you will be seeing your doctor so often, you will have plenty of opportunities to ask questions about anything that may be concerning you. Now is the time to talk to your doctor about your impending labor and delivery. If you have never been through labor, you might want to ask how you can tell if you are in labor. You may also discuss when during labor you should head for the hospital. If you've been through all this before, tell your doctor how you feel about childbirth now that you have experienced such a tragic outcome. Sometimes talking about your fears can help dispel them. You will likely receive some encouraging words in return that will help you face labor and delivery with more confidence.

Prenatal Tests of the Third Trimester

Screen for Gestational Diabetes

Early in the third trimester, you will have what is known as a one-hour glucose tolerance screening. This is to determine if you should have further testing for gestational diabetes, a pregnancy-induced form of diabetes that can have serious consequences for both a mother and her baby. The screen consists of drinking a sweet glucose solution followed one hour later by a blood test to check the level of sugar in your blood. If the reading is outside the normal range, you will have to return for a three-hour test to confirm the results. If the results show that you do have gestational diabetes, your doctor will recommend that you go on a special diet or take daily insulin injections to control the condition.

Any pregnant woman can develop gestational diabetes, but the condition is more common among women who have a family history of diabetes, have had the disorder in a previous pregnancy or are over the age of thirty-five. You are also at higher risk if you have given birth to a baby over ten pounds or have had a previous stillbirth.

Screen for Group B Streptococcus Infection

Sometime between the thirty-fifth and the thirty-seventh week of your pregnancy, you will also be screened for Group B Streptococcus (GBS). Chances are that you have never heard of GBS, or, if you have, you are not quite sure what it is or how it can harm your baby. GBS is described in chapter 1 under the causes of early infant death, but since I cautioned you not to read that section unless it specifically applied to you, it is worth discussing again.

GBS is a bacteria that is the leading cause of life-threatening infections in newborns. (It is not the same as Group A Streptococcus, which causes strep throat.) An estimated 8,000 babies contract GBS every year, and as many as 800 die, while many others are left mentally or physically handicapped. GBS is passed from mother to baby during childbirth, often by women who did not even know that they were carriers of the bacteria. But while GBS usually produces no symptoms in a pregnant woman when it is present in the vagina or lower intestine, it can have fatal consequences for a newborn if it enters the baby's bloodstream. Studies have shown that there is a higher incidence of GBS infection under the following conditions: when labor is premature, if the membranes rupture more than twelve hours before the baby is born, if the mother has a fever over 100.4° F before or during labor or if the woman has a history of GBS in previous births.

Although all this information is no doubt frightening, there is some good news, too. The Centers for Disease Control and Prevention estimates that more than 75 percent of all cases of GBS in the first week of a baby's life could be prevented if all women are screened for the bacteria between the thirty-fifth and the thirty-seventh week of pregnancy, and if those who test positive are then treated with intravenous antibiotics during labor. The screening is simple. Your doctor can do a vaginal or rectal culture that can determine if you are a carrier. Since about 10 to 35 percent of all healthy, adult women carry the bacteria in their vagina and/or lower intestine, but not all of them pass the bacteria on to their babies, doctors sometimes prefer to give antibiotic treatment only to the women who fall into the high-risk categories that we just discussed. But if you test positive for the bacteria and are worried about the possible consequences, discuss the situation with your doctor. Given your history of loss, you need to be aware of both the pros and cons of the antibiotic treatment even if you do not fall into any of the high-risk categories.

Non-stress Test

The fetal heart rate is one of the best indicators of a baby's well-being during late pregnancy. In healthy babies, the heart rate is vigorous and accelerates whenever the baby moves. If, on the other hand, a baby is in distress, the heart rate is often weak or remains unchanged with activity. A non-stress test allows a doctor to observe how the baby's heart responds to movement.

If you are required to have a non-stress test, a fetal monitor will be strapped onto your stomach and you will be asked to push a button each time the baby moves. Both the fetal heart rate and the fetal activity will be recorded side by side on a printout. If your baby does not move or if the heart rate does not increase during the thirty-minute monitoring period, further testing may need to be done to determine whether the baby is simply sleeping or in some kind of trouble. As a rule, non-stress tests are better at indicating fetal health than fetal illness. That is, good results are usually a pretty strong indicator that the baby is doing fine, but bad results do not necessarily mean that the baby is in distress. More testing is always required to be sure.

Biophysical Profile

A biophysical profile combines a non-stress test with a detailed ultrasound examination to evaluate the baby's condition. In addition to the fetal heart rate, the doctor will look at the amount of amniotic fluid around the baby, the baby's activity and how the baby is positioned. The baby will also be examined for fetal breathing movement. Even while they are still in the uterus, healthy babies move their chest and lungs in such a way to appear to be breathing. But sick babies are sometimes too weak to carry out these movements. Each of these five areas is evaluated using a scoring system that ranges between 0 and 2, with 0 being abnormal and 2 being normal. The higher the score, the better it is for the baby. The test can be repeated every week or even more often, especially if most of the scores fall in the middle range.

Stress Test

Just as the non-stress test evaluates how the fetal heart rate responds to movement, the stress test examines how the heart rate reacts to uterine contractions. It gives doctors valuable information that enables them to determine whether a baby is strong enough to make it through actual labor. In this test, which can take two or more hours, the mother is once again hooked up to a fetal monitor, but this time the focus is on contractions, not movement. If she is not having enough contractions on her own, the doctor may administer a small amount of oxytocin to induce contractions. If the baby's heart rate drops during contractions or does not maintain a normal baseline, it could indicate trouble. Since a stress test can sometimes result in premature labor, it is done only under the strictest supervision. Despite its inherent risks, the test provides information that enables the doctor to detect potential problems that otherwise might be overlooked.

Amniocentesis to Check for Lung Maturity

If early delivery is being considered, your doctor can perform an amniocentesis to determine if the baby will be able to breathe on its own after birth. The amniotic fluid obtained during the amniocentesis can be tested for substances that indicate if the baby's lungs are coated with surfactant. Surfactant is a coating that prevents the air sacs in the lungs from sticking together. Babies born without enough surfactant in their lungs may develop respiratory distress syndrome, the most common cause of death in premature babies. If you must have an early delivery for medical reasons and the baby's lungs are not yet mature, the baby can be treated before birth with steroids to mature the lungs more quickly.

Home Monitoring of Your Pregnancy

Kick Charts

From the twenty-eighth week on, it is important to keep track of the baby's movements. You can do this with a kick chart, which will get you in the habit of checking on the baby's well-being at least three times a day. That might be just before you get out of bed in the morning, again after lunch and right before bedtime. Pick a schedule that is convenient for you, but try to do it around the same time each day. Monitoring the baby's movements is easy. Simply lie down on your left side and keep track of how long it takes to feel ten movements. Record only kicks and jabs, not slight flutters. The average baby takes about twenty minutes to kick ten times, but your baby may routinely do it faster or slower. After a few days of doing this, you should begin to see a pattern of the baby's activity that will help you assess if there are any changes in fetal movement that could be cause for concern. Your kick chart might look something like the one on the next page (see page 252).

We already mentioned that "normal activity" is whatever is normal

KICK CHART

Date	Starting Time	Movements	Ending Time	Total Minutes
May 18	8:30 a.m.	ᛏᚻᛁ ᛏᚻᛁ	8:55 a.m.	25
	1:45 p.m.	ᛏᚻᛁ ᛏᚻᛁ	2:07 p.m.	22
	9:03 p.m.	ᛏᚻᛁ ᛏᚻᛁ	9:12 p.m.	9
May 19	8:17 a.m.	ᛏᚻᛁ ᛏᚻᛁ	8:36 a.m.	19
	1:28 p.m.	ᛏᚻᛁ ᛏᚻᛁ	1:49 p.m.	21
	9:20 p.m.	ᛏᚻᛁ ᛏᚻᛁ	9:32 p.m.	12

for your baby. Admittedly, that's not always easy to determine. My third baby, for example, was so erratic from day to day that I was never quite sure what was going on. Some days he was superactive and other days he seemed to be sleepy. What do you do in cases like that?

One rule of thumb uses the kick chart. If after an hour of monitoring you still haven't felt anything, eat or drink something and then monitor for another hour. If you still have not felt movement, call your doctor. The baby may just be sleeping, but it is better to err on the side of safety. You also will want to let your doctor know if you notice a dramatic slowdown in movement over a period of a day or two. This could be a sign of a problem with your placenta or an infection that is causing the baby to become lethargic. The bottom line is to trust your intuition. If you are concerned about the baby's movements, for any reason whatsoever, call your doctor.

Checking for Contractions

If you do not have a home uterine monitor, you must be very aware of any contractions that may signal the onset of labor. In fact, it is a good idea to check for contractions while you are monitoring the baby's movements. Put your hands on your belly and note whether your uterus is hardening and softening. If it is, that means you are having a contraction. Check your watch and note how long it takes the uterus to become soft again. Also write down the time between contractions. Call your doctor if you feel three or more contractions in a one-hour period or there is less than fifteen minutes between any contraction. Depending on your history, your obstetrician may ask you to continue monitoring for a few more hours, or he may want to see you immediately. If it turns out that you are in premature labor, it can often be stopped with medication. See chapter 7 for more on this topic.

Those of you who have never gone through labor before may wonder how you can tell when your delivery may be imminent. Generally, if your contractions are irregular and do not increase in frequency or severity, or they go away if you change positions, you probably are not in labor. In contrast, contractions that show a definite pattern and get worse instead of better, and do not go away if you change positions, are a sign of labor. If you're unsure about any symptoms that you are having, describe them to your doctor.

Be Aware of Danger Signs in Late Pregnancy

As we just discussed, having three or more contractions during a one-hour period is a danger sign if it happens before your due date, especially if they are less than fifteen minutes apart or accompanied by other signs of labor, such as menstrual-type cramps and diarrhea. Any sudden changes in the baby's movements should also set off an alarm. But there are other problems that we have not yet touched on which are also serious causes for concern. Heavy vaginal bleeding late in the pregnancy is one of them. This often indicates a problem with the placenta, such as placenta previa or placental abruption. Preterm labor can also cause vaginal bleeding. Call your doctor immediately if this should happen to you. You will also need to contact your doctor if you are leaking fluid from your vagina. This could be a sign that you are losing amniotic fluid or that your membranes have ruptured and that you are going into labor.

chapter seven

Pregnant Again: The High-Risk Pregnancy

MOST OF US assume that once we have had one pregnancy end in a loss, all of our subsequent pregnancies will automatically be labeled high risk. But that's not necessarily true. If your loss was due to something random that is unlikely to recur, you will be considered high concern rather than high risk. That means your obstetrician will want to see you frequently and run more prenatal tests than usual, not so much for medical necessity as for your peace of mind. In other words, even though your doctor may be convinced that the worst won't happen again, you will still need plenty of reassurance. Who would fall into this type of "high concern" category? I did, for one. There was no reason to believe that the umbilical cord problem that caused my loss would ever recur in future pregnancies. I also did not have any other major complications during my forty-week gestation. If you, too, had an otherwise normal pregnancy and your loss was due to a random event—like a knot in the cord, a bacterial infection or a rare chromosomal abnormality—chances are that you are not considered high risk, either. In that case, this chapter does not apply to you.

But many other women are indeed at higher risk in their subsequent pregnancy. That's because they had problems in their last pregnancy that have a relatively high chance of recurring. If you are one of these women, you are in good company. It is estimated that one out of every four pregnancies is high risk. Or, put another way, of the nearly four million women who give birth in the United States every year, close to one million have complications that put either their life or the baby's at risk. Remember, though, that just because you are labeled high risk, it does not necessarily mean that you will actually experience complications during your subsequent pregnancy. It only means that you are at higher risk than normal for developing problems that could result in preterm birth or pregnancy loss.

In this chapter, we'll explore some of the reasons that you might be placed into the high-risk category and what the implications will be for your medical care. We'll also discuss some of the feelings you may have during your pregnancy as well as tips for easing anxiety. Unlike the other chapters, though, we'll examine issues that most pregnant women never have to worry about—even those who have suffered a loss. These include bed rest and hospitalization and the impact they can have on your personal life and your career. Also, our tips for easing anxiety will not focus as much on activities that any woman might do in her subsequent pregnancy. Instead, we'll look at techniques that are designed to help keep you from going crazy if you're confined to your bed, or, even worse, cooped up in a hospital room.

All of us who suffered a loss and became pregnant again know firsthand how scary the subsequent pregnancy can be. Knowing that you are at higher risk for having complications makes it even scarier. Anyone who has been through the experience will tell you to prepare yourself for some tense moments in the nine months ahead. Nevertheless, keep in mind that by getting good prenatal care, monitoring your pregnancy closely yourself and possibly curtailing your activities, you will have a better chance of giving birth to that healthy child you so desperately want.

Common Reasons for High-Risk Status

History of Preterm Labor or Delivery

By far, the most common reason that women are considered high risk in a subsequent pregnancy is because of their history of preterm labor and delivery. Nearly 10 percent of all babies are born prematurely every year. That may not sound like many until you consider the actual numbers: about 380,000 babies in the United States alone. Unfortunately, if your loss was the result of a preterm birth, you are at greater risk of having it happen again in the subsequent pregnancy. Your risk may be reduced if doctors are able to determine the cause of your preterm delivery. But in more than half of all cases, doctors never find the reason why a woman delivers too early. This makes it more difficult to take measures to prevent it from happening again.

"Every woman who has had a high-risk pregnancy hopes it will not happen the next time. They just want to be normal," says Candace Hurley of Sidelines National Support Network for women experiencing high-risk pregnancies. "But women who have delivered preterm have a pretty good chance of delivering another baby preterm."

Before you get discouraged, though, consider this: although doctors may not be able to always prevent preterm labor altogether, they are getting better at determining it and then taking steps to control it once it occurs. An advance in the detection of preterm labor came with the recent government approval of two new diagnostic tests. Salivary Estriol, or SalEst, is a test designed to assist physicians in identifying women at risk for spontaneous preterm labor and delivery. Administered to women between the twenty-second and thirty-sixth week of pregnancy, it measures the levels of estriol in the saliva. That is significant because there is an increase in salivary estriol several weeks before the onset of spontaneous labor. If the test shows a woman is at risk, her doctor can then determine which course of treatment would be most effective. A second diagnostic test, Fetal Fibronectin or fFN, can be done whenever a woman between the twenty-fourth and thirty-fourth week of pregnancy reports symptoms of preterm labor or is believed to be at risk for an early delivery. If the test is positive, it alerts the doctor that intervention will be necessary to either prolong the pregnancy or prepare the woman and her baby for an early delivery.

It is also important that you recognize the early warning signs. The sooner you let your obstetrician know that you may be in labor, the quicker you can get medication that can reduce uterine contractions. Time is of essence, because once your cervix has started to dilate, it is difficult if not impossible to prevent labor from progressing. When preterm labor is detected right away, however, the chances of stopping it are very good.

"I don't think a woman should become obsessed with statistics or the possibility that something could go wrong again," continues Hurley of Sidelines, "but you should be educated about signs and symptoms of preterm labor or signs and symptoms of whatever problems you had the last time." We'll further examine early warning signs and treatment options later in this chapter.

Although it is understandable that you would be terrified at the prospect of delivering again too early, given the outcome of your last pregnancy, it is also important not to lose sight of the more promising facts. As we discussed in chapter 5, babies born at twenty-eight weeks gestation or later have a better than 90 percent chance of survival. Moreover, advances in prenatal care have also been effective in reducing the overall incidence of preterm births. This means that even though you are at higher risk of having a preterm birth, your chances of a good outcome are better today than they ever have been.

Incompetent Cervix

When doctors determine why a woman went into early labor, they often find that the cause was an incompetent cervix. About 15 percent of all second-trimester losses are caused by this condition in which the cervix, or opening to the womb, is too weak to withstand the pressure that a growing baby places on it. It then dilates and thins prematurely, leading to preterm birth and pregnancy loss.

To prevent this from happening again, your doctor can perform a cervical cerclage, a procedure whereby stitches or a band are placed around the cervix to close and reinforce it. The cerclage is most commonly put in place just after the first trimester when the threat of miscarriage is lower. In some cases, you will be required to rest in bed afterward and possibly take medication to prevent contractions. You will also be given antibiotics to prevent an infection. When the procedure is done in time and no complications arise, the chances of a healthy pregnancy are very good.

Twins, Triplets or More

The only thing better than having one healthy child is having two, three or more. Women who have suffered a loss and then become pregnant with multiples often feel that they have been doubly, or triply, blessed as a result of their trials and tribulations. But with this blessing comes additional worries. Women who are pregnant with multiples are considered high risk because they are much more likely to have complications than women who are pregnant with only one child. The most common complications are premature rupture of the membranes and preterm labor. That's largely because the extra weight of carrying multiples puts a strain on the uterus. But multiple gestation also commonly leads to conditions like hypertension and anemia.

But the news is not all bad. The risks associated with multiple pregnancies are much lower now than they had been, due to early detection through ultrasound and highly effective treatment of premature labor. You can also increase your odds of a healthy delivery by seeing a doctor experienced in multiple pregnancies. Just in case your babies do come too early, though, it's also a good idea to deliver at a hospital with a high-level neonatal intensive care unit.

History of Placental Problems

Another relatively common reason for high-risk status is a history of placental problems. If your pregnancy loss was the result of placental abruption, for example, you have about a 12 percent chance of having it happen again. While there is nothing you can do to prevent it, you can try to minimize the risks. Since high blood pressure is believed to be one of the most significant causes of placental abruption, it is important that you monitor your blood pressure closely, both at home and through frequent visits to the doctor. Cigarette smoking also increases your risk; so, if you still smoke, quit. Perhaps most important, if placental abruption is diagnosed early and the separation is minimal, the condition can usually be controlled through a combination of bed rest and medication.

Placenta previa is another life-threatening problem that can recur in a subsequent pregnancy. It occurs when the fertilized egg implants in the lower portion of the uterus, rather than in the upper portion, as in a normal pregnancy, and the placenta grows over or very near the internal opening of the cervix. When this happens there can be heavy vaginal bleeding, which can result in premature delivery and, in some cases, pregnancy loss. Most often, placenta previa corrects itself over the course of the pregnancy. The placenta simply moves up higher into the uterus. Until it does, bed rest can help stop the bleeding and lower your chances of a premature delivery. In severe cases, you may be hospitalized and closely monitored until the baby is able to survive outside the womb. Despite the tragic outcome of your last pregnancy, nine out of ten babies survive this condition. Try to keep that in mind if you have to struggle through this complication a second time.

History of Two or More Miscarriages

In chapter 1 we mentioned that if you have suffered one miscarriage, your odds of carrying the next baby to term are somewhere between 80 and 90 percent, or about the same as the general population. But once you have suffered two successive miscarriages, the odds of suffering another loss increase rather dramatically. Specifically, you have around a 25 percent chance of having another miscarriage. Needless to say, these odds place you in the high-risk category. The good news is that your chances for a favorable outcome are greatly improved if doctors can pinpoint the causes of your pregnancy loss and eliminate them.

Autoimmune disorders have been increasingly linked to recurrent miscarriages. This condition is characterized by antibodies that go haywire and start attacking normal cells instead of foreign organisms like bacteria or viruses. If laboratory tests confirm that an autoimmune disorder may have been responsible for your losses, with the right treatments, your odds of having a successful pregnancy can improve to the 90-percent range. Depending on the details of your history, you may be advised to do something as simple as taking one baby aspirin a day or as complicated as undergoing experimental intravenous immunoglobulin (IVIg) therapy.

Abnormalities of the uterus are another significant cause of miscarriages. If your doctor finds and corrects a uterine problem, it will be one less thing to interfere in the course of your next pregnancy and cause serious complications.

Since progesterone deficiency may also play a role in miscarriages, your doctor may prescribe hormone supplements if you have a history of early losses. Although the effectiveness of progesterone therapy has not been clinically proven, it is believed to be safe and could even prove beneficial.

Since no treatment can guarantee that complications won't arise, your obstetrician will want to closely monitor you and your baby throughout your pregnancy. You may have monthly sonograms to check your baby's growth. And beginning at thirty-two weeks gestation, you may also have weekly biophysical profiles and non-stress tests.

Genetic Problems

In our discussion of miscarriages, we didn't mention genetic abnormalities, which are by far the leading cause of miscarriages. That's because the vast majority of genetic abnormalities are random events that are unlikely to recur and therefore will not place you at high risk in future pregnancies. If, however, genetic testing shows that you or your partner have a chromosomal problem (known as a balanced translocation) or are carriers of any inherited diseases, your subsequent pregnancy will definitely be considered high risk.

A genetic counselor can explain the risk of birth defects in a future pregnancy as well as the options that will be available to you. But there is not a lot you can do to change your odds once you are actually pregnant again. (Before conception, you could reduce your risk by using an egg or sperm from a healthy donor.) What you can do, however, is have prenatal testing that will either put your mind at ease or help you decide whether to terminate the pregnancy or prepare for the birth of a sick baby. Chorionic villus sampling and amniocentesis can detect genetic defects, including inherited diseases.

Chronic Medical Conditions

If you suffer from a serious chronic medical condition, all of your pregnancies will be considered high risk. The actual risk depends on the type of illness and its severity. For example, if you have high blood pressure or hypertension, you are at higher risk for developing a condition such as preeclampsia or eclampsia. These reduce the flow of blood and nutrients to your baby, increasing the risk of intrauterine growth retardation, preterm birth and stillbirth. If you are an insulin-dependent diabetic, you are also at higher risk for preeclampsia in addition to episodes of high or low blood sugar levels. As a result, your baby may be either very small or very large for gestational age and at greater risk for congenital abnormalities.

Other chronic conditions that can cause problems in pregnancy include anemia, thyroid disorders, kidney disease, epilepsy, asthma, systemic lupus erythematosus and certain heart conditions. Regardless of which chronic illness you suffer from, the best thing you can do is get in good shape before you conceive. By taking care of yourself, you will be able to take better care of your unborn child.

Pregnancy after Age Thirty-Five

None of us who were over thirty-five when we got pregnant again likes to think that our age could possibly put our baby's health at risk, but that's how the medical community sees it. As most of us already know, older mothers are considered at higher risk for chromosomal defects such as Down syndrome. But what you may not know is that you are also more likely to develop pregnancy-induced hypertension and gestational diabetes.

Again, the healthier you are before you conceive, the lower your chances of developing complications during pregnancy. Good prenatal care is also important. By taking extra good care of yourself during the pregnancy, you greatly improve your chances of a good outcome.

Unexpected Complications

Sometimes you can begin the pregnancy in the "high-concern" category and end up being considered high risk before the forty weeks are over. That's because a number of conditions can develop without any prior history. In fact, some of the complications that we have been discussing—such as preterm labor and placental problems—can strike unexpectedly. So can many others, such as pregnancy-induced hypertension, gestational diabetes and intrauterine growth retardation. As long as you are under the care of a competent doctor, you can rest assured that there is a very good chance that your problems will be detected and treated as soon as they occur.

Common Concerns

Bed Rest

Since bed rest is the one of the most commonly prescribed treatments for the complications of pregnancy, it may be on your mind once you are considered high risk. There are several reasons why you may be ordered to rest in bed at some point during your pregnancy. Preterm labor, hypertension, bleeding problems, intrauterine growth retardation and a multiple pregnancy are just a few of them. Bed rest is controversial in some medical circles since there is no hard scientific evidence that absolutely proves its effectiveness. But many obstetricians firmly believe that it does make a difference and so do many patients who have healthy outcomes after resting in bed in a subsequent pregnancy.

If you are facing the threat of preterm labor, for example, getting off your feet will eliminate activity that could trigger contractions. Two additional benefits are that it will offset the gravitational pull on the baby and help lower your stress level. These are some of the same reasons why bed rest is usually recommended for women who are pregnant with multiples or those who have had surgery for an incompetent cervix.

Bed rest will also most likely be prescribed if prenatal tests indicate your baby is showing signs of intrauterine growth retardation. Lying on your left side will improve the flow of blood to the placenta, increasing the supply of oxygen and nutrients for the baby. The improved blood flow to the placenta is also why bed rest is commonly recommended for pregnancy-induced hypertension. It improves the functioning of the kidneys as well, helping eliminate the swelling that is commonly associated with high blood pressure.

Some women know that at some point in their pregnancy they will be on bed rest. For example, Cynthia, who was pregnant with twins, had been told by her doctor that she would be required to stay in bed once she hit twenty weeks gestation. To her surprise, she discovered that even though she had been dreading giving up all her activities,

What Is Bed Rest?

The term "bed rest" is a familiar one to mothers experiencing high-risk pregnancies, but they are often confused about the exact parameters of their limitations. Variabilities depend on each mother, the extent of her complications and even on the physician himself. This chart has been developed in an attempt to help mothers and their OB/GYNs mutually define needs in specific situations. Since variables change during each individual pregnancy, you may wish to make several copies of this chart, to be completed at various stages of your pregnancy.

Date

What can I do right now?

1. Activity Level

Maintain a normal activity level _____

Slightly decrease activity level _____

Greatly decrease activity level _____

2. Working Outside the Home

Maintain my full-time job _____

Work part-time
(*how many hours?*) _____

Work in my home
(*how many hours?*) _____

Stop work completely
Why: _____

3. Working Inside the Home

Continue doing all housework _____

Decrease housework including:
Heavy lifting (*laundry,
moving furniture, etc.*) _____

Preparing meals (*standing on
feet for a prolonged period
of time*) _____

Vigorous scrubbing _____

Other: _____

Why: _____

4. Child Care

Care for other children as usual _____

No lifting children _____

Have another caretaker watch
an active toddler _____

Have permanent caretaker for
children _____

Why: _____

5. Mobility

Continue normal mobility _____

Limit mobility
(*sit down frequently*) _____

Lie down each day
(*how many hours?*) _____

Recline all day
(*propped up?*) _____

Lie down flat all day
(*on side?*) _____

May walk stairs
(*how many times a day?*) _____

Stairs forbidden _____

Take a shower/wash hair _____

Eat lying down? Sitting up?
Sitting at table? _____

Why: _____

6. Driving

May drive a car _____

May be a passenger in a car
(*frequency?*) _____

7. Bathroom Privileges

May use bathroom normally _____

Should actively avoid
constipation _____

May not use bathroom
(*use bedpan*) _____

Why: _____

8. Sexual Relations

May continue normal sexual
relations _____

Should limit sexual relations
(*maximum times a month?*) _____

Should avoid sexual intercourse _____

Should avoid all types of relations that stimulate female orgasm _____

Should abstain from sexual relations _____

Why: _____

9. Maintenance of Pregnancy

Should monitor fetal activity ___ hours each day by hand, counting movements _____

Should drink wine each day (*When? How much?*) _____

Should abstain from alcohol _____

Should limit cigarette smoking (*no. per day?*) _____

Should stop smoking cigarettes _____

Should monitor fetus by home uterine monitor ___ hours daily _____

Should take (*drug*) _____ _____ times daily, dosage: _____ Reason: _____

Should take (*drug*) _____ _____ times daily, dosage: _____ Reason: _____

Should follow these dietary rules: Plenty of: Protein, vegetables, fruits, calcium, other: _____
_____

Avoid: Excess salt, excess fats, junk food, spicy foods, other:
_____

Approximate number of calories a day:
_____

What might I expect in the future?

1. Decrease in activity level _____
2. Limitations of work _____
   Stop working completely _____
3. Decrease housework _____
4. Need for childcare helper _____
5. Need to recline in bed _____
6. Limit driving _____
   Stop driving _____
7. Limit sexual relations _____

Abstain from sexual relations _____

8. Need to self-monitor fetal activity _____
9. Need to use a home uterine monitor _____
10. Need to take labor-inhibiting drugs _____
11. Need to have a cervical stitch put in _____
12. Need to stay in hospital for some period of time _____
13. Need to have amniocentesis _____
14. Need to have sonograms/ultrasounds _____
15. Need to visit OB/GYN more frequently than normal _____
16. Need to visit a high-risk specialist _____
17. Need to have fetoprotein levels done _____
18. Need to have a blood sugar screening _____
19. Need to have a non-stress test _____
20. Need to have a stress test _____

If problems arise and I go into premature labor . . .

1. When should I contact my OB/GYN? ___
2. Where will I be hospitalized? _____
3. Where might I be transferred? _____
4. Names of OB/GYN at other hospital?
   _____
5. Where would my baby be hospitalized?
   _____
6. Could my husband be present at delivery?
   _____
7. Is there a possibility of a cesarean? ___

Hospital Bed Rest

1. What position do I have to be in? _____
Trendelenberg (*head lowered*) _____
On side (*left or right?*) _____

2. Do I have to use a bedpan? _____

3. Can I reach for things, or should I use a reacher? _____

4. Personal Hygiene

Can I take a shower? _____

Can I take a bath? _____

Do I have to take a bed sponge bath? _____

Can I get out of bed to wash my hair? _____

5. Mobility

Can I walk the halls? _____

Can I walk in my room? _____

Can I sit in the chair in my room? _____

Can I take a wheelchair to the lobby? _____

Can I take a wheelchair to the nursery? _____

Can I take a wheelchair to hospital support _____

6. Visitors

When can my husband visit? _____

(If you do not have a husband:) Can I have another friend or relative visit at the times husbands are normally permitted to visit? _____

Who can visit? When _____

How many people can visit at a time? _____

If I am admitted to the labor room, who can visit? _____

Who can be present in the delivery room?

_____

7. Consults

If appropriate, may I see: _____

   a physical therapist _____

   an occupational therapist _____

   a neonatologist (*about fetal development and/or a typical preemie*) _____

   a social worker _____

   an ophthalmologist _____

   a dermatologist _____

8. Other directions:

_____

_____

_____

_____

_____

_____

_____

_____

_____

_____

_____

_____

_____

_____

_____

_____

The above chart was developed by Grace Moses, a founder of Intensive Caring Unlimited, a Philadelphia/Southern New Jersey parent support group and was reprinted from: Intensive Caring Unlimited, May/June 1986.

she was actually relieved when it came time to do it. "Since I had this deadline, I did way too much in the weeks leading up to it. I tried to get my Christmas shopping done and get the kitchen stocked, things like that," she says. "But as time passed, it was getting harder and harder for me get up and do things, so I actually was glad to have an excuse for doing nothing."

If you're like most women, though, you won't get the chance to prepare because you'll have no warning when you're put on bed rest. Pam, for instance, was caught totally by surprise. "I worked on a Saturday and the next day I went into labor and was put on bed rest, so it was this huge transition from being an extremely active person to being completely inactive," she says. "Boom, all of a sudden, I was in bed and that was real difficult in the beginning." Nancy expresses similar sentiments. "One morning I just woke up and never went to work again."

At first, the news that you will have to stay in bed can elicit negative feelings—shock, denial, fear, loss of control, even guilt that you may somehow be responsible for your pregnancy problems. You may also panic over all the day-to-day tasks you will no longer be able to do, such as work, grocery shop and drive in car pools. But once you begin your bed rest, you will quickly notice that life really does go on without you. For a while, you might even enjoy the extra relaxation. If your bed rest is prolonged, though, you will soon come to the realization that the term "rest" is a misnomer.

"There's no rest involved in lying in bed," says Maureen Doolan Boyle, who counsels many women on bed rest in her role as executive director of MOST (Mothers of Supertwins). "Your body becomes achy, many times you are on medication that will make you weepy or anxious and just the whole idea of having such a tentative pregnancy really increases your anxiety." You will also have to forego many things that women in low-risk pregnancies take for granted.

The best way to raise your spirits is to keep reminding yourself that you are doing what matters most: taking care of your unborn baby. "I thought of it as a blessing because it got me off work and totally physically committed to the pregnancy," says Nancy of her twenty-four weeks in bed. "I just think the physical demands of my job and running the household would have been too hard on me otherwise."

If your complications develop close to term, your confinement may last as little as a couple of weeks or even just a few days. On the other hand, if you bleed or have contractions early on, you may be on bed rest for most of your pregnancy. Regardless of when you are advised to begin resting in bed, it is important to know that bed rest can mean different things for different patients. For one woman, it may mean spending three or four hours a day lying on her left side on the couch, while for another it may mean staying in bed around the clock without even getting up to go to the bathroom. Grace Moses, a founder of the parent support group Intensive Caring Unlimited, and now of Sidelines, has developed a checklist that you can use to ensure that you understand what your doctor means by bed rest for you (see page 265).

Should you be resting for just a few hours each day? Or must you lie down flat on your side all the time? Is it okay to lie down on a chaise in the sun or float in the pool? What about showers or baths? Can you get up to eat? Should you be lying down even when you're riding in the car? Is sexual intercourse off-limits? These are all questions that you must ask your doctor. Also realize that the answers to these questions may change at various stages in your pregnancy.

If your condition worsens over time, you may go from partial bed rest to complete bed rest, as Pam did. "Once I started having a lot of contractions, my doctor would not let me get up and do anything at all." Nancy, on the other hand, was gradually granted privileges as she received clean bills of health at her prenatal visits. First, she moved from her bed to the couch. Later, she was able to sit at the table for meals. Eventually, she reached a point where her doctor gave her permission to go out to dinner as long as she was back home again within an hour. Whether or not you get similar privileges will depend on your own obstetrician's opinion and the particulars of your condition.

No matter what your physician recommends, it is important to follow his orders to the letter. If you ever feel like cheating a bit and getting up to go shopping or take a walk around the block, ask yourself which is worse—for you to stay in bed a while longer or for your newborn to be confined to a hospital neonatal intensive care unit. Your choice is as simple as that. Given your history, though, you might actually find it easier than most to comply with your doctor's advice. You know that this baby is alive and growing and deserves the healthiest possible start in life. That is reason enough to make whatever sacrifices are necessary. "Whatever it takes," says Nancy, who lost twins in her first pregnancy. "I knew the pain of losing babies so I was happy to lie there."

Bed Rest Survival Guide

No matter how willing you are to make the sacrifices required for bed rest, you might still find that it starts wearing on you sooner rather than later. Yes, you are willing to do whatever it takes to ensure a good outcome, but you are human and are naturally going to be frustrated as you do nothing but lie in bed day after day. You might feel like a prisoner, as you watch life go on around you while you are forced to sit on the sidelines. That you are most likely not feeling sick will make it that much harder for you to be cast in the role of the bedridden patient.

You'll also be bored. After all, there are only so many soap operas and talk shows that you can watch before you feel your brain turning to mush. When doctor appointments and *Oprah* become the highlight of your life, you'll know that you're in need of some serious distractions. Later in this chapter, we'll examine some specific tasks you can do from your bed to keep from going crazy. But in the meantime, let's discuss what you can do from the very outset to make your stay in bed as pleasant as possible.

- **Get comfortable.** Select a place in your house where you think you will feel most comfortable. Think about this before you decide. Do you really want to lie in the same bed that you share with your partner or would you rather set up quarters in a guestroom or some other favorite place in the house? Since you will be spending nearly all of your time in the room you choose, it is important that it be a place that you can make your own. Logistical considerations should also factor into your decision. If your bedroom is upstairs, you may want to pick a downstairs room so you will not overexert yourself on those rare occasions when you can leave the house.

Once you have settled on the room, rearrange it to your liking. Have the bed moved near the window or close to the bathroom if you want. Ask someone to hang your favorite pictures on the wall. Bring in all your cherished possessions, whether they be good books, treasured knickknacks or picture albums. And keep plenty of pillows around so you can prop yourself up if the doctor says it's okay. If you are free to move to other areas of the house on occasion, set up several spots where you feel comfortable: a cozy den sofa, a chaise in a sunroom or a futon in your home office are all good choices.

- **Eat right.** Since you probably won't be allowed to fix your own meals, consider keeping a small refrigerator near your bed with some of your favorite foods inside. If you don't want to invest in a fridge, use a small ice chest instead and make sure it's restocked every morning. You'll want to have plenty of water on hand for drinking (preferably in an insulated thermos), especially if you're at risk for preterm labor or suffering from high blood pressure. Healthy snacks for in-between meals are also nice. A tray table will come in handy when you're eating food that requires a fork and knife, and you can use it later as a writing desk.

- **Find links to the outside world.** When you are cooped up at home all day, you will definitely want links to the outside world. A cordless phone, along with your personal phone list and a city telephone directory, will do wonders for your morale. If you are allowed to prop yourself up, a laptop computer with access to the Internet is another lifesaver. You can e-mail friends and acquaintances and chat with other women who are in the same boat, even if they happen to be halfway around the world. The high-risk pregnancy group, Sidelines, provides e-mail support as well as supervised chat rooms.

- **Take care of yourself.** Imagine needing to blow your nose and not having a tissue, or having dry, itchy eyes and no contact lens solution. If you don't prepare in advance for your bed rest, these kinds of things could very well happen to you. Essentials you should have on hand include a mirror, a hairbrush, cosmetics, contact lens solution and eye glasses, moist towlettes, makeup and earrings for the days when you feel like dressing up a bit. In case you are not even allowed to get up to go to the bathroom, a bedpan or rented bedside commode is obviously required. Keep a change of clothes handy, too. Whether you lounge around in nightgowns or make the effort to wear street clothes, there will be times when you want to freshen up and change into something else.

- **Keep track of time.** Although it may not be such a good idea to mark off each passing day on a calendar (which could just make your bed rest feel eternal), it is nice to have a weekly calendar or book that describes exactly what your baby looks like at each stage of the pregnancy. It will be gratifying to know when your baby has reached major milestones. It's also a good idea to keep an alarm clock by your bedside to remind you when to take any medications that may have been prescribed for you or when it's time to do your home monitoring for contractions.

- **Arrange for entertainment.** Most pregnant women who are confined to bed become very dependent on their television. To keep from getting bored with the same old shows, you might want to have a video cassette recorder so you can watch your favorite movies. A CD or tape player is nice for playing soothing music, and you might want to invest in some audio books so that you can drift off to sleep while listening to a good story.

- **Call for help.** For the first, and perhaps only time in your adult life, you will be waited on hand and foot. So be sure you have a bell or intercom to summon help when you need it. And don't hesitate to call the doctor if you ever have any questions or concerns about your condition. It doesn't matter whether it's day or night, obstetricians are used to dealing with emergency calls; it's their job even when the crisis turns out to be a false alarm.

- **Put it all together.** Once you have gathered all the things you need, you will want to keep them all on a large table within arm's reach. It's best if the table has wheels so you can move it out of the way when necessary. Another option is to use an ironing board as a bedside table. It holds a lot, but doesn't take up much room. Cover it with a pretty tablecloth and then adjust it to whatever height you need.

Hospitalization

For some of the same reasons that you are ordered to rest in bed, you may at some point end up in the hospital. For example, if you are having premature contractions that have not been brought under control by bed rest at home, you will be hospitalized so that tocolytic drugs can be administered intravenously. Hospitalization is also the only option for conditions that require twenty-four-hour surveillance, like placental abruption, premature rupture of the membranes and severe pre-eclampsia. Occasionally, women have to be hospitalized to undergo surgery, either on themselves for conditions like an incompetent cervix, or, more rarely, on the baby in utero.

It probably goes without saying that being hospitalized for any reason other than delivering your baby at full-term is a pretty scary experience. But if you consider that you will be in the best possible place for both your health and the baby's, it may help ease your mind. As Linda says about her nine-day hospital stay, "I felt totally at peace because they were monitoring me so closely, and I felt like I was in very good hands."

If your hospital stay is expected to be lengthy, some of the same tips that we just discussed for bed rest will help make the experience more bearable. In particular, you should ask someone to bring you a few of your favorite things from home so you can personalize your room a bit. Find out whether you can eat something besides the hospital fare. Get a small stereo with headphones to listen to music or audio books. Be sure to wear your own nightgowns. And invest in a good pair of eye shades and ear plugs to shut out the rest of the world.

As you can imagine, there will be plenty of times when, try as you might, you cannot shut out the world. Anyone who has ever been hospitalized knows all about the constant interruptions to check vital signs, get urine and blood samples and change IVs. These regular intrusions will only add to your stress. On the positive side, however, you will know that you and your baby are being closely watched for any sign of trouble. Fetal monitoring and regular non-stress tests and sonograms will also give you much-needed reassurance.

Doctors and nurses in the obstetrics ward are usually good about relaying the information they gather from all this testing. But if you are not getting the answers you need, keep asking until you do. That is the only way to gain a sense of control over a very difficult situation. And just in case you end up in a hospital that pairs you up with a new mother as a roommate, ask to be moved. In fact, if you prefer, find out whether you can distance yourself from the regular maternity floor altogether. I'll never forget seeing all the telltale signs of new babies in my room when I was hospitalized after losing Patrick. You will relish all those things when your baby actually arrives, but for now, you should not have to be subjected to it.

The Impact on Your Family

Whether you're in the hospital or at home in bed, a long convalescence can wreak havoc on family life. Your partner may have to go from husband, father and provider to cook, housekeeper, errand boy and babysitter. And he may not be very experienced at any of his new roles. Meanwhile, you will be cast in a role that you don't much like either: the role of the helpless patient. Realize that your house won't be run the same without you, but be patient if you can. It will be much easier on your partner if you have older children or close family members that can pitch in and help as well. Mothers, mothers-in-law and sisters can make a huge difference—assuming you can all manage to get along under one roof. But realize that no matter how much assistance you have, your bed rest will be almost as great of a challenge for the rest of your family as it is for you.

If you have children at home, they especially will miss having you around to do things with them. But while you may not be able to go to your children's soccer games or school plays for a while, there are still plenty of things that you can do to continue mothering them. Read them a story or watch television together. If you can sit up, color or play games with them. Help them with their homework or let them eat their meals with you. If you cannot do much, just cuddle them or take a nap together. You're planning to welcome a newborn to your family very soon, and that won't leave nearly as much time for your older children. So consider this your special time together.

The Impact on Your Career

Even though you are willing to do anything necessary to ensure the birth of a healthy baby, it can be difficult to put your career on hold or, in some cases, even jeopardize your job altogether because of the pregnancy. By law, employers cannot discriminate against you for being confined to bed for health reasons. You are entitled to sick leave and disability pay just as you would be with any other medical condition. But legislation can't protect against the ill feelings that could develop among your colleagues if you are off the job for a long time, especially if this is your second or even third round of bed rest. It also can't alleviate the disappointment you might feel if you're forced to put off the fast track for the foreseeable future.

Even if you are not under doctor-prescribed bed rest, you may have to limit your work activities in order to improve your chances for a good outcome. This is especially true if your job entails physical labor or other duties that could be harmful to your baby's health. In that case, find out if you can work from home occasionally or job share with someone else who wants to work part-time.

Whether you're reducing your workload or not working altogether, this will be a major adjustment for you. It might also put a strain on your family's budget. Although you may be receiving disability payments, they usually are only a fraction of your regular salary. Meanwhile, your medical bills may be mounting, especially if your insurance has high deductibles and copayments. Despite the stress this type of situation normally causes, most couples find they are able to keep things in perspective. They know that they cannot put a price tag on the pregnancy, and one way or another they will dig their way out of debt after the baby is born.

Cynthia and her husband are a case in point. During her high-risk pregnancy, she was forced to quit her job so she could go on bed rest. She was also given the option of undergoing expensive treatment that her insurance company considered experimental and refused to cover. Rather than forgoing the potentially life-saving treatment for financial reasons, Cynthia and her husband decided to proceed with the treatment and charge the medical expenses on a low-interest credit card. She explains: "We know I'll have to go back to work eventually, and we're really struggling right now on just my husband's income. But it would be much worse if I didn't do it and something happened. I would rather double the debt and have two little babies in my home."

If you had trouble conceiving and underwent fertility treatment, you already know how quickly medical bills can add up. But you also probably decided long ago that your medical care was worth the cost. The same will be true during your pregnancy. Your health and the baby's will always come first.

That the Worst Might Happen Again

Every one of us who has ever been through a pregnancy after a loss has feared that the worst might happen again. It may be something that you haven't even admitted to yourself, but nonetheless the fear exists. For me, books on pregnancy loss and my support group brought those fears to the surface. I remember one book I read shortly after losing Patrick, which told the story of two women who had lost babies very late in their pregnancies to seemingly fluke events. At first, I was outraged. How dare the authors feature these examples so prominently in a book aimed at women who so desperately needed hope? But then I got scared. Did this mean that the same thing could happen to me?

I had a similar reaction a few months later when I attended a support group meeting that featured a panel of parents who had successfully been through a pregnancy after a loss. One of the couples who spoke that night told of losing two babies. By then I was pregnant again, and my fear was even greater. But why, I thought, would they ask a couple to speak who had had the misfortune of having it happen twice?

The fact is that the worst can—and sometimes does—happen again no matter how hard a woman and her doctor try to prevent it. Those women must then relive the nightmare of grieving over another baby, searching for answers and later agonizing whether they are willing or able to try again. But it is also true that the overwhelming majority of women do go on to have a successful pregnancy after a loss, especially if the problem that caused the loss was something that doctors consider unlikely to happen again.

If you're like me, you think that you would not be able to endure another loss. But couples who have had that misfortune sometimes find that they have more strength than they expected. As one mother says, "You know the darkest day of your life is not going to stay that way. Where before, you were working through your grief blind—you didn't know what to expect—the next time, you're working through it with your eyes open." Diane, who suffered a late first trimester miscarriage after losing a son shortly after birth, says she also found it easier to come to terms with her grief the second time. "I had already had to answer the hard questions for myself," she says.

If you're concerned about a second loss, understand that these feelings are normal as long as they are not obsessive. Naturally, it would be better if you could think positively, since the odds are most likely very much in your favor no matter how high-risk your pregnancy. But sometimes that is just not possible. And if you've already suffered more than one loss and fear having it happen yet again, try to remember that no matter what happens, you are a survivor. You've been through it before and you have made it. Somehow, some way, you will find the strength to do it again.

Selective Reduction

When most of us worry about the worst happening again, we think of miscarriage, stillbirth or early infant death. In other words, things that are beyond our control. But as more and more women are becoming pregnant after using ovulation-inducing fertility drugs or assisted reproduction techniques such as in vitro fertilization, another type of loss is becoming prevalent: multifetal pregnancy reduction. This is the medical term for women who are pregnant with triplets, quadruplets or more and undergo a procedure to abort one or more of the babies to give the others a better chance of surviving. The procedure is typically done in the second trimester to avoid triggering a miscarriage of all the babies. This choice is agonizing for any couple, but nearly unfathomable for someone who has lost one or more babies before.

"In many ways it is a 'Sophie's choice' because the vast majority of these pregnancies are not only planned but desperately wanted pregnancies where families have been trying to conceive a baby for years," says Boyle of MOST. "These are people who are emotionally and financially invested in the pregnancy."

Couples who opt for selective reduction often do so because of the high-risk nature of being pregnant with multiples. Triplets, quads and quints are twelve times more likely than other babies to die in their first year of life, mainly because they are often born too early and suffer from respiratory and digestive complications that are common among preemies. Depending on how early the babies are born, they also are prone to more serious problems, like blindness, cerebral palsy and mental retardation. But there are some couples, especially those who are approaching their forties, who choose selective reduction because of the parental and financial demands of raising several children.

Research has shown that mutiple pregnancies reduced to twins usually proceed as if that were the number of babies originally conceived. But since selective reduction is an invasive procedure, it can also result in the loss of the entire pregnancy as well as considerable emotional distress among couples who see it as their "least bad alternative."

In the book *A Time to Decide, A Time to Heal* by Molly A. Minnick, Kathleen J. Delp and Mary C. Ciotti, couples who have undergone multifetal reduction share their feelings about the procedure. The differences in how they view their decision in retrospect speaks volumes about the divisiveness of this issue. One woman, who became pregnant with quadruplets after fertility treatment, knew from the beginning that she wanted the procedure. She says, "We of course knew the risks of reduction, but we never even second-guessed the decision. It was the only answer for us, as we were unprepared to deal with four potentially unhealthy babies. We just wanted it over with, so we could go on with the twins' pregnancy."

This woman ended up giving birth to full-term, healthy twins and claims to have no regrets. "We made the right decision. We have no doubts," she says. "If we had not had the reduction, our perfect children would not be what they are now, and I just can't imagine them any other way."

But another mother, whose pregnancy did not have a happy outcome, has an entirely different perspective on the procedure. She, too, chose selective reduction after undergoing in vitro fertilization and becoming pregnant with triplets. But her two remaining babies were born prematurely at twenty-seven weeks gestation and did not survive. She says:

> *In the wake of these tragedies and a year of mourning, rational and irrational questions still run through my mind. Was it a healthier fetus that was terminated? Could that baby have made it though the others didn't?*

Was I somehow being punished for the reduction through the loss of the other babies? Did by-products of the termination contribute to the complications that followed? (Our doctors speculate that may have been possible.)

When she got pregnant a second time through in vitro fertilization, she was relieved to know that she was expecting twins and would not have to make the decision about selective reduction again. She reflects:

If I could turn back time, would I choose the selective reduction or not? I don't know. I do know that I've learned an important lesson. Pregnancy situations are not always black and white. There are gray areas between success and failure, and those gray areas continue to haunt me in the middle of the night.

If you are pregnant with multiples, only you and your partner can decide whether selective reduction is an option for you, especially given your history of loss. Do you see it as a way to avoid losing any more babies to prematurity or ill health, or do you consider it playing God and deciding which one of your babies will live or die? These are hard questions with seemingly impossible answers. The best thing would have been not to become pregnant with so many babies in the first place. But if you are already expecting three or more babies, the next best thing you can do is seek counseling—both medical and spiritual—before making a decision. By carefully weighing all the options, you will know that your choice is one that you can live with no matter what the outcome.

Common Feelings

Concern

Although all of us who have suffered a loss worry a lot in our subsequent pregnancies, women in the high-risk category usually have even more reason than most to be concerned. Your fears will not be based on imagination, but on hard facts. You know that you are statistically more likely than most to develop complications during your pregnancy. You may also experience actual problems that keep you on pins and needles. Margo, for example, developed placenta previa, which forced her to be on bed rest for most of her pregnancy. Everytime she gained the confidence that perhaps all was well, she would have another bleeding episode, which is symptomatic of this condition. And then, her baby started showing signs of intrauterine growth retardation—the same problem that caused her first baby to die in utero. Although she ultimately gave birth to a healthy child, she describes it as "the pregnancy from hell."

I went to the hospital three times with bleeding, and every time there were big clots. As long as I was on bed rest, things were okay. But as soon as the doctor said it was okay to start getting up, it would happen again. I woke up one night with blood all over the bed and passed a clot in the bathroom. So I had to stay in bed for most of my pregnancy, and my husband did it all. Right before my due date, I had some more bleeding so I called the doctor and said "I'm having this previa mess again," but that time it turned out to be my plug and I went into labor. But all the way up until the very end, it was never relaxed.

If you are on bed rest, your worries may also be heightened by you having too much time to focus on nothing but the baby's well-being. As Judy says: "I felt like all I did was sit in bed all day and all night wondering if the babies were okay. I had too much time to think, and most of what I thought was not positive." Anytime you feel the worries start to overwhelm you, remind yourself that you are doing everything you can to ensure the birth of a healthy baby. And resolve once again to worry only about the problems you are actually facing, not those you fear could develop in the future. Remember, too, that you never would have gotten pregnant again if you did not believe in your heart that this time things would be different. Hold on to that thought in your darkest moments, and it will bring you comfort.

Isolation

Going on bed rest, leaving your job and cutting back on outside activities can make you feel isolated from the rest of the world. If family and friends are there to support you, however, they can help to fill the void in your life during your pregnancy. But when those closest to you disapprove of your decision to become pregnant again given the high-risk nature of your problems, your sense of isolation can be even greater. You may sometimes feel that you and your partner are the only ones in the entire world who really believe that your baby has a chance.

This was the situation Marian faced when she got pregnant again after suffering two losses. Since she already had two surviving children, she was met with outright hostility by her extended family, who seemed to believe that "enough was enough." Although her mother did agree to help around the house when Marian was hospitalized briefly to undergo surgery, her disapproval was palpable. Marian remembers that "My mother's attitude was basically, 'How in the world can you put us through this again?' My husband said he felt like she was mostly mad at him for allowing me to get pregnant again. She even told him once, 'You're endangering the life of my child.' "

Some women who are high-risk actually go against their own doctor's advice when they get pregnant again. Leslie, who also had suffered two second-trimester losses and nearly lost her own life, fell into this category. She says: "My doctor said I should not get pregnant again, but I knew I was going to go into this one with my eyes open. We knew what to look for. And my husband stressed from the very beginning, my life is coming first."

If you are feeling as isolated as Marian and Leslie were because of the high-risk nature of your pregnancy, surround yourself with friends who support your decision. If you are seeing a doctor who advised against the pregnancy, switch to someone who specializes in high-risk cases and has confidence that a good outcome is possible. And talk to other women who have been in the same position and beaten the odds. Marian and Leslie did: they both gave birth to healthy babies after complicated pregnancies.

Another excellent source of encouragement is Sidelines, the organization that provides support for women going through high-risk pregnancies. Ask to be paired up with one of their telephone counselors. They are all volunteers who were once in a similar situation themselves. Talking to them will do wonders for your frame of mind, especially if you are matched with someone who had a loss and then went on to give birth to a healthy baby. When you're feeling your worst, you'll know that help and encouragement are only a phone call or a mouse click away.

Stress

Women who face daunting odds are not the only ones who feel stressed during a high-risk pregnancy. Stress can come from a wide range of sources. Bed rest can be stressful, especially if you are accustomed to being an independent and active person. Doctor appointments can also be stressful, since you may often find yourself fearing the worst. Even seeing women who are having care-free pregnancies can be stressful. Says Cynthia, "I'm so jealous of anyone who can enjoy a normal pregnancy where they can be happy and excited." In other words, you probably will find many things stressful during this very trying period in your life.

Later in this chapter, we'll talk about tips for easing anxiety. Many of the suggestions will help lower your stress level as well. The bottom line is that if you can control stress before it controls you, then stress does not necessarily have to be negative. Stress is a natural reaction to any risky situation, even one where the stakes are not nearly as high. The key is to take the negative energy and turn it into something positive.

Feeling stressed about staying in bed? Get relief by tackling projects that you never had time to do before. (Assuming you can do them from your bed.) Are your nerves frayed because your next doctor appointment is coming up? Check out some pregnancy books from the library so you can read up on what's supposed to be happening in your pregnancy. That way you can go in to your appointment armed with knowledge and concrete questions. Feeling sorry for yourself because everyone else seems to have it so easy? Look into whether you can do telephone counseling for a church or any other organization that runs a crisis line for people in need. By turning challenges into opportunities, you will look back on this time and realize that a lot of good was mixed in with the bad.

Weakness

Although there are plenty of positive things you can do during your pregnancy, even if you are confined to bed, you may find that extended bed rest will zap your strength. The longer you rest in bed, the more muscle tone and overall strength you will lose. Your neck and back may be stiff, your feet and hands may swell, and you may feel light-headed at times. Getting up to go to the bathroom may make you dizzy. If you are on strict bed rest and are unable to get up at all, you will be even weaker and may have trouble walking once the pregnancy is over.

One way to combat these symptoms is to hire a physical therapist. That may sound strange considering that you are not allowed to get out of bed, but a trained professional can teach you how to move and change positions in bed without increasing pressure on your abdominal muscles. A therapist can also give you massages and offer suggestions on positioning pillows to reduce muscle pain. Make sure, however, that the therapist is trained to work with women in high-risk pregnancies and communicates with your doctor about what you are allowed to do.

If you don't have a physical therapist to turn to for advice, listen to your body instead. On days when you just don't feel like doing anything, don't. Watch television, read and take naps instead. Tomorrow you may feel more energetic and do more. Staying active is a good idea because it will enhance your strength and boost your morale as well. But even if you just laid around and did absolutely nothing for nine months, you would still be doing the most important thing in the world: growing a baby.

Gratefulness

Assuming that your family and friends accept your decision to get pregnant again, you will probably be amazed by how much they reach out to help you during this difficult period in your life. Phone calls, visits and offers to help will make the months go by much more quickly and will give you a sense of how fortunate you are to be surrounded by people who care about you.

You will also undoubtedly feel grateful for simple things: the baby's kicks, positive reports from the doctor and each week that brings you closer to the birth of your child. In her best-selling book *Simple Abundance*, Sarah Ban Breathnach says such a sense of gratitude has a transforming power. "Real life isn't always going to be perfect or go our way," she writes, "but the recurring acknowledgement of what *is working* in our lives can help us not only survive but surmount our difficulties." A high-risk pregnancy is difficult, but there is no denying that you also have much for which to be grateful.

Tips for Easing Anxiety

Hire Help (If You Can Afford It)

When you first found out you would be on bed rest during your pregnancy, you probably worried mostly about the big things. What would you do about work? How would you arrange to get your meals during the day? Who would care for the kids after school? But did you also consider who would scrub the toilets and mop the floors? Probably not. All of us like having a clean house, but when you're dealing with concerns about your baby's health and the prospect of nothing but bed rest for weeks or even months, housework is usually not at the top of your list of priorities. It's one of those things that you usually only start to notice when no one is doing it. So when your sheets are stained with yesterday's lunch, and the trash is overflowing, and the bathtub is lined with mildew and soap scum, that's when you start worrying about the housework.

If you can afford it, one of the best investments you can make during this time is to hire a housekeeper. Having someone come in and clean once or twice a week can boost your morale. You might even be able to find a housekeeper who will run errands and prepare something for dinner. It's true that your partner could take on the tasks and save you the money, but unless he is used to doing more than his fair share around the house, he may already be pushed to the limit by having to grocery shop, cook meals, and otherwise attend to your every need. You could ask your mother or another close relative to help, but that might make you uneasy. Preparing meals for you is one thing; cleaning your bathroom is quite another. So while hiring a housekeeper might be something that you would normally consider a luxury, right now it may very well be a necessity.

Try Not to Dwell on Your Predicament

Let's assume you have all your outside help in place. There are people responsible for cleaning your house, cooking your meals, babysitting your children, running your errands and doing your work at the office. Now what are *you* supposed to do? You could spend your time watching daytime television, but you'll soon tire of it. Reading is nice, but again, there's a limit to how much reading you can do in a day. That leaves naps, meals and doctor appointments to look forward to, and they will quickly lose their luster.

But of course, there can be much more to bed rest than that. If you make the effort to compile a list of things to do, you'll be amazed at how much more quickly the days pass. Here are some suggestions to add to your list:

- **Stimulate your mind.** The main purpose of bed rest is to give your body, not your mind, a break. By keeping your mind active, you will not have as much time to dwell on your predicament, so your outlook may improve. Fortunately, you can exercise your mind without ever lifting a muscle. Keep a journal. Log on to the Internet. Play the stock market. Do volunteer work by phone. Work crossword puzzles. Read up on child care. If you're really motivated, study a foreign language or take a correspondence course. Learn a new art or craft. Anything that gets your focus off of yourself and your baby and on to something else will do you good. Since it is inevitable that you will still spend lots of time thinking about your pregnancy, be sure that some of it is spent in quiet meditation or prayer. That will usually give you a refreshing, and more positive, perspective on your situation.

- **Shop**. Treat yourself to a shopping spree. These days, you can find nearly everything you want for sale in catalogs, on the Internet or on cable home shopping networks. Or you can clip newspaper ads and send someone out to do your shopping for you. If money is a concern, not to worry. You can make a wish list and comparison shop so that when your finances improve, you will know just what to buy. So, start your Christmas shopping early. Redecorate your house. Assemble a wardrobe for your postpartum body. Or if you're not superstitious, pick out things for the baby's room. Splurge. You deserve it . . . even if it's only in your dreams.

- **Invite friends to visit**. Everyone needs friends, and you'll need yours more than ever now that you're cooped up in the house all day. Too many visitors might tire you out, but if a few close friends get in the habit of dropping by, it will give you something to look forward to and brighten your day. Ask them to call ahead, so you can arrange for them to visit when it's most convenient for you. Occasionally, ask them to run an errand for you on the way over. They won't mind and, in fact, will probably be happy to know that they can help.

  If you're like me, you've been meaning to see more of your friends anyway but just haven't had the time. Well, now you do have the time and they will make time for you. Arranging to see a few close friends on a regular basis works best for me. For example, you could meet a good friend every Wednesday morning for breakfast, or have a standing dinner date with a coworker every third Tuesday of the month. But since the purpose of bed rest is for you to get as much rest as possible, don't hesitate to ask them to leave if you're tired. They'll understand.

The telephone can also keep you in touch with those you care about. Use it to catch up on what's been happening at the office or to check in with family members who live too far away to visit. If your phone bills start getting out of control, recapture the art of letter writing. If you can sit up in bed, use a laptop computer to send e-mail.

- **Get counseling.** As helpful as friends can be, they will not always understand what you are going through, and they may grow tired of hearing you complain about the miseries of bed rest. If this happens, one alternative is to talk to a counselor. As we discussed, Sidelines can match you up with another woman who has experienced a complicated pregnancy. She can offer peer support and practical suggestions from the perspective of someone who has been there. In the magazine *Left Sidelines*, women describe what a difference telephone counselors made in their pregnancy. One woman writes:

> *In my case, my Sidelines volunteer was always there to listen and to lift my spirits. I also enjoyed the packet of information and the articles I received. I know that it was this support that I received that helped me deliver two healthy babies, a boy and a girl, at thirty-six weeks (the day I went off all of my medication).*

You also can arrange for professional support. If you are already seeing a therapist, for example, there's no reason why you cannot continue to seek counseling over the phone.

- **Work.** Depending on what kind of job you do, you may get your doctor's approval to work from bed. If you enjoy doing it, and it takes your mind off your problems, that's great. But you may find that your motivation is limited when you're lying around all day. Pam tried working from home while she was on bed rest but soon discovered that her heart wasn't in it. "I need adrenaline and deadlines to really get me motivated," she says. "But when I was in bed, I felt brain dead. My brain just wasn't functioning correctly, so I just started doing little projects where I didn't have to think, like cross stitch." If your job is stressful, it probably is not a good idea to work from home anyway. Talk to your doctor about these details before you make a decision.

- **Get organized.** Who doesn't have pictures to put in photo albums, or recipes to index? Now is your chance to finally get organized. There are myriad things you can do to put your affairs in order. Update your address list. Pay the bills. Fill out your tax return. Respond to unanswered letters. Write thank-you notes. The possibilities are endless. Just think of all the things you've been meaning to do but have been putting off, and then do them.

Stick to a Schedule

Now that you have your list of things to do, create a schedule and try to stick to it every day. That's right, a schedule. Decide what time you are going to eat meals, take naps, make phone calls, monitor contractions, watch television and work on your activities. If you don't make a schedule, you risk drifting in and out of sleep all day and lying awake half the night. Before long, you will be in a vicious cycle that leaves you feeling bored and depressed.

Needless to say, your schedule can be extremely flexible. If naptime is at two o'clock and you get sleepy an hour earlier, by all means go to sleep. The point is to provide some structure to your day, not force you to do what you don't want. A typical schedule for a woman on bed rest might look something like this:

9:00 A.M.	Wake up. Have breakfast. Read the newspaper and watch the news.
10:00 A.M.	Shower (if permitted). Change into a fresh nightgown or get dressed. Put on makeup if you're in the mood.
10:30 A.M.	Monitor for contractions, transmit the information to the nursing staff. Use this time to read a book, watch television or listen to music.
Noon	Have lunch with a friend.
1:30 P.M.	Nap.
2:00 P.M.	Do an activity. It doesn't matter what it is, as long as it's something besides watching television or reading.
3:30 P.M.	Make phone calls or send e-mail.
4:30 P.M.	Have a snack.
5:00 P.M.	Watch the news.
5:30 P.M.	Spend the evening with your partner talking, watching television, monitoring for contractions or just being together.

If you're a morning person, you may want to get up earlier and schedule your activity in the morning. Or maybe you prefer doing things after everyone has gone to bed at night, and then sleep late in the morning. Devise a schedule that suits your body clock. Some days no one will visit you, and it will be harder to find ways to pass the time. But there will be other days when you get out of the house for a doctor appointment and feel like time has flown. But no matter how hard you try to stay active and interested, you will still have days when you feel like you are going stir crazy. You'll desperately wish that you could go somewhere, anywhere: the mall, a restaurant, the hairdresser, the park. All the things you took for granted or even dreaded (like grocery shopping) will suddenly look very appealing.

But just keep reminding yourself that you are staying in bed for your baby's health and that getting up could seriously jeopardize the pregnancy. That should give you all the incentive you need to overcome your moments of weakness.

Keep Your Eyes on the Goal

One of the fringe benefits of being on bed rest is that you will get the opportunity to know your unborn baby more intimately than most mothers ever will. You will know which times of day she is most active and when she likes to sleep. You'll know just how she kicks and perhaps even what position she is in. Since you'll be going to the doctor a lot, you will get to know her through sonogram images, too. Seeing and feeling the baby who is the reason for all of your efforts will make your sacrifices seem small in comparison. You already know that every day that you stay in bed is one less day that she potentially will have to spend in the NICU nursery. It should help your attitude if you try never to lose sight of that fact.

Another good tip is one that all of us who have been through a subsequent pregnancy have tried to follow, although not always successfully. Take it one day at a time. Don't think about how many more days you will be in bed, or how long it will be until you deliver. And try not to worry too much about tomorrow. As one wise person once said: "Today is the tomorrow that you worried about and all is well."

Prenatal Visits

Early prenatal care will significantly improve your chances for a full-term pregnancy, so it is important that you contact your obstetrician from the moment you suspect you are pregnant. Depending on your complications, you will probably see a perinatologist in addition to your regular obstetrician. The main advantage to seeing a specialist is to receive medical care from someone who is experienced in managing complicated pregnancies. If you live in a large city, find out whether you can go to a major medical center where you will have access to a perinatologist, genetic counselor, nutritionist, radiologist and other specialists in a single location. Since those of you who live in a small town or rural area will not have that luxury, it is vitally important that you find an obstetrician who has experience dealing with high-risk pregnancies.

If you are on complete bed rest and must lie down twenty-four hours a day, there is a possibility that your obstetrician may arrange to make housecalls on occasion. But most of the time, you will be going into the office where the doctor has access to the equipment needed to adequately monitor your pregnancy. Because the office staff won't always be aware of the particulars of your situation, make it a point to ask whether you can go into an exam room and lie down while you are waiting to see the doctor. And be sure that you are dropped off at the entrance and keep your walking to a minimum. You might even want to check if a wheelchair is available.

Prenatal Tests in the High-Risk Pregnancy

Your prenatal tests will not necessarily be any different from those of someone whose pregnancy is not considered high-risk. You will probably just have more of them. Sonograms will be frequent—perhaps at every visit—along with non-stress tests and biophysical profiles. If you are having contractions, the doctor will also check you frequently for signs of the onset of preterm labor.

Home Monitoring of Your Pregnancy

Signs of Preterm Labor

Although your doctor will monitor you closely if you are at risk for an early delivery, it is still critical that you know the signs of preterm labor. As we already discussed, you are at higher risk for a preterm birth if you have delivered early before. But you also have an increased chance of going into preterm labor if you have complications such as gestational diabetes, pregnancy-induced hypertension or placenta previa.

The key to preventing a preterm delivery is early detection. Usually, once you are two centimeters dilated, there is no turning back. The challenge that you will be facing, though, is that some of the symptoms of preterm labor are not that different from common discomforts of pregnancy. (What pregnant woman hasn't had an occasional backache or contraction?) Although we already discussed the symptoms of preterm labor in chapter 5, they are worth reviewing again here. And remember, when in doubt, check with your doctor. The overwhelming majority of early deliveries occur because women do not seek medical attention until it is too late for tocolytic drugs to be effective.

- Low back pain that is either constant or rhythmic and is not relieved by a change in position.

- Abdominal or menstrual-like cramps with or without diarrhea. The cramps may be rhythmic or come in waves.

- Abdominal pressure or contractions. The contractions may feel like a tightening and relaxing of the uterus, but they are sometimes painless during preterm labor. Three or more contractions in a one-hour period should be reported to the doctor.

- An increase or change in vaginal discharge. For example, if the discharge becomes watery, bloody or mucous or if the color changes, it could be cause for concern.

- Vaginal bleeding, no matter how slight.

- A feeling of pelvic heaviness or that the baby is coming out.

- Diarrhea.

- A gut feeling that something is wrong.

Sometimes, the onset of labor is obvious because there is a premature rupture of the membranes (PROM). In other words, your water breaks. When this happens too early, preventing labor is difficult, as evidenced by the fact that PROM is responsible for about one-third of all cases of premature birth in the United States. But it is sometimes possible to extend the pregnancy through complete bed rest in a hospital where doctors can keep a close watch for any sign of infection. One of the best tools that doctors have for this purpose is the biophysical profile. By using this combination of ultrasound and non-stress testing, they can distinguish healthy babies who can safely remain in the womb from those who are infected or at high risk of infection and should be delivered immediately.

Home Uterine Monitor

A woman can easily be in the early stages of preterm labor and have no symptoms whatsoever. That's why doctors sometimes recommend a home uterine monitor for their patients who are at high-risk for an early delivery. It can alert a woman to any silent contractions she may be having and enable her to get in touch with her doctor while there is still time to prevent a preterm birth.

If you are given a home uterine monitor, you will probably have to use it for one hour twice a day. You simply strap a belt around your abdomen so that the transducer can detect possible contractions. The information is then stored in a monitor. At the end of the hour of monitoring, you transmit the data by modem where it is evaluated by a specially trained nurse assigned to your case. This twice-daily contact with a trained professional means that you have someone to turn to when you have questions about your pregnancy or just need emotional support.

Although a recent study concluded that home uterine activity monitoring failed to prevent early deliveries, advocates of the monitoring say they are a valuable tool in the earlier detection of preterm labor. In some cases the pregnancy can be prolonged so that premature babies have a higher birth weight and spend less time in the neonatal intensive care unit.

Treatment for Preterm Labor

If the home uterine monitor indicates that you are having three or more contractions per hour, that is usually cause for concern. You may be advised to empty your bladder (since a full one may cause contractions), drink two twelve-ounce glasses of water and lie on your left side. The theory is that lying on your left side, along with drinking the extra fluids, will increase the blood flow to the uterus and help it relax. Drinking plenty of water is also believed to reduce the adverse effects of the hormone oxytocin, which can cause cramping.

When these types of home remedies are not effective, women are hospitalized so that fluids can be administered intravenously. In most cases, bed rest and fluid therapy alone are enough to stop the contractions. But there are cases when tocolytic drugs must be administered. When these drugs are administered in the very early stages of labor, they are very effective in prolonging pregnancy. The first dose might be administered by IV in the hospital. Once back at home, a woman might either give herself injections, take pills or use a tocolytic pump that regulates the timing and amount of medication going into her system.

While tocolytic drugs are often effective in stopping labor, they can also have uncomfortable side effects. These include shakiness, nausea, headaches, heart palpitations and nervousness. The good news is that the side effects often diminish over time and are not believed to be harmful to the baby. In fact, the babies of women being treated for preterm labor tend to grow more quickly and have more mature lungs at an earlier gestation. The drug of last resort in stopping preterm labor is magnesium sulfate, also known as IV mag. Any woman who has taken it before dreads the prospect of taking it again because of the painful side effects. It can leave a woman feeling excruciatingly hot, weak and disoriented. But it, too, can have a positive effect on the baby. Evidence suggests it might prevent brain bleeds in premature babies.

Once delivery appears inevitable, corticosteroids are usually given to speed up the maturation of the baby's lungs and reduce the risk of respiratory distress syndrome. This can be given anywhere from two to forty-eight hours before birth. Thyroid hormones have also been shown to promote a good outcome in early births.

chapter eight

Labor and Delivery

WITHOUT QUESTION, ONE of the happiest moments of my life was when my son Andrew was born. For months, I had wondered if I would ever see the day when I would give birth to a living, breathing child. I had wanted to believe it with all my heart, but many times during my subsequent pregnancy I wasn't sure it was possible. Then, when it did happen, it seemed almost too good to be true. Could it be that this beautiful baby was actually mine? Was everything *really* all right? After a while, reality sunk in, and I was overwhelmed with joy. The long ordeal of the pregnancy was over, and, for the first time in more than a year, I felt truly happy again.

But it didn't take long for the old doubts and anxieties to come creeping back. Even though the pregnancy was over, many of the feelings I had experienced were still present. I soon realized that I was still extremely worried about my new baby's well-being and still grieving the loss of Patrick. The first indication that those feelings would linger for a while came the next day when the pediatrician informed us that Andrew's collarbone had been fractured during de-livery. Although the doctor assured us the problem was minor, to me it seemed monumental. All of a sudden I realized that I still had no assurances that this baby would be all right. Sure, he had lived through the pregnancy, but what next? I felt that anything could hap-pen.

That night, I had a nightmare that the baby had died, and woke up terrified that it was not a dream. Even after I called the nursery and was told that Andrew was sleeping soundly, I couldn't relax. In the middle of the night, all alone in my hospital room, I cried like I had never cried before—not even when Patrick had died. Now that I had another baby, I understood exactly what had been taken from me. And no matter how irrational it was, I was terrified that the worst could happen again.

As you look forward to your own labor and delivery, you may be convinced, as I was, that the birth of a healthy baby will mark the end of all your fears and anxieties. As long as you can make it through the pregnancy, you tell yourself, everything will be just fine. Although that may be true in the long run, some obstacles need to be overcome first, especially right before and shortly after your baby's birth. Most notable of these are labor and delivery itself, which can lead to anxious moments and sometimes even flashbacks of your last experience. And even after your baby is born, anxiety may linger that something could still go wrong.

In this chapter, we'll explore those feelings and others you may be having right now and discuss ways that you can ease your anxiety. We'll also look at the various issues that may concern you, such as whether you can be induced early or whether your doctor will be on hand for the delivery. Finally, we'll explore what you can expect if your baby is born with health problems that require treatment in the neonatal intensive care unit.

Regardless of whether your baby needs a little extra care or goes home with you right away, you will probably soon come to the same realization that I did: just as your feelings of grief and anxiety did not magically go away once you got pregnant again, they will not suddenly disappear after the birth of your next child. The journey we started on the day our babies died is a long one, with many twists and turns. And just when you think you've reached the end of the road, another curve appears ahead.

Common Concerns

Inducing Labor

As your due date approaches, you may wonder whether it's possible for your doctor to induce labor. If you are having serious complications that put your baby's life in jeopardy, there is no question that you will deliver sooner rather than later. But if everything is going well, inducing labor is typically not an option until thirty-eight or thirty-nine weeks. At that point, though, you may find that your past history factors into the doctor's decision. Diane's obstetrician, for example, was sensitive to her desire to avoid giving birth to her second baby around the same time that her first one had died. "I requested to be induced two weeks early so we wouldn't get into the anniversary dates, and my doctor didn't have a problem with that." Melinda wanted an early delivery because she had no explanation for why her last pregnancy ended in a loss at thirty-eight weeks gestation. Her doctor also agreed to deliver two weeks before her due date. "I would have been an absolute wreck if I had had to wait any longer," she says.

If your doctor decides to induce labor, you may be admitted to the hospital in the evening so that you can be given prostaglandin gel or suppositories to soften your cervix overnight. If your cervix is already showing signs of dilating, your doctor might rupture your membranes or administer oxytocin to help start contractions. Then it may take anywhere from half an hour to eight or more hours for labor to begin. If your wait turns out to be long, fetal monitoring can help ease your mind. "My doctor knew how nervous I was, so he let me keep the strap on my belly all night so I could listen to the baby," says Carli. "Of course, I didn't sleep at all."

If your labor is not induced, it will be up to you to judge when to go to the hospital. Although women are sometimes advised to wait until their contractions are about five minutes apart, you may want to leave for the hopital as soon as you suspect you are in labor. That way, you too can have the reassurance of hearing the baby's heartbeat on the fetal monitor. This can be especially helpful if you had to go through your last delivery knowing that the baby had already died. Talk to your obstetrician beforehand to find out whether it's okay for you to go directly to the hospital when labor begins or if you should call ahead first. Keep in mind that labor often progresses much more quickly when you have already given birth before. But if you are more comfortable staying at home until the contractions become more intense, you should still be able to time your delivery so that you reach the hospital with plenty of time to spare.

Delivery by Another Doctor

You may recall that one of the questions in the interview with your new physician was whether or not the doctor could arrange to be present for your delivery. If the answer was "maybe," now is the time for you to start preparing yourself for the possibility that someone else may be stepping in. If that turns out to be the case, your physician can make the experience less stressful for you by planning ahead to ensure that the doctor delivering your baby is sensitive to your needs. Heather's obstetrician, for example, alerted everyone on his staff that she would need special attention. She recalls:

> A female doctor delivered, whom I had never met before, but the wonderful thing was that my doctor knew he was going to be out of town so he made sure everybody knew I was coming in. He had three other doctors in his practice and every single one of them checked in on me before Samuel was born. When she came in, she took my hand and said, "I hear we're going to have a baby today. I know about your history. I know about your last baby and we're going to make this a special time." I just fell in love with her.

You can also do your own planning by hiring a doula or labor support professional to be in the delivery room with you. Since you will meet with her several times before the birth, she can be your advocate in your doctor's absence. Keep in mind, too, that it may be just as difficult for another physician to step in and handle your delivery as it is for you to trust anyone besides your own obstetrician. As Brooke, who had previously given birth to a baby with a chromosomal abnormality, remembers, "The same partner was on call when I went in again and I could tell that he was a nervous wreck because of what happened the last time."

Labor

Labor is difficult under any circumstances, but it may be especially hard on you because of your fears for the baby's well-being. It is not unusual for women who have suffered a loss to have flashbacks during the subsequent delivery. You may remember every excruciating detail of your miscarriage or of giving birth to a baby you knew was no longer alive. Or maybe you keep thinking back to the moment when you found out that your newborn was going to die. Even if you are not dwelling on the details of the last delivery, you may nonetheless expect another bad outcome. Brooke, whose third baby had died within hours of birth, says she could not help but fear the worst when she went to deliver her fourth child.

> *I always deliver my babies very quickly, so I knew that I was going to have a short labor. In fact, even before I got to the hospital, I was already feeling like I needed to push. But the nurse kept trying to tell me that it wasn't time yet, and was saying, "I can handle it." And I was like, "No, you can't. There's going to be something wrong with this baby and I've already lost one, so get the doctor here now."*

Despite her fears about the baby's well-being, Brooke did have the advantage of knowing a little bit about what to expect during labor itself. But if you've not been through labor, you will have the additional anxiety of facing the unknown. You may worry about everything from how painful the contractions will be to whether you will embarrass yourself during the delivery. Even if you did go through labor last time, you may find that everything is different this time. Your contractions, for example, may be much more intense at full-term than they were if you delivered a preterm baby that weighed only a pound or two. And even if you went full-term before, your labor won't necessarily be the same. Just as every pregnancy is different, so too is every labor.

Your feelings will also be different this time around. In fact, some women say their feelings changed even from one stage of labor to the next. Some started out confident that all was well and then gradually became more fearful as the contractions intensified. Others felt just the opposite, scared at first but later too immersed in labor to worry about anything else. For me, it was always the epidural that triggered my most anxious moments. I would start shaking (a common side effect of the drugs) and then proceed to lose all control of my emotions. I remember one nurse telling me it was just a case of hormones, but I knew it was so much more than that. Other women told me they were most afraid when it came time to push. That may be because in their particular case pushing is what brought them face to face with death the last time.

If you find yourself getting anxious during labor, try to relax and think positively. Remember, too, that the hardest part is nearly behind you. Before long, your baby will be here, and your pregnancy will be only a memory. You'll find other tips for easing your anxiety later in this chapter.

Cesarean or Vaginal Delivery

The vast majority of us went into our first pregnancy hoping and preparing for a vaginal birth. We may not have been sure whether we wanted to go the completely natural route or have an epidural for pain relief, but we *were* certain that we wanted to avoid a cesarean section if at all possible. After all, anyone who has been pregnant knows the advantages of delivering vaginally. Every pregnancy book talks about it, every doctor stresses it and every childbirth class extols it. Given all the build-up, it is not unusual for women to feel disappointed when a cesarean turns out to be necessary.

But now that you have had a pregnancy end in a loss, you may not care at all how the baby is delivered as long as he or she comes out alive. You may even wonder whether an elective cesarean is an option so that you can get the baby out as quickly as possible this time. In most cases, the answer is no. C-sections are considered major surgery. Not only do you run the risk (albeit small) of complications, such as infection or internal bleeding, you will also require a relatively lengthy recovery.

Sometimes, however, vaginal delivery is not an option. Such situations include serious complications in the mother, such as diabetes or active herpes infection; pregnancy complications, such as placenta previa or placental abruption; and fetal distress. But if you don't fall into any of these high-risk categories, you will almost certainly have to go through labor. Occasionally, however, you may be allowed to opt for a surgical delivery if your labor does not progress as expected. Melinda is a case in point. She remembers:

We induced in the morning, and my doctor kept checking me to see if I was dilated and I wasn't, so he gave me a choice. He said, "You can come back in a couple of days or you can have the baby with a C-section at the end of the day, whatever you want." And I said, "Let's have the baby. I don't want to come back." I didn't see any reason to wait. The baby was ready, so why not take it?

If you are not as open to the idea of a cesarean as Melinda was, you might want to try jump-starting your labor in the event that you run into any problems. Sometimes walking or changing positions can help. You can ask your doctor or obstetrical nurse for other tips. Even if you end up having a surgical delivery despite your best efforts, a trial of labor can still be a good thing. Babies who are exposed to the natural hormones released during contractions tend to have fewer breathing problems than those born to mothers who did not go through labor, and they are usually better prepared to face life outside the womb. Knowing that all your pain will result in gains for your baby will undoubtedly make the experience more tolerable.

If your previous delivery was a cesarean, you may still have the option of delivering vaginally this time. If that possibility interests you, talk to your doctor about VBAC, or vaginal birth after cesarean. As the term implies, VBACs have debunked the "once a cesarean, always a cesarean" myth. Not only will a VBAC help you avoid another major surgery, it will also ensure that your subsequent delivery is not anything like your last one. That was one of Glenda's main goals when she requested a VBAC. "With Nicholas I had a c-section, and I told the doctor I wanted to go VBAC the next time because I wanted a totally different birth experience," she says. "He said as long as the baby wasn't over 8 pounds it wouldn't be a problem." Check with your doctor to see what he recommends in your case. Before making your decision, though, find out your doctor's success rate with VBACS and the possible risks. You can then decide whether you want to undergo a trial of labor or schedule an elective cesarean.

Bonding with the Baby

When the nurse finally puts your newborn baby in your arms, you will be overwhelmed by all kinds of feelings: joy, sadness, relief and gratitude, to name a few. You may even have trouble believing that this tiny infant is really yours. In fact, it may take some time before you feel close to the baby. While you may worry that it is somehow abnormal not to feel maternal right away, it actually makes sense. After all, you may have just spent most of the last nine months trying *not* to bond, and changing course can take time. Kim says, "When Chelsea was born, part of me was overjoyed to see her, but part of me felt very distant to her. I really had not had a chance to get attached to her." Margo felt even more distant when she awoke from the general anesthesia that had been given to her during an emergency c-section.

*They told me it was a girl, and I had wanted all boys, so I just said, "Oh,"
and went back to sleep. My husband thought I didn't love her, but I think
the reason I acted so strange is that I was still so scared. I just knew*

something was not going to be right. But after a while, I wanted to see her and hold her.

Researchers have found that this hesitancy to bond usually lasts only a short while. Before long, your feelings for the subsequent baby will be as strong as those experienced by any other mother. But feelings of anxiety are usually not so easily dismissed. Parents are often apprehensive for months or even years after the birth of their subsequent children. As a result, they tend to be more overprotective than most, at least in the short run. We'll talk more about this and other parenting issues in the next chapter.

Breastfeeding vs. Bottle Feeding

To help facilitate early bonding, mothers are usually allowed to hold their newborns immediately after birth. They are also encouraged to breastfeed their baby right away. If you've never nursed before, you may find that this does not necessarily come naturally. Like so much else, it must be learned. Don't hesitate to ask your nurse for assistance or see a lactation specialist if you feel like you need extra help. Persevering may be easier if you keep in mind that breast milk is the best source of nutrition for your newborn. In fact, the American Academy of Pediatrics now recommends breastfeeding for at least the first year of life. That's partly because research shows that in addition to being a better source of nutrition than infant formula, human breast milk can also decrease the incidence of certain infections and allergies in the baby. Some evidence suggests that breastfeeding may offer protection against SIDS as well.

But the advantages of nursing go beyond nutrition and health. Breastfeeding is convenient and cheap—two advantages that formula doesn't offer. It can also give you a sense of pride to know that you are providing your child with everything he or she needs to grow up healthy. Given all these benefits, why would anyone ever bottle-feed their baby? Some women change to bottle-feeding when they return

to work. Others prefer to pump their breastmilk and bottle-feed occasionally to give the father more opportunities to bond with the baby.
Still others quit breastfeeding if they have trouble making it work. A
few won't even try breastfeeding because they see it as continued
responsibility for keeping the baby alive. "I feel like my body has
done all that it can do," says one new mother. "I can't even imagine
being my baby's food supply."

Just as so many decisions during the pregnancy were only yours to
make, the decision to breastfeed is also a uniquely personal one. Try
not to feel guilty if you ultimately decide that nursing is not for you.
Yes, breastfeeding is best for the baby, but feeding babies formula
also suffices.

The Baby's Health

If life were even the least bit fair, all of us who have suffered a
pregnancy loss or the death of a newborn would somehow be ensured
of having perfectly healthy children in the future. Since we've already
experienced such a tragedy, we shouldn't have to endure any more
heartache with our children. But we all know that life is not fair.
Subsequent babies are sometimes born with health problems, or they
occasionally get sick after birth. And those of us who have suffered
complications know that any kind, no matter how minor, can send us
into a panic. When I heard that Andrew's collarbone had been fractured, I started imagining all kinds of worst-case scenarios, such as
my baby being in a cast or even crippled. After the doctor explained
that the fracture would heal itself without any kind of medical intervention, I breathed a small sigh of relief, still worried that the story
wasn't over. It was only when the pediatrician confirmed several
weeks later that the bone had indeed healed that I finally began to
relax.

When I started interviewing women for this book, I quickly discovered that my reaction was not unusual. Problems that would cause
only passing concern in most parents become major crises for those
who have suffered a loss. Brooke, for example, became hysterical
when her baby ingested meconium during the delivery.

The doctor wanted me to stop pushing so that he could suction the baby's lungs, but I couldn't stop. So he came all the way out and they had to call neonatal in, and I'm sitting there screaming, "I've killed my baby." For a good thirty seconds—and it may have been longer than that—I thought he had died and that I had done it. I thought I had killed my baby because I couldn't stop pushing.

Brooke was relieved once her baby started breathing on his own and no other complications developed. You'll recall she was the woman who told the nurse during labor that there was going to be something wrong with the baby. Like so many women who have suffered a loss, she expected her baby to have problems because she could not believe that she could be fortunate enough to have a healthy child. Sharon felt much the same way. When her preterm baby developed respiratory syncytial virus (RSV) a few days after birth, it confirmed what she had most feared. As she explains, "Those first few days, I told my mom and my husband both, 'It seems too good to be true that we have this beautiful perfect baby.' So when he got sick, I said to my husband, 'I told you so.'"

In both Brooke's and Sharon's case, the babies did not require extended stays in the neonatal intensive care unit. But that didn't make these episodes any less traumatic for the mothers. In instances when babies are born with special needs that require lengthy hospitalization, the situation can be even more overwhelming. We'll address that issue later in this chapter.

Common Feelings

Calmness

Calm is not a word most of us would use to describe our feelings during our subsequent pregnancy. In fact, many women continue to be wracked by fear right up until the umbilical cord is cut. But a few say that by the time their labor finally began, an inexplicable calm came over them. Perhaps it's because at that point they knew they had done all they could, and the rest was in God's hands. Or it could be that they were so focused on getting through the labor itself that they no longer had time to be apprehensive about the baby. Some, like Margo, say they just couldn't explain their eerie sense of calmness. She remembers:

> At one point while I was in labor, we all of a sudden lost the baby's heartbeat. The doctor came running in and he couldn't find it so he said, "C-section, stat," and all of a sudden there were fifteen nurses and doctors on top of me. They wouldn't even let my husband go in because they thought the baby had died. But I can remember them putting me under and I had the calmest feeling and I thought, "This is going to be okay." And my parents are out there thinking this baby has died; [my husband] is thinking the baby's died; the doctor probably thought so, and I just had the most peaceful feeling that everything was gong to be fine. I'm not sure why, but I just did.

Fortunately for Margo, she turned out to be right and the baby born that day under the most frightening of circumstances is now a healthy, ten-year-old girl. We can only hope that your delivery will be nowhere near as dramatic, but breathing exercises and other relaxation techniques may help you achieve the same sense of calm. You may also want to try the visualization exercise described later in this chapter. If you can't manage to calm yourself down or think positively, try not to worry about it. That doesn't mean there is anything wrong with your baby. Some women are just better at mastering their emotions than others.

Joy

When you finally do give birth to a healthy child, nothing can match the joy you will feel. Hearing your baby cry for the first time or holding your newborn in your arms will provoke feelings that are simply indescribable. The joy is often even sweeter coming as it does on the heels of such great pain, as Rita, whose first baby died from complications related to prematurity, recalls.

There was so much joy when Trevor was born. Even my doctor cried because he was so happy. It was funny, because the first thing the baby did was pee all over the doctor, and we thought that was the greatest thing that ever happened because our baby who died at times would not urinate. Now we had this healthy eight-pound, fourteen-ounce boy, and there was a whole lot of joy that God had given us a healthy baby.

Undoubtedly, you are looking forward to a delivery like Rita's, one with lots of laughter and celebration. If you gave birth before in a shroud of silence and grief, it is no wonder that you would want the experience to be ideal this time. But even if the circumstances surrounding the subsequent birth are less than perfect, it will probably not be enough to put a damper on things. Kim, for example, delivered her next baby in the same room at the same hospital where her daughter was stillborn. "It didn't matter," she says. "I was just so relieved and so happy to have my baby. You feel like it's never going to end, like you'll never be happy again, but then you are happy."

Relief

Like Kim, you, too, will feel enormously relieved that your pregnancy is over and you have given birth to a healthy baby. It will also give you a sense of confidence to know that you are capable of having a successful pregnancy, even though at this point you may not care whether you ever go through it again. Says Sharon: "I never ever thought I would be so glad for a pregnancy to end because I loved every minute of my first pregnancy. But I think you don't realize what a gift it is to enjoy being pregnant until you lose a baby. Then you wish things could go back to the way they used to be. I know both my husband and I held back a little bit of ourselves right up until the cord was cut and we had a baby." Try to savor that feeling of relief while it lasts, because it probably won't be long before it's replaced by still more anxiety.

Anxiety

Even though you were under the impression that all of your anxiety would disappear after the birth of a healthy child, you may discover that you remain anxious long after you take your newborn home from the hospital. Some women are unable to shake the feeling that if it happened once, it could happen again. If the hospital does not allow the baby in the room with you round-the-clock, your most trying moments may come when the baby is in the nursery at night. Leslie describes how she felt about allowing her baby to go to the newborn nursery:

> I kept the baby in my room the first night and didn't sleep at all, so the second night I let the nurse take him and then I lay there for hours thinking she had abducted my baby. I slept maybe thirty minutes. The rest of the time I kept thinking, "Where was her tag? Where was her picture?" I knew in my head that he was fine and I needed to get some sleep. But it's just that mother thing—you worry.

Susie was so apprehensive that she refused to allow her baby to go to the nursery, even though the hospital didn't allow rooming in at night. "Since they told me the baby couldn't stay with me while I was asleep, I just stayed awake the whole night. I flat out didn't sleep. The nurses got mad at me because I wouldn't let her go."

Why all this anxiety once the baby is safe and sound? Some apprehension is normal among all new mothers, but women who have experienced a loss are painfully aware that life offers no guarantees. As Kelly says, "I was horribly worried because I thought, 'Now I have him here in my arms, but that doesn't mean he's going to live past tomorrow.' "

Sadness

Your subsequent pregnancy will be one of contradictions. There will be the joy of expecting another baby, but also sadness over the one that you lost. The birth of your subsequent baby is no different. It, too, will be marked by contradictions. Like many women, you may find that the birth of your next child resurrects much of the grief over your loss. "For some women, the birth of the subsequent child is a reminder of what they lost and a renewal of grief for a while," says Dr. Judith Lasker, coauthor of *When Pregnancy Fails*. "They're sad at first when they expected to be deliriously happy."

Others may have a hard time understanding why you are sad at a time when they, too, are convinced you should be happy. But having another baby often makes your loss all the more real. In some cases, postpartum depression only serves to heighten your already sad feelings. Julie's reaction is typical: "I thought, 'What, am I crazy?' I'm holding this baby and I'm crying for Gina. I guess seeing him just made me realize how much I missed her. And I think in a way, I was waiting for him to die, too. I just couldn't believe he could be okay after grieving for so long."

Sharon, who had lost a baby girl, experienced similar emotions when she first laid eyes on her newborn son. "He filled so much a part of me, but so much of me was still with her," she says. Margo found the memories of her stillborn son most overwhelming when it came time to leave the hospital with her new baby. "When I was being wheeled out with Katie, my head was down the whole time. All I could think about was how awful it had been to leave the hospital without Matthew. I think it hits everybody in different ways, and that's how it hit me."

It is understandable that you would feel some sense of sadness over your loss once your next baby is born. You know all too well that this baby has a sibling who should be there with you, too. But the grief you feel now is one more step that will help you work through the pain.

Feeling Overwhelmed

If this baby is the first one you will actually care for, you may feel a lot like all new parents: overwhelmed by the awesome responsibilities that await you. Sheila describes how she felt immediately after the birth of her baby boy: "I had worked so hard to have this baby, but I remember being in recovery and thinking, 'What do I do now?' Now that I had the baby, this was a whole new chapter that I hadn't even thought about."

I, too, had focused so much of my energy on learning everything possible about pregnancy that I hadn't even thought about how I would care for my baby. Unfortunately, I didn't have much experience, either. Although I had sometimes baby-sitted older children, I had never taken care of a newborn before. All I really had to fall back on was advice from other mothers and a little hospital booklet entitled *My Baby's Here . . . Now What Do I Do?* That pretty much summed up how I felt.

I don't think the reality of the situation really hit me until the day we took the baby home from the hospital. Things were tense from the moment we got in the car. Somehow we had propped the car seat up so much that I spent most of the ride home trying to keep the baby from sliding out. Then as soon as we got home, the tears started— both mine and the baby's. At the hospital, Andrew had slept pretty soundly, usually only waking up to eat. Now, not only was he wide awake, he was refusing to breastfeed. I tried everything from holding him in different positions to taking warm showers to let down my milk supply, but nothing seemed to work.

By morning, I was desperate and frantically searching the phone book for the number of anyone who could tell me what to do. Finally, I got through to my support group leader who also happened to be a lactation specialist. I tearfully explained that I was afraid my baby was starving to death. He hadn't eaten in hours and his diapers were dry. Although my fears were legitimate, I apologized at the time for overreacting. Maybe I was being neurotic, I told her, because my other baby had died. But I was just so scared. She quickly reassured me that my reaction was perfectly normal. The first night home from the hospital is hard on most new mothers, she said, even those who have never had a loss. (I've since discovered how right she was.) She then invited me to take the baby up to the hospital so she could help me with breastfeeding.

That was the first of many similar situations in the days and weeks that followed. I worried about everything from how often he nursed to whether or not he was breathing. What made it worse for me was that I thought I was somehow strange for feeling that way. I didn't know how very normal it is for parents who have lost a child to be anxious in the early weeks, especially if they have never cared for a child before. So don't be surprised—or discouraged—if you are a basket case for a while after you take your baby home. It seems to go with the territory. Although it probably won't be long before you begin to feel like a pro, it may take some time before your apprehension disappears completely. We'll talk more about the parenting issues you are likely to face in the next chapter.

Tips for Easing Anxiety

Go Back to the Hospital

One of the best things you can do to prepare yourself for the experience of labor and delivery is to visit the hospital where you plan to give birth. This is especially important if you are returning to the same place where your baby died. By facing some of your memories beforehand, they are less likely to overwhelm you during the birth itself. If you have been in counseling in the months since your loss, consider talking to your therapist before you make the trip to the hospital so you can better prepare yourself for any emotional fallout. Even if you are going to a different hospital, it is still a good idea to see where you will be giving birth. Although the facility may be different, the basic setting will be the same, and that may trigger painful flashbacks. Again, those memories will be easier to handle if you deal with some of them before you even go into labor.

Sherokee Ilse, author of *Empty Arms* and numerous other books on pregnancy loss, says she felt compelled to return to the hospital on the first anniversary of her baby's death. She asked to go back to the room where she had given birth and then took time to reflect on everything that had happened on that tragic day a year before. She recalls: "It helped me to cry, remember and relive the experience, which I think was a necessary part of the healing. It also gave me some peace. I was less afraid to go back to the hospital when it came time to deliver my next baby."

Although a hospital tour is a standard part of any prepared childbirth class, you may want to go on your own as Sherokee did so that you have time to reflect privately. If you don't have the courage to go directly to the labor and delivery floor, consider approaching it in stages. Drive by the hospital a few times first. Then go into the building, but stay in the lobby area. That in itself can be difficult because it may remind you of when you left the hospital without your baby. Once you feel comfortable, continue to labor and delivery. Besides cutting down on the number of flashbacks you're likely to have during the birth, returning to the hospital can remind you of any special requests you want to make. If your loss was a late one and you recognize the room where you delivered before, for example, you can ask to be put somewhere else.

Since my doctor's office was in a building adjoining the hospital, I could have toured the facility at any time. But for months, I kept walking straight through the lobby and on to my car. Then one day, I mustered the courage to go to the floor where I would be delivering my baby. The experience was both painful and exciting. I knew that in a few weeks I would be getting a second chance to give birth, and yet I couldn't help but remember the tragic details of my last delivery. After standing in one of the labor and delivery rooms for a while, I walked over to the nursery to look at the babies. While that might not sound like a big deal to most people, it was actually a major breakthrough for me because it marked the first time since Patrick's death that I had come face-to-face with a newborn. As difficult as that experience was, I think it helped me better prepare for the day when I went back to deliver my own baby. Since I had already dealt with the initial shock of returning to a labor and delivery ward, it was one less thing for me to cope with on the day I gave birth.

Make Sure the Staff Knows Your History

Another advantage to touring the hospital before you have your baby is that it will give you the opportunity to make the labor and delivery staff aware of your history. Ask to talk to the head nurse and tell her about your loss. Request that a note be attached to your chart so that everyone involved in your delivery will also know that you have special needs. If the staff knows your history, they are likely to be more sensitive to your feelings and help you from unwanted comments and questions. It's hard enough to answer questions such as, "Is this your first baby?" when you're standing in line at the grocery store. But when you're in labor, it's totally unacceptable. Leslie describes what a difference it made for her to have a supportive nurse during her subsequent delivery:

> The nurse practitioner knew me, and she knew about my baby who had died, and she was like an angel from heaven. She bent over backwards to make the delivery everything I ever dreamed of. She handed my baby to me right away, and I kept him with me a long time before they even took him to the nursery. Then since she knew I would be paranoid about the baby going to the nursery, she let my husband go with him.

You'll find that the medical team's joy nearly matches your own when the baby is safely delivered. They know what it's like for a pregnancy to end in a loss; they see it all too often. Just as they share in a woman's sadness when the worst happens, they revel in her happiness when all goes well.

Get Support

Others who may be able to help during labor and delivery are counselors from any support group you may have attended after your baby died. They will be in tune with your feelings and can help you deal with painful memories. It will be especially reassuring to hear them tell you that it is normal for you to be thinking about your other baby at this time. All of us who have given birth again following a loss have had the same thoughts. Nancy credits her counselors with making an otherwise nerve-wracking situation better.

A couple of counselors recognized me and so they came in and gave me suggestions. They said if you know what room you were in, you can asked to be moved; if you want something or don't want something, you have to let it be known. Someone else may not know, so you have to tell them what is comfortable for you.

In many cases, the counselors work full-time at the hospital, so they will be nearby should you need them. But if your support group meets at a different location, you can always make arrangements beforehand for a counselor to meet you at the hospital for the delivery.

Ask for Explanations and Reassurance

Later in this chapter we'll examine the different types of fetal monitoring you can have to keep track of your baby's well-being during labor. But as wonderful as technology can be, it's not perfect. Equipment can malfunction, and the baby's heartbeat can show signs of distress or disappear altogether, even when all is well. That's why it is extremely important for an obstetrical nurse or a professional labor assistant to talk you through each stage of labor and give you clear explanations of what is happening. You need to know precisely what to expect and when it will end so that you can be an active participant in the process.

Relax and Visualize

Whether you took a prepared childbirth class during your last pregnancy or you have just recently completed a round of instruction, you undoubtedly learned a lot about relaxation during labor. Some common techniques that women have found helpful through the years include breathing exercises, laboring to music, warm baths and massages. But considering that you have spent most of the last nine months feeling tense, you may need a little extra help to relax your mind and body. The visualization exercise developed by Joann O'Leary of Abbott Northwestern Hospital is designed especially for women who have experienced a loss (see page 318). Consider using this script to prepare for labor and then take it to the hospital with you so that your partner or labor support professional can read it aloud when your nerves start to get the best of you.

Medical Issues during Labor and Delivery

Fetal Monitoring

Given the tragic outcome of your last pregnancy, your biggest concerns during labor may not be so much about yourself as about the baby you are carrying. One way doctors have of keeping track of the baby's well-being during childbirth is through fetal monitoring. Using special equipment, they can check to see how the baby's heartbeat responds during contractions. If the monitor shows an irregular pattern, it may indicate that the baby is in distress and in need of immediate medical attention.

The use of such technology during labor is controversial, since some experts believe that fetal monitoring is largely responsible for the rise in the cesarean rate in recent years. The theory is that monitoring leads to far-too-many false alarms and unnecessary surgical interventions. But if you had to deliver your last baby already knowing that the doctors could no longer detect a heartbeat, you may consider fetal monitoring essential to your mental health. This will be espe-

Visualization Script to Help Parents Prepare for Labor

Settle back into your pillow/chair. . . . Rest your head and body and sink into relaxation. Take a deep breath, breathing in . . . and out. Breathe slowly . . . and purposefully, as naturally as you can. Let your emotions slowly release bit by bit.

Think about the baby you are carrying now in your uterus. This baby, with each breath you take, is moving up and down, gently rocking to your breaths. This baby feels comfortable . . . warm . . . and secure . . . rocking with each breath, hearing your heartbeat, feeling your worries and concerns, but knowing the worry is because of the baby who was here before he/she was . . . the baby you loved and wanted, but whose life with you was too short.

This baby here with you today has listened to your stories, has felt your pain, and knows your love is given cautiously, not because you don't love him/her, but because you love him/her so much. This baby feels deeply the concern and protection you have clung to during this pregnancy, to want him/her to feel safe.

Breathe in and out . . . visualizing this baby inside loving you and the other voices in the family that your baby hears. This baby is waiting to come out to show you his/her own unique personality and will help you believe again that life can be good and beautiful. Continue to breathe in and out at your own comfortable rate, letting go of as much as the fear you can for this baby.

You have nurtured and cared for yourself and this baby all these long months. Now begin to allow your body to prepare for labor and birth . . . let go of the tension . . . let go of the fear. Let the contractions come when the baby is ready . . . start slowly and build up your strength, opening your cervix, allowing this baby to come into your life. Let the children who came before celebrate with you this new life that will begin to heal your wounds and nurture your continued journey into parenting.

cially true if your baby was among the few who died due to complications related to the birth.

Remember, though, that the benefits of fetal monitoring come with some drawbacks. As we've already discussed, there is always a risk that the equipment could malfunction and indicate a problem where none actually exists. The jury is also still out on the effectiveness of electronic monitoring. At least one study concluded that it is no more effective than listening to the heart rate periodically using hand-held devices. It will be up to you to decide whether the disadvantages outweigh the advantages. To help you make the most informed decision, let's look briefly at the different kinds of fetal monitoring that are available.

External Fetal Monitoring

Most of the time, fetal monitoring is done externally, using two belts that are strapped around the mother's abdomen. One belt monitors the fetal heartbeat, while the other one records uterine contractions. The results appear on a printout. Typically, a baby's heart rate will speed up with movement and either remain stable or drop slightly during a contraction. As long as the baby is getting enough oxygen, the heart rate will quickly return to normal levels once the contraction is over. But if the heart rate remains low or does not show the normal pattern of deceleration and acceleration, it may be a sign that the baby is in distress or not getting enough oxygen.

Normally, external fetal monitoring requires that you stay in bed, but you may want to ask whether your hospital has telemetry, a system whereby vital signs are transmitted with radio waves. This would give you the freedom to walk around during labor while still keeping track of your baby's well-being.

Internal Fetal Monitoring

If the results of external monitoring show cause for concern, your doctor may opt to monitor the baby internally. This can provide an even clearer picture of what is happening inside the womb. With internal monitoring, an electrode is inserted through the vagina and attached to the baby's scalp to track the fetal heart rate. Another device is placed in the uterus to record the strength and duration of contractions. Internal monitoring can only be done once the membranes have ruptured and the cervix has started to dilate. Because it is an invasive procedure, it also carries a higher risk of infection.

Fetal-Scalp Blood Sampling

Fetal-scalp blood sampling is an even more sophisticated way of checking on the baby's well-being. In this procedure, which is only done when there is reason to believe that the baby is not getting enough oxygen, a blood sample is drawn from the baby's scalp so that it can be checked for oxygen concentration. Although the results are usually available within a few minutes, you might find it difficult to wait that long when your doctor suspects your baby may be in distress. Consider talking to your obstetrician now about what criteria will be used to determine when a surgical delivery is necessary.

After-Birth Care

When your child has finally made his or her way into this world, there will be a flurry of activity as the cord is cut and clamped and the baby's condition is evaluated. Using what is known as an APGAR scoring system, your doctor or nurse will check the baby's activity or muscle tone (A), pulse (P), grimace or reflex (G), appearance or skin color (A), and respiration (R). Scores in each category range from 0 to 2. A total score of 7 to 10 is considered normal. Newborns who score 6 or below usually need some kind of assistance, which can range from suctioning their mouth and throat to more drastic lifesaving measures. The APGAR is done at one minute after birth and repeated at five minutes after birth. Most babies do better on the second evaluation since they have had time to recover from labor and get used to life on the outside.

Depending on the standard practice at your particular hospital, your baby may be wrapped in warm blankets and handed to you immediately after birth, or only after the evaluation is completed. (If you have had a cesarean, the baby will be brought to you later in your recovery.) Either way, it will be a moment that you cherish for the rest of your life. In fact, you may be reluctant to ever let go. But at some point, the baby has to be taken to the nursery to be bathed, weighed, measured and footprinted. Usually additional evaluation is done there. Depending on hospital policy, your partner may be able to stay with your baby until the three of you can be reunited.

The Neonatal Intensive Care Unit

Occasionally, babies are born with such serious health problems that they must go directly to the neonatal intensive care unit. Although we hope this won't happen to your newborn, in case it does, it will help if you have planned ahead for it. As we already discussed in Chapter 3, the easiest way to prepare is to deliver at a hospital that has a high-level neonatal intensive care nursery. Otherwise, your critically ill baby would have to be transferred to another hospital, and you would be unable to visit until you were released. In the meantime, your partner would have to shuttle between the two facilities, as Glenda's did after the birth of her son who later died. "I had never realized that I had to look at the neonatal level of a hospital before, so Nicholas had to be transferred to another hospital, and my husband was having to go back and forth. I vowed that would never happen again." And it never did. When Glenda gave birth to her subsequent child, she made sure it was at a hospital with an NICU.

Assuming that you *are* delivering at a hospital with an NICU, what can you expect if your baby ends up in one? You may not even want to think about this prospect, but looking back, don't you wish that someone had prepared you for the possibility that your baby may have died? Wouldn't you have done some things differently if you had known then what you know now? I certainly would have. I would have spent more time with my baby and taken pictures of him and kept everything that ever touched his skin. But as it was, I had no clue what to do. So just in case your subsequent baby needs extra care in the NICU, let's go over some things that will help you cope better with the situation.

For starters, you should know that if your baby is born with health concerns, it may be difficult for doctors to immediately determine what is causing the problem. A neonatologist—a pediatrician who specializes in the care of newborns—will consider many possibilities and eliminate them one by one. Many of them will sound scary, but that doesn't mean they are more likely to cause the baby's problems.

When Michael was born, for example, the neonatologist literally recited a list of possibilities that could be causing his breathing difficulties. "It could be a heart defect or an infection," he said. Just in case it was the latter, they were going to give him antibiotics. "It could also be fluid in his lungs or lung immaturity," he added. There was just no way of knowing without running some tests. Fortunately, it turned out that Michael had fluid in his lungs as well as some lung immaturity, two fairly routine problems that babies have when they are born too early. But during the hours it took to figure that out, I had to lie in my bed wondering whether I was about to lose another child.

Even once the doctors isolate the problem, they sometimes continue to paint worst-case scenarios to avoid getting your hopes up in the event that things do not go as planned. This is what my doctor did. For instance, he never volunteered that he had ruled out a heart problem or infection. I had to ask him. And when he saw that I was relieved by the news that Michael's problems were related to his lungs, he told me, "Mrs. Lanham, you have a very sick baby." He did not bother to add that it was probably unlikely that my baby was going to die from his problems since, at thirty-seven weeks gestation, he had none of the other complications generally related to prematurity. It was only a couple of days later that my husband mustered up the courage to ask another doctor in the NICU, "Do you think he's going to die?" The doctor looked flabbergasted by the question and responded with an emphatic, "No!"

Unfortunately, there will be times when the news is not as good. And if that happens to be the case with your subsequent baby, you will once again be walking a tightrope, wondering whether your child will live or die. What are some other things that will help you cope during what will be a very trying few days or weeks? Here are some suggestions gleaned from my own experience and those of other women who have had babies in the NICU.

Brace yourself. If you have never seen a baby in the NICU, it may help if you know what to expect when you first lay eyes on your child. If your baby is premature, she will probably be in an incubator to help maintain her body temperature. Otherwise, she will be lying on her back on a tablelike bed with bright lights overhead to keep her warm. She will be clad only in a diaper. Her head may be shaved so that an IV can be inserted into her scalp where the veins are larger and easier to access, or she may have a catheter in her navel. She will also have electrodes attached to her chest to monitor her heart rate and breathing. She may have a small tube running down her nose to help remove mucus. If she cannot breathe on her own, she will be on a respirator. Otherwise she might have what is known as a CPAP (continuous positive airway pressure) or simply be placed under a clear plastic hood filled with oxygen. Periodically, the nurses will be taking small amounts of blood for tests. She will also likely be under very close supervision, with one nurse assigned to her and just one other baby.

Learn the ropes. If you think it's bad to see your baby hooked up to so many wires and monitors, it's even worse to walk into the NICU and not be able to find her at all. And yet, this happens all the time. As new infants are brought into the unit, other babies are moved to different places within the nursery or to other nurseries within the hospital. If you know that this is a possibility, you won't be as surprised when it happens. It can also be disconcerting to hear all the warning bells that will be sounding almost continuously from your baby's monitors. Although the equipment is designed to help the nurses keep track of vital signs such as the baby's heart rate, respiration rate and blood pressure, alarms do not always mean that something is wrong. Ask the nurse to explain them to you, and then do your best not to become obsessed by them. If you stay focused on how your baby looks, that will usually give you the best indication of her condition.

Ask questions. As my own experience illustrates, doctors do not always come back to tell parents when a serious illness has been ruled out. In other cases, physicians simply do not know what the long-term effects of a baby's illness will be. They can only make educated guesses based on their experiences and the facts they have at hand. The best way to deal with this uncertainty is to follow the same course you took during your pregnancy. Ask questions and keep asking until you get answers that satisfy you. Remember, no question is a dumb question. By being as informed as possible, you will be able to make the best decisions for your baby.

Bond with your baby. At first, you won't even be able to see your baby, much less hold her. But as time goes on and her condition improves, the nurses will usually be willing to rearrange all the wires and tubes so that you can hold your newborn in your arms. At that point, you can also ask whether you can participate in some of her care. Bathe her, if they'll let you, and change her diaper. It's also important to stroke and talk to your baby. She will recognize your voice and be comforted by your touch. Ask if you can put pictures in her incubator and bring toys from home, especially any that play soft music. Since it can be taxing for some babies to be overstimulated, there may be a limit to the things you can do. Heed the nurses' advice so that you can do what is best for your baby.

Encourage immediate family to visit. When babies are born sick, there is obviously not the same joy and celebration that follows a normal birth. But it is still important to encourage those closest to you to visit the baby. Maybe this is obvious to most of you, but among members of my family there was a feeling that they should wait until my son was better to come visit. Both my mother and brother stayed away for several days because they did not want to see Michael when he was hooked up to equipment. But if he had died, I would have been faced with having another baby that those I cared most about had never seen. Don't take that risk with your family and friends.

Take pictures of your baby. When the NICU nurses first asked my husband and me whether we had taken pictures of Michael, we were aghast. We were so distraught by the sight of him hooked up to so many tubes and wires that the last thing we wanted to do was take a picture. Thankfully, a wise and very kind nurse brought her own camera in at one point and snapped a picture of me holding my baby. To this day, I remain grateful to her because she was right: once Michael was out of the woods, I wanted a picture of how he had started out his life. And if, God forbid, something had happened to him, I would have treasured that picture all the more.

Try to arrange to stay at the hospital after your release. Since you have already left the hospital once without a baby, it can be heart-wrenching to do so again, even if this time your child is alive and breathing in the NICU. If you have reason to believe that your baby will only be in the hospital for a few days, find out whether you can stay as well. Some hospitals have rooms set aside for mothers who are nursing their NICU babies. I slept in a private room at no charge for several days after I was released. So, when I finally went home, it was not alone but with Michael. If no such rooms are available at the hospital where you deliver, check to see if there is a section for people who have loved ones at the hospital who are critically ill.

Take care of yourself. If your baby's hospital stay drags on for weeks or even months, it will be important for you to take care of yourself. Although you may never want to leave your baby's side, you need to spend some time away every once in a while so that you can clear your head and avoid an emotional collapse. Remember, too, that you are planning on taking this baby home with you this time, and you will need all your strength to care for her.

The Follow-up Visit

While some of the details may have faded from your mind, you no doubt still remember what it was like to go back to the doctor for your follow-up visit after your loss: the pain of seeing a lobby filled with happy mothers-to-be, the fear of what your physician was going to say about your prospects for another pregnancy, the grief of returning to a place where you had once listened excitedly to the baby's heartbeat. But as difficult as that appointment was, it will enable you to appreciate the joy of the next follow-up visit all the more.

The doctor's appointment that follows the birth of a healthy child is always a time of celebration. In your case, it will also give you, the doctor and the staff a much-needed sense of closure to what undoubtedly was a difficult experience for everyone. Consider taking your baby along. Your obstetrician will enjoy seeing how much your newborn has changed in the weeks since the birth, and it will give the staff the opportunity to see your baby. Don't worry too much about keeping your baby quiet during the exam—you'll no doubt find plenty of people willing to lend a helping hand.

As much as you may have looked forward to the end of the pregnancy, you may actually feel a little sad when you leave the office for the last time. After at least nine months of regular visits (and much longer than that for women who stayed with the same doctor after their loss), you will feel strange knowing that you probably will not be returning again until your annual checkup. Saying good-bye will be even harder if you think this baby may be your last. An important part of your life will be coming to an end, and it will take time to get used to that idea. But as close as you may feel to your doctor and staff right now, you probably won't miss them for long. Soon you will enjoy having your body and your time back to yourself. And while you will always be grateful to your doctor for the care he provided during your pregnancies, it will feel good to move on with your life.

Select a Pediatrician

Ideally, you should have selected a pediatrician during your pregnancy so that the doctor would be available to visit your baby in the hospital. But some women who have had a loss are simply too superstitious to interview pediatricians before their baby's birth. Just as it can be difficult to prepare a nursery or buy things for the baby in advance, it can be hard to choose a pediatrician when you still find it hard to believe you will actually need one. Whether you look for a pediatrician before or after your baby's birth, it is important to keep in mind that—at least at first—your needs will be similar to those you had while you were pregnant. You will need to find someone who understands that you may be even more apprehensive than most new mothers. Your doctor should be willing to take your phone calls, spend extra time explaining things to you and not discount your fears and concerns. Consider choosing a pediatrician who has a nurse practitioner on staff since they often are available when the doctor is not.

I was fortunate to find a sensitive doctor in my sons' pediatrician. He always spent plenty of time with me and my baby at each appointment and never hesitated to personally return my phone calls. If I ever had the slightest cause for concern about my child's health, he would urge me to go into the office immediately. Tragically, years later, he came to an even deeper understanding of the special needs of bereaved parents like me when he lost a granddaughter who was born sixteen weeks prematurely. The baby had a twin sister who miraculously survived, and my doctor witnessed first-hand the effect that the loss had on his daughter and son-in-law. Fortunately, doctors do not have to experience the death of a baby in order to understand your special needs. Just be sure that they know your history and are willing to provide the extra level of care that you require.

chapter nine

After the Next Baby's Arrival

YOU'VE MADE IT. The pregnancy is over. Your newborn is home from the hospital. Your prayers have been answered. You finally have a baby to hold and nurture and raise. No more worries about fetal heart rates or kick counts. No more visits to the obstetrician or hospital. No more concerns about overexerting yourself or doing the wrong thing. No more reluctance to bond or dream about the future. From now on, you can be just like those "other women" we talked about back in chapter 1—the ones who seem to have it so easy. Now it's your turn to sit back, relax and enjoy being a mother.

If only life were that simple.

Although it is true that a very difficult period is behind you, it is unlikely that you will ever regain the innocence you had before your loss. And if your last baby died after coming home from the hospital, your biggest worries may be just beginning. Without a doubt, you will treasure your child, but you will also have a new awareness that life is fragile and offers no guarantees, not only during pregnancy but also following birth. But what implications will this have for you and your family? Specifically, how has the loss changed you? Has it made you a different parent than you otherwise would have been? How has it affected your outlook on life and your other children? These are some of the questions we'll try to answer in this chapter.

As discussed in the last chapter, I noticed a difference between me and most other new mothers almost right away. I know that all parents worry, but I could not seem to shake the feeling that my baby was going to die. For months, I continued to have recurring nightmares along those lines. It almost became a ritual. Every night, I would wake with a start and frantically shake my husband, saying, "Where's the baby? What happened to the baby?" He would point reassuringly to the bassinet near our bed and say, "He's right there. Everything's fine." But even though I could see the baby in the crib, I was never convinced that he was really okay. I had to put my hand on his chest and feel him breathe before I could lie down again and try to go back to sleep. On the positive side, every moment with my baby was precious. I loved holding him and feeding him and just looking at him. I even enjoyed getting up with him in the middle of the night because it was a special time we had all to ourselves. I truly felt blessed in every way.

Three years later, the differences between me and most other mothers of young children are a little less obvious. While I love my boys very much, and still feel incredibly blessed to have them, I no longer enjoy sleepless nights. Taking care of a three-year-old and a one-year-old is hard work, and I find that by the time they go to sleep at night, I am ready for a break. And although I used to think that I could never leave them in anyone else's care, I now rely on a trusted babysitter while I work part-time from home, and I look forward to those rare evenings when my husband and I can go out alone. I even let the kids spend the night at their aunt and uncle's house every once in a while—all things that I could never have imagined doing a couple of years ago.

Yet some fundamental differences remain. For starters, not a single day goes by that I don't think about Patrick and what might have been. In a sense, my family will always feel incomplete to me. And I have never been able to forget that my other two children could be taken from me at any time. As a result, I am still enormously grateful for everything that I have. For those reasons and many, many others, I consider myself a completely different person—both as a woman and as a parent—than I would have been had my first-born son not died.

What about you? What can you expect in the weeks, months and years that lie ahead? Let's start by exploring parenting issues that tend to be unique to those of us who have experienced a loss and continue with examples of how your outlook on life may have changed. We'll conclude by looking at ways that we can choose to remember our babies, because no matter how brief their time on this earth was, they will always live on in our hearts.

What You Can Expect

Anxious Parenting

As you've realized by now, most of us who have suffered a pregnancy loss or experienced the death of a newborn continue to feel anxious long after our next child is born. Especially during the first year, we tend to be gripped by an all-consuming fear of Sudden Infant Death Syndrome. "For six months I worried that he would die of SIDS," says Brooke. "I was almost afraid to go in and check on him sometimes because I thought I would find him blue." Athough worries about SIDS are nearly universal, they can take many different forms. Melinda, for example, became so dependent on the nursery monitor that it bordered on an obsession. She explains:

> The nursery was upstairs, and when I would put the baby to bed, I would always turn on the monitor in his room. But if I got downstairs and found that the other part of the monitor was turned off, I would run back upstairs to be sure that nothing had happened to him during those few seconds it took me to turn on the other monitor.

Suzanne's behavior was even more extreme by most standards. She literally held her baby every single night for the first six weeks of her life. As she remembers, "I slept in a bed with her and held her in my arms constantly. I couldn't sleep; I didn't get a good night's sleep for a solid six weeks. I watched her breathe; I literally watched her take every breath. So my greatest worry came after she was born."

Those who lost their previous baby to SIDS usually have the benefit of a device that monitors the baby's breathing or heartbeat or both, but these parents struggle nonetheless. One mother says, "At first I didn't even trust the monitor, but I couldn't have lived without it." While the monitor can be comforting, it can generate false alarms as well. It also cannot provide absolute guarantees that a baby will not die of SIDS. That was the reason why Traci, whose first-born son died of SIDS, constantly checked her son's breathing even when he was connected to the monitor. "At least once a day for the first eight months I would look in his crib and literally think he was dead. Poor Trent was jerked up out of his bed so many times during a deep sleep, I'm now surprised he can even sleep at all." Many mothers can only breathe a sigh of relief once their child has reached their first birthday, which is when there is no typically more risk of SIDS.

Even after the fear of SIDS has subsided, other anxieties often remain. A fever or other illness can send you running to the doctor in a panic. Any problem, no matter how minor, may lead you to fear the worst. If your child was born with health problems, that too may only serve to heighten your sense of anxiety. Martha, whose subsequent pregnancy ended with the delivery of a baby who was ten weeks premature, continued to worry that her son would stop breathing long after he was out of the high-risk category. "For the first two or three years of his life, I got up to check on him several times a night. And it wasn't enough to see him breathing, I had to feel him. Even now that he is four, I still get up sometimes at night to check on him and my oldest daughter."

It is not unusual for other members of your family to feel the same way. Even though your partner might not say it, he probably worries, too. And children are often deeply affected as well. Kim's son, for example, was delighted at the birth of his baby sister, Chelsea, a little over a year after his other sister died. But even though he was only six years old, he, too, had the sense that anything could happen. As Kim explains, "One day Chelsea was crying and her face turned all red and she couldn't catch her breath and he said, 'Oh well, there goes another baby.' "

These types of feelings tend to diminish over time. As your child grows stronger and more independent, both you and other members of your family will gain a greater sense of confidence about the future. And if you later give birth to other children, you may find that you are a little more relaxed with them. I know I was much less anxious with Michael than I had been with Andrew. In a way, that surprised me, since I thought the breathing problems Michael had in the hospital would make me a real basket case once we got home. But thankfully, that wasn't true. Maybe seeing that Andrew survived his infancy unscathed gave me the confidence to believe that Michael would be all right, too.

Overprotective Parenting

Largely as a result of the anxiety that some parents feel, those who have lost a baby tend to be overprotective with their subsequent babies and any other surviving children. Some simply keep a more watchful eye on their child than they otherwise might have. Others find that their concerns about their baby's well-being pervade every area of their lives. While it is true that most new parents are overprotective to some extent, it can be more pronounced among those who have experienced a loss. Why this difference? Kim sums up how many bereaved parents feel: "I think I'm a little more overprotective as a parent because the thought of losing them is more real."

There are as many examples of overprotectiveness as there are mothers. Ashley, whose first baby died of a congenital heart defect shortly after birth, still keeps a nursery monitor in her daughter's room even though she is seven years old. Ginger routinely takes antibacterial spray with her when she goes out with her premature baby so she can discreetly spritz away germs if anyone should happen to touch her. Dinah is reluctant to leave her child with a baby-sitter, even if it's just for an evening out. Janet is having trouble finding daycare that will enable her to go back to work. Chris decided to quit her job altogether because she could not stand the thought of being away from her baby.

I found it especially hard to move my baby out of my bedroom and across the hall to the nursery. In fact, I put it off until Andrew was so big that he basically would no longer fit in the bassinet. Even then, I probably would have just moved the baby bed into my room if it hadn't been for it being too wide to fit through the door. Forced to let him go, I slept for the next several months with the monitor turned up high enough so that I could hear his every breath. Sound crazy? Maybe. But as I interviewed other bereaved mothers, I discovered that I was not alone. Traci would wheel her baby from room to room with her all day, even when he slept. And when he outgrew his bassinet, she bought a portable crib so he could remain in her bedroom. Julie stopped sleeping in her bedroom altogether so she could spend the night by her baby's bedside: "I quit sleeping with my husband for eight months, and I went and slept with my son, Timothy. Fortunately, my husband was very understanding. He just said, 'Do what you have to do.' I couldn't help myself. I had to be sure he was alive and breathing."

Just as anxiety diminishes over time, so too does overprotectiveness. One mother I talked to says she becomes a little more relaxed with each passing year. "A lot of people would still say that I'm overprotective, but I'm learning to let go as my children grow up." In her book *Empty Cradle, Broken Heart*, Deborah L. Davis observes that some parents are concerned about their overprotectiveness and try to hide, disguise or control it. But she stresses that it is important to avoid overcompensating for protective urges by ignoring signs of illness or neglecting hazardous situations that could endanger a child's life. As Davis explains, the best approach is to try to strike the right balance between a child's dependence and independence:

> *Especially during infancy and toddlerhood, there is a lot of protective parenting that is nurturing and not stifling. However, by holding on too tightly,*

you give your children the impression that the world is a dangerous or unmanageable place. By letting go, yet remaining available, you give your children the security to become independent, the confidence to meet challenges and the courage to overcome difficulties. It helps to remember that attending to your children's need for dependence and independence is part of being a responsive parent.

As we all know, so much about life is beyond our control. But as you watch your children become more independent, you will gain the confidence you need to gradually let them go.

Better Parenting

When tragedy strikes, some people take comfort in looking for anything positive that may have come out of the experience. When it comes to the loss of a baby, a silver lining is almost impossible to find. But if there is one, it may be that those of us who have had a baby die, often go on to become exceptional parents. We appreciate our children just a little bit more and have that extra bit of patience that others sometimes lack. Gail, whose first baby was stillborn, put it this way in an address to a grief support group at her church:

I believe a mother cannot truly appreciate holding a baby in her arms, unless she has once left the hospital with empty arms. She cannot appreciate a baby's cry unless her house has been silent. She cannot appreciate hearing mommy for the millionth time in one day, unless she once thought she would never hear that word. She cannot truly appreciate a baby unless she has known what it was like to have lost one.

This sense of appreciation can make the more trying aspects of child rearing a little easier. According to Nancy, "When I got up and nursed in the middle of the night, I didn't feel bad. I was so honored to be able to get up with a baby. Even now that she's reaching a little more demanding age, I think I'm more tolerant when I wipe up the floor for the tenth time." That kind of attitude sometimes even rubs off on family and friends who have been touched by your experience. As Diane says, "We have friends who have told us: 'We used to be upset about sleepless nights and now we are so thankful.' And that was a neat thing. I was thankful that our experience could have a positive effect on them.' "

Those women who had given birth to other children before their loss often notice a difference in how they parent their subsequent children. Glenda says the loss of her infant son changed her for the better: "I'm a very driven person, but I really try now to make the effort to play with my children more. I realize that's more important than having a clean house or finishing a particular project. They are only little for such a short time."

They *are* only little for a short time, and those of us who have lost a baby understand that better than most. Because we were deprived of the joy of raising at least one of our children, it is only natural that we would want to savor every moment of raising the others.

Normal Parenting

No matter how grateful you are to have your baby and how much you appreciate the privilege of parenting, you are still human. This means that times will arise when you lose your patience or crave time to yourself or wonder how you will ever make it through the toddler years. Melinda admits that "I never thought I would feel this way, but this terrible twos thing is very trying on me." Although it's hard for me to admit, there are times when I, too, get frustrated and angry with my children. You'd think after all I went through to have them that I would treasure them every moment of every day. But life just isn't that way, at least not for me. Raising children is no easy task, and, as we've already learned, the challenges begin from the moment of conception.

So as you look at your own angelic newborn today, realize that there may soon come a day when that child is no longer quite as cooperative. Eventually, you will reach a point when you start losing your temper and have to impose ground rules. When that happens, try not to feel guilty about it. If we all treated our subsequent children with kid gloves their whole lives, they would grow up to be terribly spoiled adults. Discipline can be a good thing, even when it is doled out to a very precious child.

Continued Sadness

Just as pregnancy does not magically erase your grief, neither does having another baby. Painful feelings may continue to strike unexpectedly for months and often years. As you rock your baby to sleep, you may cry for the one you never got to hold. When you see someone who has the same number of children that you have, it may serve as a bitter reminder of the one you no longer have. Maybe you find it hard to go to baby showers and see the naivete of those who are seemingly unaware that pregnancies can end in a loss. Perhaps you only have a hard time on certain days, such as your child's birthday, your due date, holidays or the first day of school. Heather, for example, found that her own birthday was difficult after the loss of her newborn daughter. "My birthday was devastating to me for a couple of years," she says, "because it made me sad that I could be growing older when she couldn't." Rita sums up how many of us feel years later:

> I have found that there's a difference between grieving and being sorrowful. It's two different things. It's okay for me to be sorrowful about it the rest of my life; to be sad that I can't see her. It's not okay to get stuck in a stage of grief. For a long time, I thought I was screwed up because I wasn't getting over the sad part about it.

Can you really ever *get over* the loss of a child? I don't think so. Because when a baby dies you don't just lose someone you love and want so dearly, you lose an entire future. And each time you look around at your family and realize someone is missing, you'll be sad. That doesn't mean you'll dwell on it every day or spend your life grieving, but it does mean that a part of you will always wonder how things might have been.

Introspection

One of the ways that we imagine what our children might have been like is to look at the ones who survive. You can expect that as you watch your subsequent child grow up, you will find yourself wondering whether your other baby would have shared some of the same characteristics. Would she have smiled the same way or had the same color eyes? What sorts of things would she have liked to do? These kinds of thoughts are even more likely if your new baby is of the same sex or looks a lot like the one who died. At the beginning, you may even mix up their names on occasion. Understand that this type of behavior is normal and not at all harmful unless it becomes obsessive.

I decided early on that I wanted all of my subsequent children to be boys so that each one would give me a glimpse into what Patrick would have looked like. After all, I reasoned, brothers do often look alike. Well, I got my wish and gave birth to two more boys after Patrick, but they look about as different from each other as two children can. Andrew has dark hair, brown eyes and very light skin, while Michael has blondish hair, blue eyes and dark skin. Who might Patrick have looked like? I'm not sure now.

Maybe you won't wonder as much what your child would have looked like as what he or she would have done. You may sometimes find yourself imagining the kind of life they might have lived. As one woman who lost a newborn son who would now be in his thirties told me:

> I have raised my son in my mind all these years. I knew exactly what he would have looked like and what he would have done. Every year, I knew what grade he would have been in in school. I even imagined which college he would have gone to and what he would have majored in. My son may not have been here with me physically, but he has never been far from my thoughts.

It would be unhealthy if these kinds of thoughts dominated your mind and forced your subsequent children to live in the shadow of the sibling who died. But it is normal for you to stop sometimes and wonder what your life might have been like had your baby's life not been cut short.

A New Outlook on Life

There is no doubt that our lives would have been different had our children lived, but they also are different because they died. As we've been saying all along, the loss of a child changes people. Some of those changes are good, while others are not so good. For example, in chapter 5 we discussed the reluctance that many women have to bond with their child during pregnancy. That means they don't make plans and dreams for the baby or look forward to a future with them. For some people, that feeling carries over after the birth of their subsequent child. Nancy, who lost twins in her first pregnancy, describes how her loss changed her perspective on life:

> With my twins, I pictured everything. I knew they were going to wear their khakis and button-downs to school. And I thought, "We're going to go fishing, and they're going to have their fishing vests." I had visualized everything. With Amy, it was completely different. I didn't plan anything when I was pregnant. Now she's one and a half, and I can't imagine her being two. With the boys I had all those images and they were crushed and ripped away from me, so now I can't allow myself to think ahead. I don't picture her in any situation in the future.

A psychologist might argue that Nancy's inability to visualize her daughter's future indicates a problematic relationship. Nancy couldn't disagree more. She says she loves her daughter very much and cherishes every moment with her. She simply no longer thinks as optimistically as she once did.

Sharon also says the loss of her baby changed her basic outlook on life.

I don't have that assurance anymore that everything works out for the good, and that always used to be my motto. Any time anyone was going through anything hard, I was always thinking there is a reason for this. It wasn't a callous thought. It was really something I believed—that there was something down the road that you can't see now that will be wonderful. But of course when I was thinking that, the worst thing had never happened to me.

While your loss may have taken away some of your optimism and innocence, it may also have resulted in more positive changes in your life. Maybe you are more sensitive now to the needs of other bereaved people and can give them much-needed support. Perhaps you have reordered your priorities, slowed down your pace and started to appreciate the little things in life. One of the biggest changes of all may be that you no longer fear death as you once did. As Virginia says, "I know that my daughter's first memory is of seeing God; how much better can it get? And I know she'll be there when I get to heaven. She'll be the first one to come running to welcome me."

If you, too, believe in life after death, you can take comfort in knowing that your baby is up there somewhere watching over you and your family and will be waiting to welcome you when you get to the other side.

Divine Moments

Most of the time, you have to take it on faith that your child is in a better place. But occasionally, you may be given a sign or reassurance that your baby is indeed still alive in spirit. In the book *Angelic Presence,* parents and grandparents recount how their lives have been touched in a special way by babies who have died. One mother writes of the day she saw an image of her son who had died of SIDS. Though the vision was fleeting, she describes how she received a message from him that clearly said, "Please don't worry about me, Mom. I'm okay." Although his "angelic presence" never appeared again, it has given her strength to carry on with her life. She writes, "I had cried many tears because I never had the chance to say goodbye, but I smile now when I think how blessed I am to have been given another chance to say hello."

Another mother describes what she calls her "angel experiences." One happened the first Christmas after her daughter Rachel's death. She and her husband had decided to light a luminary at their daughter's grave on Christmas Eve. The wind was particularly strong that night, and they tried to convince themselves that it didn't matter if the candle blew out right away. Since the flame was already flickering as they drove away, they avoided looking back. Amazingly, though, when they returned the next night, the candle was still burning. "Our eight-hour candle had burned in the winter wind for twenty-four hours," she writes. "We decided to leave it so it could burn itself out. The next morning we returned and were again shocked to discover the flame still alive, the candle nearly gone. . . . With tear-streaked faces, we reached for one another as we watched the flame disappear. This was Rachel's Christmas gift to us."

I, too, have been blessed with what I consider divine moments since my son's death. One was when I found out that I would be taking my son Michael home from the hospital on what would have been Patrick's third birthday. I saw that as a sign that he was making his presence felt in our lives. Another thing that has brought me great comfort is the fact that in the four years since Patrick died, I have had three good friends give birth to baby boys on St. Patrick's Day. The first year it happened, I didn't find it comforting at all. It had only been ten months since my loss, and it hurt me to the core to see my friend give birth to a boy on that particular day and name him Patrick. As selfish as it was, I was devastated that her Patrick was here while mine was not. Two years later when it happened again, it started to feel like serendipity. I thought that maybe my Patrick was trying to tell me something. When the same thing happened yet again a third time, I couldn't believe it. I just looked at the birth announcement and burst into tears. I don't know what the chances are of three baby boys being born on St. Patrick's Day to three close friends, but I would put them at about one in a million. Outside the realm of human understanding, I feel like my son is reminding me that he is very much alive and still an important part of our lives.

Keeping the Memories Alive

Even after we have given birth to a healthy child, all of us who have lost a baby continue to look for ways to keep the memories of our child alive. Most of the time, this takes the form of very personal gestures. We might visit our baby's grave, plant a tree in our child's name or look at our precious keepsakes. Other times we might choose to do something more public, like attend a memorial service or reach out to someone else who has had a loss. In the remainder of this chapter, we'll look at both the private and the very public ways that parents have chosen to remember their babies. My hope is that by adopting some of these ideas as your own, you will find comfort and healing in the years ahead.

Make a Baby Book

If you haven't done so already, consider making a baby book for your child. This can be a very therapeutic process and provide one more avenue for bringing a sense of closure to an extremely painful period in your life. Even if your loss was relatively early, you may discover that you have far more mementoes of your baby than you think. Aside from pictures of your baby, which you may or may not have, your book can include sonogram images, photos of you pregnant, even if you weren't showing yet, photos from your baby showers, cards sent by family and friends, hospital bracelets and anything special that you or others may have written. Take the time to record everything you remember about the pregnancy. How did you find out you were expecting? When did you tell others? What was their reaction? How did you feel during the months that ensued? What special plans did you have for your baby? These details may fade from your mind over time, especially as you go through subsequent pregnancies. But if you write things down now, you will enjoy being able to look back and remember that the pregnancy brought you much joy in addition to great sorrow.

As you put your book together, take special care to ensure that your treasured keepsakes are protected from the ravages of time. One option is to use a memory book with acid-free paper. Not only will you be able to write personal notes and descriptions beside each photo, you will avoid the damage that can occur when you mount pictures on self-sticking pages with plastic covers. If you have any Polaroid pictures of your baby, consider taking them to a trusted photo lab for reproduction. Otherwise, they may crack, yellow and even fade over time. If you cut a Polaroid, the photographic image could disappear altogether. Also make copies of any other photographs you have. Or scan them into a computer and keep a digital archive. Then store the originals in a safety deposit box or some other secure spot.

Keep Mementoes of Your Baby

Anything that will not fit in your baby book can go in a shadow box or other special place. If you can find one, a small cedar chest is ideal because it will help protect everything that's inside. If you miscarried early, you will not have many keepsakes. Perhaps your only memento is the positive pregnancy test that revealed you were pregnant. But if your loss came later in the pregnancy, you may have the tiny outfit your baby wore, or the blanket that was used to wrap your child. You may want to use the chest to store your original photographs or the baby's lock of hair. I have a small box where I keep the infant gown, diaper and receiving blanket that we had planned to use to bring Patrick home from the hospital. It also contains the pictures from my baby shower, the cards we received after our loss, and a tiny book with the baby's handprints, footprints and a lock of his hair. It may not be much, but they are among my most treasured possessions. Every so often I like to pull everything out and reflect on what was and what might have been.

Consider displaying some mementoes in your home, if you have them, rather than stowing them away in a box. You could frame a picture of your baby, if one was taken. If not, frame any handprints or footprints that may have been made. Since Patrick's prints were smudged and off-center, I had a graphic artist scan them into a computer and lay them out with his name, birthdate and a poem. They now hang on the wall beside my bed.

If your loss came too early to have any tangible reminders of your baby, you can create one of your own. Get a charm to wear around your neck. Engrave a bracelet with your baby's initials. Wear an angel pin or start your own angel collection. If you dried any of the flowers that you received when your baby died, you can press them on velvet and frame them. Another alternative is to use them to make potpourri. Then you can add to it every time you buy flowers for your child's birthday or some other anniversary date.

Start Family Traditions

Because your baby is still very much a member of your family, you may want to establish traditions that reflect your sentiments. Many parents find that their child's due date or birthday is a time when they want to do something special. Kim, for example, always bakes a cake on her baby's birthday. Martha and her family go to the tree they planted in her son's memory and release balloons. Heather visits the cemetery with her husband and surviving children and goes through a ritual that has become an annual rite.

We always get a candle with the number that she would have been. Then we light it and sing happy birthday and let the wind blow it out. We think of it as the wind blowing from heaven. We always take a camera, too, so we can take a picture of how big the other kids are getting. To someone who hasn't had a loss, it may sound really morbid, but for our kids it's no big deal to go to the cemetery.

Many find comfort in religious rituals. Catholics, for example, can request that a Mass be said in memory of their baby. They can also light candles in church that symbolize their special prayer intentions on behalf of their child. Mourners of the Jewish faith can light a Yahrzeit candle on the anniversary of their loved one's death. It burns for twenty-five hours from sunset to when the stars come out the next night. "It's a silent and dignified and moving symbol," says Rabbi Nina Beth Cardin, author of *Out of the Depths I Call to You: A Book of Prayers for Married Jewish Women.* Since the Yahrzeit candle is only appropriate for babies who lived outside the womb, you can get a candle that burns for fewer hours if you lost an unborn child. Another Jewish rite for those whose baby died after birth is the Mourner's Kaddish, a prayer that is recited on the anniversary of a family member's death. It is also customary to give charity on that day.

Christmas and Hanukkah are other times when families choose to honor their child in a special way. Some attend holiday candlelight services organized by grief support groups. At the service I go to, for example, there is singing, poetry reading and a few comforting words from a minister. But the highlight of the evening comes near the end when each parent walks to the front of the church and lights a candle as their child's name is read aloud. For many of us, it is the only time that we ever get to hear our son or daughter's name spoken in public. It is even more touching coming as it does in such a beautiful setting with all the white candles flickering in the darkness.

The Compassionate Friends, an organization based in Oak Brook, Illinois that assists those who have lost a child of any age, organizes a different kind of candlelight vigil on the second Sunday in December. They invite bereaved parents to light a candle in memory of their child for one hour beginning at exactly 7:00 P.M. no matter where in the world they happen to be. "As candles are lit in each time zone at 7 P.M., imagine a wave of light that moves around the globe marking the entire twenty-four hours of that day," writes Diana Cunningham, the organization's executive director. If you later use that same candle in your table centerpiece, you will have a visible reminder of your child during the many festive holiday meals that follow.

Another holiday idea is to collect Christmas ornaments or other seasonal pieces in memory of your child. You can then add to your collection every year. Each of Kathi's surviving children, for example, has his or her own box of special ornaments that they will take with them one day when they leave home to start their own family. Kathi also has a box of ornaments for her baby daughter Lauren, who died several years ago. Those are special to every member of the family. "The children always know which ornaments are Lauren's when they hang them on the tree. It means so much to us to have a visible reminder that she is a part of us."

Tell Your Other Children about Their Brother or Sister

Whether your only surviving child is the one who was just born or you have older children who remember the pregnancy that ended in a loss, it is a good idea to talk openly to them about their brother or sister who died. By telling them about their sibling from the beginning, you can make the baby a part of their lives, too. It's best to use plain language rather than euphemisms like "we lost the baby," otherwise a child might respond "well, let's go look for him." "Difficult facts are best dealt with simply, using language that is concrete and not mystifying," says Dr. Charles A. Corr, who has written several books with particular emphasis on death-related issues associated with children and adolescents.

Use the same approach to answer questions as they arise. Don't worry about saying too much, since children will either ignore what they don't understand or ask for an explanation. Remember, too, that it is all right to cry. Your children may not be able to fully comprehend why you are sad at first, but they will come to a deeper understanding over time. "Adults need to role-model for kids. They need to show them that it's okay to have those feelings," says Dr. Corr.

This is quite different from the approach parents took in the past. Years ago, people either never spoke again about a baby who died or did so only in the vaguest of terms. One woman I know regularly accompanied her mother to the cemetery as a child to visit "the little angel." It was only as an adult that she realized the little angel was actually her brother who had died at birth.

By sharing your own feelings about the loss, you will find that your surviving children naturally come to understand that the baby is indeed a member of the family. Diana's children, for example, never fail to include an angel when they draw a picture of their family. Heather's children correct her if she doesn't count the baby she lost when someone asks how many kids she has. As one mother whose baby died a few hours after birth says, "In a lot of families they just don't talk about it, or if they talk about it, it's a hush-hush thing or everyone gets upset. But my children accept it. It's a fact of our life. It's a fact of our family, and even though it is sad, it doesn't change the fact that it happened."

As time passes, your child having a sibling who died will take on new meaning. There may even come a time when your children surprise you by showing how much they care about their sibling whom they may have never met. Heather describes a particularly touching moment with her surviving children:

Anytime my children get a balloon, they'll send it to their sister. Then one day we saw a rainbow and one of my sons said to me, "Mom, I just figured out what Anne does with all those balloons we give her. She makes them into rainbows." And I was just like, "Wow, isn't that cool?" They all remember her even though my two youngest ones weren't even born. They all remember her in a special way.

In addition to telling your children about your baby, you may want to share your history with new friends who may not have known you at the time. They will be able to relate to you better if they understand what you have been through. Try not to be discouraged, though, if the subject of your baby never comes up again. As you know by now, most people are uncomfortable talking about anything that has to do with death and dying. They fear they might upset you by mentioning your baby or even acknowledging that the loss ever happened. All of us could cope better with these kinds of slights if we adopted Julie's perspective: "No one ever mentions my first child except friends who've had a loss themselves. But that's okay. She is alive and well where it matters most: in her mommy's heart."

Visit a Place That Reminds You of Your Baby

Because the world does not always recognize the significance of our baby's life, we sometimes have to be alone in order to reflect on what our child means to us. "It's so important for people to have a place where they can go and remember," says Sister Jane Marie Lamb, founder of SHARE Pregnancy and Infant Loss Support. An obvious place to do this is the baby's grave site. But what if your loss came too early for you to bury your baby? One option is to ask whether your hospital has a memorial garden or an unmarked grave where they bury babies who were miscarried. Many do. If the thought of that kind of grave site makes you uncomfortable, consider creating your own memorial garden. Plant a tree in your baby's name and go there whenever you need time to yourself. A Bradford Pear tree is a good choice because it does well in both intense heat and bitter cold. Aside from its physical beauty, the tree is also a wonderful symbol. It shapes itself and blossoms every year but does not bear fruit.

Another idea is to create a special garden in your own backyard. Diana Sundwall, for example, planted a white rose bush in memory of her son Derek Joseph and put other flowers around it that represent her four living children. She has since been amazed to see the rose bush survive twelve years of harsh Minnesota winters. But Diana didn't stop at her own personal garden. She also helped establish a place where every parent who has lost a child can go to remember and reflect.

In 1986, she devised the idea of putting a marker in a public park to memorialize all the babies who had died in her hometown of Faribault, Minnesota. City officials initially refused her request. But later, they changed their minds and offered her an entire park to establish any memorial she saw fit. Diana and other members of the organization she founded—Infants Remembered in Silence (IRIS)—were allowed to pick out the name of the new park as well as the playground equipment. They also got the marker they wanted—a shoulder-high memorial that honors children who are gone but not forgotten. Bereaved parents now go to the park to plant trees or flowers and remember their own babies.

We decided to call it Kinder Park, from the German word for "children." At any point, parents can have a tree planted in their child's name, or they can plant it themselves. They can also plant flowers anytime they want. At Christmas time we find wreaths out there and flowers and small toys. And it's interesting because other children come and play with the toys sometimes, but they always put them back without being told.

By helping others we help ourselves. Maybe you, like Diana, have an idea that would be comforting to other bereaved parents. If you do, don't be afraid to explore the possibilities. The worst that can happen is that someone will say no to you. But as Diana discovered, you can end up doing far more than you ever imagined.

Make a Donation in Your Baby's Name

Another way to help others, and in turn help yourself, is to make a donation to your house of worship, a school or any local organization and ask that whatever project you fund be dedicated in your baby's name. For example, one couple I know funded a new church library named after their baby. Another decided to sponsor scholarships in their child's name. I always like to buy Christmas presents for a needy child through a program organized by the Salvation Army during the holidays. I select a child who is the same age as mine would have been and shop for him as I would have for Patrick.

Like some of the other ideas that we discussed, this also can be done on a larger scale. Becky and Jeff Thompson, for example, started Our Precious Angels, a nonprofit organization in Plano, Texas that helps bereaved couples pay for their baby's funeral expenses. Support group counselors at a local hospital contact Our Precious Angels whenever they encounter a couple in need of financial assistance. The group also helps with child care, meals and other needs during the days immediately following the loss.

In addition to its service to individual couples, Our Precious Angels also helps arrange public memorial services at certain times of the year. In May, the group provides the headstone for a ceremony held in memory of babies lost in early pregnancy. In October, it organizes a memory walk for families to gather and reflect on how the loss has affected their lives. Like most non-profit organizations, Our Precious Angels is funded entirely by private donations. But anyone who makes a contribution in memory of their child can have their baby's name and birth date engraved on a plaque that hangs in a hospital chapel.

Help Others Who Have Suffered a Pregnancy Loss

Like the Thompsons, many of us feel a need to reach out to others who have suffered the loss of a baby. Even a simple gesture on our part can have a profound effect, both on us and on the people whose lives we touch. Allison, for instance, met a woman whose baby died on the very same day as hers. She discovered that helping that woman was good for her own soul. "Instead of feeling sorry for myself, she was my cause," she says. "We worked together on scrapbooks and went to memorial services together. I think it did us both good." If others know of your willingness to help, you'll be amazed at how many phone calls you receive from friends who know of someone who would like to talk to another woman who has walked in the same shoes.

By allowing your heart to lead you, you will find plenty of ways to reach out and help others. For me it was clear within a few weeks of my loss that this book was to be my calling. Others have left jobs in unrelated fields to work full-time assisting those who have lost a baby. Most of those who serve as directors of major pregnancy loss organizations, for example, have lost one or more babies themselves. Many support group leaders have also personally experienced the same tragedy that they counsel others about. In some cases, I met researchers

who decided to study the topic of pregnancy loss only after they themselves had lost a baby.

Reaching out to others does not have to be complicated or time
consuming. It simply has to come from the heart. One of the women
I met who best illustrates this point is Gail Fasolo. Before she was
interviewed for this book, she sent me a handmade white felt heart
lined with tiny beads and a lace border. Stitched in the middle was
the word "HOPE." Gail told me that she started making her "Hope
Hearts" when she was pregnant again after a loss. She explained that
she was Christmas shopping one day when she noticed a small, gold-
sequined heart that said "HOPE." It caught her eye, she said, because
she was in such desperate need of some hope herself at the time. She
ended up buying the heart and hanging it in her living room. It still
hangs there today.

In the years since then, Gail has been making her own Hope Hearts
and giving them to women all over the world. In the letter she sends
with her gift, she explains:

> When I was so depressed, wondering if I'd ever be happy again—it gave
> me hope. As I kept trying to get pregnant again (for a year)—it said hope.
> When I did get pregnant again and wondered if this baby would live—it
> was always there telling me to have hope. Now I'm giving you a heart
> because I care . . . always have hope.

Once they have given birth to their subsequent child, many of the
women who have received a Hope Heart from Gail send her a picture
of their babies. She has mounted them all on a poster that she calls
the Hope Heart Babies poster. "It gives me immense joy every time
I add a new picture. I get a warm feeling looking at them, knowing
how much heartbreak their moms endured, and how much they are
loved," she says. "I also know that for every baby on the poster, there
is also a very special one in heaven that will live on in their mom's
heart forever."

The number of babies on Gail's poster grows every year. And while it is by no means statistically significant, it is heart-warming to see how many women who have lost a baby have gone on to have healthy children. In describing what motivates her to keep her Hope Heart collection going year after year, Gail quotes Emily Dickinson: "If I can stop one heart from breaking, I shall not live in vain."

Appreciate the Good Things Since the Loss

Many parents believe that their baby's life, no matter how brief, changed the course of their own lives. In some cases, family members who had been feuding for years were reunited, or couples were brought closer together. "There was a reason for my son's life. He brought the family together in an unbelievable way," says Michelle. Often, the most profound changes of all have occurred within people's hearts. As Nancy says, "I think I'm a different person. I value life a lot more as a gift and I think of parenting as a privilege." Heather expresses similar sentiments:

> Even though I'm not perfect, and never will be, I think my loss has made me more understanding and made me care more for other people. It really puts things into perspective—what's important in life and what's not. Everybody has times when little things bother them, but it doesn't happen to me as much anymore.

In this chapter, we've examined how our loss may have deepened our sense of gratitude for our surviving children. Knowing that our subsequent child might never have been born had it not been for the loss of our baby only adds to our appreciation. As Sharon, whose daughter died before she gave birth to her son, says:

> I don't think anything good can come from losing a child, but my biggest thing is what has been good since it happened and not because of it. For me, it's that I'm experiencing this mother–son relationship that is awesome and that I otherwise would not have had. And that's what I keep telling

myself. It's more comforting some times than others. But I think it's im-
portant to try to focus on the good, and not just let what happened com-
pletely devastate you.

It is devastating to lose a baby, but most of us do manage to gradually pick up the pieces of our lives. You have. In the months since
your loss, you have found the strength to try again and you now have
another child. Although the birth of this baby cannot erase your pain,
it can bring much-needed joy back into your heart. But where will
you go from here? Will you try to put the past behind you as much
as possible? Or will you look for ways to give your baby's life meaning
on this earth? Will your child's legacy be one of tears and sorrow or
will it be one of gratitude and good will? Only you can decide what
comes next. Just know that the greatest tribute you can pay to your
baby is to live a life that is even more meaningful than it otherwise
would have been.

chapter ten

The Father's Perspective on Pregnancy after a Loss

ANY MAN WHO has had to endure the pain of losing a baby knows from first-hand experience that his feelings are often overlooked. "How is your wife?" his coworkers might ask. "What can we do to help her?" relatives want to know. "Is she feeling any better?" friends inquire in the weeks after the tragedy. Very rarely, if at all, do men ever hear, "How are *you* doing?" What's true in the bereavement period is even more true in a pregnancy after a loss. The focus continues to stay on the woman. Doctors, relatives, friends, coworkers, neighbors, store clerks—just about everyone—will want to know how *she* is doing? In many ways, their concern is well placed. No one will feel the pain over the loss quite as intensely as the woman who carried the baby. And no one has more at stake in the next pregnancy than she does.

But fathers have feelings, too, even though they may not always show it. The baby who died was their child, too, and the baby on the way now is every bit as important to him as it is to his wife. So it is worth taking a closer look at the father's perspective on the pregnancy after a loss. Not only will understanding your partner's feelings help you be more empathetic—filling the void that others leave—it will also help you relate better as a couple. This will enable you to support each other during what is no doubt an extremely difficult period for both of you.

Common Feeling

Men are notorious for hiding their true feelings, and your partner is probably no exception. This means that even during a high-stress pregnancy like yours, he may not offer a whole lot of clues into what he is thinking. Perhaps he fears that he would upset you were he to share his fears and concerns about the baby. Maybe he is uncomfortable with displays of emotion and prefers to "take it like a man." Or it could just be that he does not want to make himself vulnerable to you by revealing his innermost thoughts. In that respect, he may not be acting any differently now than he normally does. But unless you know him well enough to understand the reasons why he is not sharing his feelings during your pregnancy, you might take it to mean that he does not care about you or the baby.

It might comfort you to remind yourself, though, that you most likely wouldn't be having a child together if he did not care about you. And, as a rule, expectant fathers care very much about their unborn babies, too. In fact, some men's involvement in the pregnancy goes so deep that they actually experience the same physical symptoms as their wives. Nausea and vomiting, indigestion, changes in appetite, food cravings, weight gain, constipation and headaches are all symptoms that have been reported by fathers-to-be. Researchers have given this male counterpart to pregnancy a name—couvade syndrome. The term, which was coined back in 1865, was derived from the French word for "hatching."

Estimates on the incidence of couvade syndrome vary widely, but it is thought to affect to some degree anywhere from 22 percent to 79 percent of expectant fathers in the United States. Although there is no known physiological basis for the condition, there are many theories as to its psychological basis. For example, some hypothesize that it may be an expression of the expectant father's anxiety over the pregnancy. Others suggest that it is simply a man's way of showing that fathers matter, too. Whatever the cause, the existence of couvade syndrome is evidence that men often do have very strong feelings about their partner's pregnancy, even though they often are reluctant to talk about them. Let's take a closer look at what your partner may be feeling during your subsequent pregnancy.

Fear

A man frightened by pregnancy? Not a chance, you might say. My husband is like a rock. Nothing fazes him. He doesn't think the way I do. But you might be surprised at the intensity of your partner's fears were he ever to open up to you. His heart may skip a beat everytime he hears you get up in the night, or he may become alarmed whenever he sees you grimace from one of the many aches and pains common in pregnancy. In addition to being concerned about the baby's well-being, he may worry about you. He may fear that he will hurt you or the baby if the two of you have sex. Or he may wonder whether you are physically and mentally ready for this pregnancy. Above all, he may fear that the worst may happen again. "I had a lot of stress and anxiety, but some days were worse than others," recalls Richard, whose wife became pregnant again after their second child died at birth. "Like the days when she didn't feel well, I thought maybe something was wrong with the baby."

Like your fears, his may not always be rational. Sam, for example, could not shake the feeling that his baby's death was somehow retribution for something he had done wrong in his own life. "When my wife was pregnant the next time, I wondered if maybe there was something else that I might have done that was going to cause something to go wrong again," he says. These types of irrational fears often continue even after the birth of a healthy baby. James and his wife willingly took turns staying up with their newborn the first few days home from the hospital so that someone could always watch over him. "I didn't feel I could go to sleep because I was afraid he'd stop breathing or I'd have to pull the blanket off his face," he says.

Sound familiar? As these men's comments reveal, expectant fathers often have feelings that are not unlike those of mothers-to-be. But there is one major difference: he can put the pregnancy out of his mind much more easily than you can. His fear may lift when he goes to work and gets wrapped up in his job. Even when he is home, he does not have to live with the constant awareness of whether your baby is moving or not. As Bob says, "When I was at work, it was not a constant concern. I was only worried if I stopped and thought about it. But as soon as I walked in the house, everything changed. It was not a negative feeling like doom, but there was definitely tension there."

On occasion, women manage to gain insight into their husbands' unspoken fears. As Martha remembers, "My husband hurt more than he showed. Sometimes I'd wake up in the middle of the night and he'd be up sitting in the den and I'd see tears in his eyes, but he was really quiet about it." Diane started to see a pattern develop that revealed when her husband was upset: "The way I released the pain was to cry; the way he released it was to go work in the garage." If you're wondering whether your own partner is feeling anything at all, look for these kinds of subtle clues and use them as an opportunity for opening the lines of communication. Later in this chapter we'll discuss some of the best ways to do that.

Feeling Overwhelmed

Your partner's fears may go beyond your health and that of the baby's. He may also be concerned about how to cope with mounting medical expenses, the loss of a second income, higher costs associated with running the household or other financial difficulties that may have resulted from your complicated pregnancy. If you are on bed rest, he may be worried about how to handle the additional responsibilities that have suddenly fallen on his shoulders. In addition to caring for you, he will be looking after the house, your other children and everything else that your family needs. He may also not be getting

enough sleep from having to squeeze these extra duties into his otherwise busy day. On top of that, you will be needier than usual. You
may be moody or lonely and see him as your primary link to the
outside world. All of this can add up to make even the most helpful
father-to-be feel completely overwhelmed.

The situation will be even worse if you have other setbacks in your
life during this period, as can sometimes happen. Richard, for example, felt that outside circumstances were conspiring against him
and his wife:

> In January, I found out I was being transferred to another job. In March,
> a cousin who was my same age died. The next month, I totalled my car.
> The month after that, my wife's grandmother died. Then, we totalled the
> new car. Every month, something major happened. Everyone kept saying,
> "God doesn't give you more than you can handle," and I was like, "God
> must know us better than we know ourselves."

Although there has not been much research on how pregnancy
affects expectant fathers, there are studies that support the contention
that a high-risk pregnancy can take a very real toll on fathers-to-be.
In particular, research has shown that fathers experience extreme
stress when their wives are on bed rest, especially when it is prolonged. Some men are able to be lighthearted about it, as Katharyn
May described in a study of expectant fathers that appeared in a
nursing publication:

> One [father] was able to joke in retrospect about his "first triumphant return
> from the grocery store," having done the weekly shopping for his family of
> four, only to have his partner explain that it had taken him "two hours to
> forget milk, eggs, and bread, and to buy all the wrong things."

But for many, the consequences are much more serious. May found
that "as the pressure of managing jobs, household duties and an increasingly stressed couple relationship mounted, some men worried

that they would just 'lose it,' either by forgetting to do something important or doing something wrong because they were too tired or distracted."

Although you may feel that you are the one who needs all the support during this pregnancy, it does not hurt to show your appreciation for what he is going through as well. Compliment him on what he does right, while keeping your criticism to a minimum. He will not be able to do things the way you do, but he deserves some credit for his efforts. Also, try to reassure him when the opportunity presents itself, whether it's about the baby's health or your financial situation. If the result is a happier relationship with each other, it will be well worth your effort.

Helplessness

In addition to feeling overwhelmed by all the extra burdens he is carrying, your partner may be experiencing something else as well: a feeling of helplessness. Accustomed to being the one who protects the family, he will suddenly be faced with a situation that is beyond his control. Men sometimes react to losing control in one of two ways. They either bury themselves in their work or in something else that they can control, or they try to regain some sense of control over the situation, no matter how futile the effort.

Suzanne's husband is a classic example of a man who tried to keep his focus on what he could control. When she became pregnant again after losing their second child near term, he started staying late at the office nearly every day. He frequently scheduled out-of-town trips. And even as her due date approached, he made no effort to rearrange his schedule to ensure that he would be around for the big day. "He just absorbed himself in his work. He had a tendency to be a workaholic anyway, but this was much more extreme than usual," says Suzanne. "But I know he cared because almost every day when he did come home from work, one of the first things he would say is 'How's the baby doing?' And he would always ask me if the baby had been moving."

There are other men who take the opposite approach and try to regain what control they can over the actual pregnancy. Charlie, for example, developed an almost obsessive fear about leaving his pregnant wife alone. He was so worried that something would go wrong when he was not around that he went to great lengths to make sure he was constantly accessible. He got himself a beeper and his wife a cellular phone. He urged friends and neighbors to drop in and check on her while he was at work. He called frequently while he was at the office and often asked how she was feeling when he was at home. Some women might welcome this kind of behavior because it shows that he cares, but it can become almost as annoying as the behavior of the man who buries himself in his job.

If your partner is at one of these extremes try to look beyond his actions to what is motivating him. Pregnancy is nearly as life-changing for him as it is for you. It is only natural to expect him to find ways to cope with the situation. If his coping skills are not compatible with yours, talk to him about it in a nonjudgmental way. Instead of nagging him about coming home too late, ask him whether he sees work as a way of relieving some of his stress over the pregnancy. Then explain that you have needs as well, and that there might be room for compromise. If it's overprotective behavior that is getting on your nerves, tell him how much you appreciate his concern but reassure him that you can get by with a little less oversight on his part. Then let him know how he is actually helping you during this difficult period. That may be one of the best remedies of all for counteracting his helpless feelings.

Frustration

For some men, a feeling of helplessness can also translate into a sense of frustration. He may be frustrated by just about anything: that your last baby died, that you have to go through another pregnancy, that you are going back and forth to doctors again or that you are in emotional—and perhaps even physical—distress. Since he is well aware of how difficult the pregnancy is for you, he may be especially frustrated that there is not much he can do to ease your pain.

The changes that will occur in your everyday life during the pregnancy may cause him frustration as well. He may miss the usual intimacy you share as a couple, especially if sex is off-limits for a while. He may feel lonely as you turn in early night after night or spend long afternoons napping in bed. And since you will be more preoccupied than ever with your baby, he may feel neglected. These feelings may be more pronounced if this is your second pregnancy in a relatively short time period.

As often happens with feelings of frustration, he may take them out on you or others. Knowing what lies at the source of his feelings may make it easier for you to understand when he blows up at the doctor for not doing more or gets upset with you over something you've done. Try to remember that he is no more prepared for the subsequent pregnancy than you are. There are no rules on how he is supposed to act or what he is supposed to say. Frustration simply comes with the pregnancy.

At Odds with You

As you probably realized during the bereavement period that followed your loss, crises bring some couples together and drive others apart. I'll never forget the doctor who delivered Patrick telling me and my husband that night that we should consider seeking counseling. Couples often tend to break up after the loss of a baby, she warned. We were offended by her suggestion at the time (needless to say, her timing could have been better), and you may also beg to differ with the suggestion that you and your partner could be at odds now. After all, many couples do not grow farther apart after a loss; they grow closer. We did.

But being at odds does not necessarily mean that your relationship is in danger. It could just mean that you are thinking and feeling different things at different times. For instance, you may be fearful about the outcome of your pregnancy when he is confident that everything will be just fine, or vice versa. There may be days when he comes home in a good mood, only to find you in a depressed state made worse by raging hormones. You may feel a constant need to talk about what you're feeling, when his only desire is to be left alone. Bed rest may be pushing you to the brink of insanity, while he has the gall to joke that he wishes he could spend the whole day in bed.

"Everything was very hard on the marriage—the loss, the infertility, the bed rest during the next pregnancy," says Kelly. "My husband did not feel the same connection with the baby that I did, so he was able to go about things as usual, and he didn't understand why I was always moping around." Says Beth: "He was not as anxious. His anxiousness came from my anxiousness." As another woman remembers, "I think I talked more about my feelings with others than I did with my husband."

These kinds of sentiments are normal, even in otherwise healthy relationships. Occasionally being at odds during the nine months of your pregnancy, does not mean that you will be at odds forever. Strive to agree about what matters most: your commitment to doing everything in your power to bring a healthy baby into your family.

Happiness

Just as you are happy for the second chance that this pregnancy is giving you, your partner is undoubtedly happy, too. New life brings new hope, and who wouldn't be happy about that? He may have even developed a new appreciation for the wonder of pregnancy and childbirth. As a result, the subsequent pregnancy can turn into a life-changing experience, as it was for Brooke's husband. As Brooke explains:

> When I was pregnant with Dylan, he was still kind of wanting to run around with his buddies and hang out. He was a good husband and a good father, but he was not always there. After the loss, he was home all the time. He became very much a family man, very much a Christian. He became so much closer to our children and really developed a different

outlook on life. He realizes, and so do I, what a true miracle little babies are.

Like you, though, he may sometimes still have a hard time believing that it is actually possible for you to have healthy baby. "I didn't feel like we'd ever make it to that point," says James. "It was always something out there that we couldn't quite get to." But when it finally does happen, as it did for James and his wife, the sense of appreciation and happiness will be that much greater.

Tips for Easing His Anxiety

As you read the heading for this section, you may have thought: "Why should I be trying to ease *his* anxiety? I'm having enough trouble taking care of myself." No one would argue that you don't have enough to worry about right now. But many of the tips you are about to read will ultimately help you, too. If you can encourage him to communicate his feelings, for example, you will probably get along better as a couple. If you can get him involved in the pregnancy, you will have an ally who is looking out for your best interests. And if you can show him ways that he can help, you will have a better chance of getting the support you so very much need. So let's examine some of the ways that you can ease his anxiety. In a roundabout way, you will be easing your own anxiety as well.

Find Ways to Communicate

As we've already discussed, men often have a hard time expressing their feelings. They are inclined to think that talking will not change anything, or they are embarrassed to reveal their sentiments. If you push them too hard, they tend to look for ways to escape. Maybe you noticed this tendency after your baby died. He may have put in more hours at the office or started a major home improvement project that kept him busy in the garage for long stretches. "Society has different views about what is proper for a man and a woman," says William Reinhart, who serves on the National Board of Directors of SHARE Pregnancy and Infant Loss Support. "He may think he will look weak if he cries, or he may be trying to support his partner, so he becomes like a rock. He isolates his own feelings as much as he can and winds up quite often not communicating and expressing them."

Usually, men are just as reluctant to share their feelings with their male friends as they are with you. One man who participated in a study that researched the effects of miscarriage on expectant fathers recounted this conversation he had with a coworker whose wife had also recently lost a baby: "He asked how things are going and I said that she was in [the] hospital . . . because of a miscarriage. Now his wife had one two weeks ago. Well all I said is, 'Well, shit like this happens.' He just nodded and we never mentioned anything else about it."

The men I interviewed told similar stories. Typically, once they had shared the news of the loss with a coworker or friend, the subject never came up again. If your partner also has trouble communicating his feelings, why should you try to make him act any differently? One reason is because pent-up feelings have a way of coming out in other, more destructive ways. Anger, hostility and depression can all be signs of repressed emotions. And if you do not know how your partner is really feeling, there is a lot more room for misunderstanding between the two of you.

Experts suggest that one of the best ways to open the lines of communication is to find the right place and the right time to talk. Don't bombard him with questions the minute he gets home from work or when he's in the middle of doing something else. Choose your moments carefully. You may even want to schedule some time each day for the two of you to sit down together and talk. Be sure to reassure him that you want to hear what he has to say, no matter how trivial he may think it is. Then listen to each other. Sometimes solutions to problems become clear only after the problems are discussed. At other times, a particular fear loses its power once it's communicated. Try to remain non-judgmental if you can, keeping in mind that feelings in and of themselves are neither right nor wrong. But by talking through those feelings, whatever they may be, you can ultimately improve your relationship and your peace of mind.

Suggest Ways He Can Find Support

Some couples find it impossible to communicate no matter how hard they try. Others have problems that they feel they cannot solve themselves. In these kinds of situations, a licensed professional counselor may be able to provide much-needed guidance and advice. Another option is a support group for bereaved parents. "I didn't even want to go to the first support group meeting," says Richard. "It was kind of like, 'I'm a macho man, I don't need that kind of support, I'll deal with this myself,' and then once she took me there they couldn't shut me up." Attending support group meetings together has additional benefits. The meetings can serve as a springboard for talking when you get home. Going together also avoids a situation in which you come home feeling better, while he is still dealing with unresolved issues. Other alternatives are to talk to a clergy member or another couple who has been through a similar experience.

Get Your Partner Involved in the Pregnancy

Something else that can improve communication between the two of you is to get your partner involved in your pregnancy. If he knows what is going on every step of the way, your conversations will not be one-sided exchanges, with you doing all the talking. By being a participant rather than an onlooker, he will know almost as much about the pregnancy as you do and be in a better position to offer you valuable insight and opinions. It will also keep him from feeling left out, which, as we discussed, often happens among expectant fathers.

The most obvious way to get him involved is to encourage him to go with you to your doctor appointments. This can have a number of benefits. He can get the questions he wants answered directly and not have to depend on you to serve as an intermediary. Since men usually like to deal with hard facts and data, your prenatal visits will give him both. He may also be more comfortable with certain aspects of your medical care than you are. You may not want to know all the risks involved in prenatal testing, for example, while he might be eager to learn every detail. Another plus is that he will be reassured, as you will be, by seeing ultrasound images of the baby and hearing positive reports from the doctor. If a crisis should develop, he can be your advocate and play a key role in making decisions. James describes how going to the prenatal visits helped him during his wife's subsequent pregnancy:

> I tried to make every doctor's appointment because I always had questions and I liked hearing the answers directly from him. It also helped me to be there when we hit certain milestones—like when we could first hear the baby's heartbeat, or we could see that the level-two sonogram showed no abnormalities. Barbara and I always tried to make a list of questions before the appointment, so it wasn't like the questions were from me or from her; they were from both of us. When I did miss an appointment, she would tell me what the doctor had to say, but since I wasn't there to play off his answers, it was kind of hard for me. I just preferred to be there whenever I could.

By getting your partner involved from the very beginning of your pregnancy, he will get to know the doctor almost as well as you do. While his relationship with your obstetrician may never be the same as yours, at the very least he will not feel like an outsider.

Your husband can also do plenty at home to be an active participant in your pregnancy. He can help you keep charts of fetal movement or uterine activity. He can read up on any complications you may be having or brush up on the details of a particular stage of your pregnancy. You can ask him to review certain sections of a book that explain what you are experiencing. Or ask him to read things that make you uncomfortable (such as passages that discuss the causes of pregnancy loss). While this may take some prodding on your part, both of you will ultimately benefit. "We tend to get our information largely through osmosis from our spouse," says Reinhart of SHARE. "But usually we will read what they bring home, especially if it's shoved at us and they say, 'read this.'"

Of course, one of the nicest ways to get him involved in the pregnancy is to let him feel the baby move. Some couples make it a ritual each night before they go to sleep, or first thing in the morning when they awaken. Share details of the baby's activity with him, too. Tell him when the baby has the hiccups or is having a particularly rambunctious day. All of this will serve to help him develop a closer connection to both you and the baby.

Encourage Him to Take Time Out for Himself

A subsequent pregnancy can be exhausting, for him as well as for you. Worrying about the baby's well-being is so stressful that you both will probably need a break every now and then. Unfortunately, breaks for you are hard to find. No matter where you go or what you do, the baby is always with you and so are your worries and concerns.

But your partner can really get away occasionally, and he may come back refreshed and ready to support you even more. Suggest that he have lunch with a friend, see a movie or play a round of golf. If you have other children whom you would have a hard time caring for alone, arrange for baby-sitting during his time away. These simple acts of kindness will pay off in the long run in the form of a happier, more relaxed mate.

Let Him Know How He Can Help You

We've just discussed several ways that you can help your partner during the pregnancy, which, in turn, helps yourself. But considering that you will have more needs than usual right now, it is also critical that you directly tell him how he can help you. Since he cannot read your mind, if you want certain things done, you have to tell him.

Maybe you need relief from physical activities: housework, grocery shopping, taking care of other children. Make a list and be specific about what you would like done. Perhaps it's your emotions that need stroking. In that case, ask him to plan a special evening for the two of you. Maybe you need a massage every now and then. No matter what it is, be sure to let him know. Usually your partner will be so glad to know that there is actually something he can do to help that he will be more than happy to oblige.

This Too Shall Pass

As stressful as things may get during your subsequent pregnancy, keep reminding him—and yourself—that the situation is only temporary. Pregnancy never lasts more than around forty-two weeks. So, never forget that this too will pass, and your pregnancy will one day be only a memory. And there is no greater reward for all of your tribulations than the birth of a healthy baby.

Resources

Pregnancy and Infant Loss Support Groups

Amend (Aiding a Mother and Father Experiencing Neonatal Death)
4324 Berrywick Terrace
St. Louis, MO 63128
314-487-7582

Bereavement Services/RTS
(Formerly known as Resolve Through Sharing)
1910 South Avenue
La Crosse, Wisconsin 54601-5400
800-362-9567, ext. 4747

Compassionate Friends
For parents who have lost a child of any age
National Headquarters
P.O. Box 3696
Oak Brook, IL 60522-3696
630-990-0010

Pregnancy Loss Support Program
National Council of Jewish Women
New York Section
9 East 69th Street
New York, NY 10021
212-535-5900

Share Pregnancy & Infant Loss Support
St. Joseph Health Center
300 First Capitol Drive
St. Charles, Missouri 03301-2803
800-821-6819
www.nationalshareoffice.com

High-Risk Pregnancy Support Group

MOST (Mothers of Supertwins)
Support Information and Resources for Families of Triplets, Quadruplets and More
P.O. Box 951
Brentwood, NY 11717
516-859-1110
www.mostonline.org

Sidelines National Support Network
A Support Group for Women with Complicated Pregnancies
P.O. Box 1808
Laguna Beach, CA 92652
949-497-2265
www.sidelines.org

Triplet Connection
A Support Network for Multiple Birth Families
P.O. Box 99571
Stockton, CA 95209
209-474-0885

Subsequent Pregnancy Support

Pails of Hope Newsletter
Pregnancy & Parenting after Infertility and/or Loss Support
Pen-Parents Inc.
P.O. Box 8738
Reno, NV 89507-8738
775-826-7332
www.penparents.org

Parent Education Program
Information on organizing subsequent pregnancy support groups
Abbott Northwestern Hospital
800 East 28th Street
Minneapolis, MN 55407
612-863-4427

Infertility Support

Resolve Inc.
1310 Broadway
Somerville, MA 02144-1731
617-623-0744
www.resolve.org

Internet Resources

Hygeia
An On-line Journal for Pregnancy and Neonatal Loss
www.hygeia.org

Childbirth.org
Pregnancy and childbirth information
www.childbirth.org

InterNational Council on Infertility Information Dissemination
www.inciid.org

Obgyn.net
Resource for professionals in obstetrics and gynecology and the women they serve
www.obgyn.net

SPALS
Subsequent Pregnancy after a Loss Support
www.inforamp.net/~bfo/spals

Pregnancy Resources

American College of Nurse-Midwives
818 Connecticut Avenue, NW
Suite 900
Washington, DC 20006
202-728-9860
www.midwife.org

American College of Obstetricians and Gynecologists (ACOG)
409 12th Street, SW
Washington, DC 20024
202-638-5577
www.acog.org

Doulas of North America
1100 23rd Avenue East
Seattle, WA 98812
206-324-5440
www.dona.com

International Childbirth Education Association
P.O. Box 20048
Minneapolis, MN 55420
612-854-8660
www.icea.org

La Leche League International
1400 N. Meacham Road
Shaumburg, IL 60173-4048
847-519-7730
www.lalecheleague.org

March of Dimes Birth Defects Foundation
1275 Mamaroneck Avenue
White Plains, NY 10605
914-428-7100
www.modimes.org

Books and Other Information on Loss and Subsequent Pregnancy

A Place to Remember
1885 University Avenue, #110
St. Paul, MN 55104
800-631-0973
www.aplacetoremember.com

Centering Corporation
1531 North Saddle Creek Road
Omaha, Nebraska 68104-5064
402-553-1200
www.webhealing.com/centering

Pregnancy and Infant Loss Center
1421 E. Wayzata Boulevard, #70
Wayzata, MN 55391
612-473-9372

Wintergreen Press
Publisher of *Another Baby? Maybe* and numerous books on pregnancy loss
3630 Eileen Street
Maple Plain, MN 55359
612-476-1303

Permissions